The Performer's Voice

The Performer's Voice

Michael S. Benninger, MD

Thomas Murry, PhD

PLURAL
PUBLISHING
INC.
SAN DIEGO
OXFORD
BRISBANE

MW

5521 Ruffin Road
San Diego, CA 92123

e-mail: info@pluralpublishing.com
Web site: http://www.pluralpublishing.com

49 Bath Street
Abingdon, Oxfordshire OX14 1EA
United Kingdom

Copyright © by Plural Publishing, Inc. 2006

Typeset in 10/13 Garamond by Flanagan's Publishing Services, Inc.
Printed in Hong Kong by Paramount Printing

For permission to use material from this text, contact us by
Telephone: (866) 758-7251
Fax: (888) 758-7255
e-mail: permissions@pluralpublishing.com

Every attempt has been made to contact the copyright holders for material originally printed in another source. If any have been inadvertently overlooked, the publishers will gladly make the necessary arrangements at the first opportunity.

Library of Congress Cataloging-in-Publication Data

The performer's voice / [edited by] Michael S. Benninger, Thomas Murry.
    p. ; cm.
  Includes bibliographical references and index.
  ISBN-13: 978-1-59756-067-2 (hardcover)
  ISBN-10: 1-59756-067-7 (hardcover)
  1. Voice—Care and hygiene. 2. Voice disorders—Treatment. 3. Singers—Health and hygiene.
I. Benninger, Michael S. II. Murry, Thomas, 1943-   .
  [DNLM: 1. Voice Disorders—therapy. 2. Voice—physiology. 3. Voice Disorders—diagnosis.
4. Voice Training.   WV 500 P438 2006]
RF511.S55P47 2006
616.85'5—dc22

                                                              2006006643

Contents

Preface

The Performer's Voice brings together a group of dedicated professionals from disciplines related to the care and treatment of individuals who use their voices in professional settings. Otolaryngologists, speech-language pathologists, psychologists, singing voice specialists, singing teachers, and performers have contributed their knowledge and offered insights on the various aspects of professional voice care and management.

In this book, the focus is primarily on the singer and actor; however, other performers are included— voiceover artists, dancer/singers, and instrumentalist/ singers, to name a few. Each type of performer brings specific issues to the treatment team and requires special attention from various members of the team. This book identifies these individuals, presents reports on cases with special needs, and offers myriad solutions designed to preserve the voice and prevent further damage.

All of the contributors to this volume have shown a dedication to the care of the performer through their academic training, research interests and experience, and clinical and/or performance backgrounds. Most of the contributors have been on stage as a performer at some point in their lives and bring that performance history to their specialty. The contributors range from current day performers to choral conductors to past rock and roll musicians.

The book is divided into six sections. Part I presents an overview of the world of performance artists— who they are and why they are important. In addition, a short review of the vocal anatomy and physiology is presented.

Identifying and diagnosing singers' voice problems follows in Part II. Problems that require medical care, voice training, or adaptation to the performance world are described.

Part III describes pharmacologic treatments for the performer. The information in this section is particularly important for singers as many medications may have negative side effects that alter the voice temporarily despite their beneficial effects.

Part IV considers nonsurgical treatments for the performer. In this section, speech pathologists and singing voice specialists offer a broad range of treatment options for the performer, both for the acute and long-term care of the singer.

Part V describes surgical considerations for the performer. These chapters are specific to the performer's voice. Types of surgery, when to do it, and how to avoid damage to the vocal mechanism are all considered in these chapters.

Part VI addresses the needs and training involved in building a professional voice practice. Professional singers are not the most common patients seen by the speech-language pathologist, the psychologist, or the otolaryngologist. Thus, in this section, important guidelines are provided to direct individual practitioners on how to build and develop their practices to accommodate performers.

In summary, *The Performer's Voice* is a comprehensive book for those who treat the performer and for those who perform. The information brought to this volume by those who have cared for performers during their careers is an invaluable reference for everyone who cares for singers and other performers.

Contributors

Jean Abitbol, MD
Ancien Chef de Clinique
Faculty of Medicine of Paris
Oto-Rhino-Laryngologiste
Phoniatrie—Chirurgie
Paris, France
Chapter 5

David M. Alessi, MD, FACS
Assistant Clinical Professor
University of California Los Angeles
Former Chief, Division of Otolaryngology
Cedars Sinai Medical Center
Los Angeles, California
Chapter 14

Mara Behlau, PhD
Director, Center for the Study of Voice
Professor of Voice
University of Sao Paulo
San Paulo, Brazil
Chapter 16

Michael S. Benninger, MD
Chair, Department of Otolaryngology–Head and
    Neck Surgery
Henry Ford Hospital
Detroit, Michigan
Chapters 1, 7, 20, 25

Thomas F. Cleveland, PhD
Director, Singing, Arts and Sciences
Department of Otolaryngology
Vanderbilt University Medical Center
Nashville, Tennessee
Chapter 23

Audrey Crummey, BS
Weill Medical College
Cornell University
New York, New York
Chapter 14

Seth H. Dailey, MD
Assistant Professor
Division of Otolaryngology
Department of Surgery
University of Wisconsin Hospital and Clinics
Madison, Wisconsin
Chapter 21

Philippe H. DeJonckere, MD, PhD
Professor
University of Utrecht
The Netherlands
Visiting Professor
Catholic University of Leuven
Belgium
Chapter 9

Janet Madelle Feindel, MFA, ATI
Associate Professor Voice/Dialectics and
    Alexander Technique
School of Drama
Carnegie Mellon University
Pittsburgh, Pennsylvania
Chapter 17

Charles N. Ford, MD, FACS
Chairman, Division of Otolaryngology
Department of Surgery
University of Wisconsin
Madison, Wisconsin
Chapter 21

Glendon M. Gardner, MD
Laryngology Airway and Voice Disorders
Department of Otolaryngology–Head and Neck
   Surgery
Henry Ford Hospital
Detroit, Michigan
Chapters 12 and 22

Jack Jiang, MD, PhD
Associate Professor
Division of Otolaryngology–Head and Neck Surgery
University of Wisconsin-Madison
Madison, Wisconsin
Chapter 4

Philip J. Lanzisera, PhD, ABPP
Senior Bioscientific Staff Psychologist
Director, Psychology Intern Program
Henry Ford Behavioral Health
Detroit, Michigan
Chapter 19

Jeannette L. LoVetri
Director, The Voice Workshop
Consultant and Faculty
Steinhardt School of Education
New York University
Adjunct Professor
Teacher's College
Columbia University
Singing Specialist for the Brooklyn Youth Chorus
   Academy
New York, New York
Chapter 18

Nicholas E. Maragos, MD
Associate Professor of Medicine
Mayo Clinic
Rochester, Minnesota
Chapter 3

Albert L. Merati, PhD
Associate Professor
Chief, Division of Laryngology
Department of Otolaryngology and
   Communication Sciences
Medical College of Wisconsin
Staff Surgeon, Zablocki VAMC
Milwaukee, Wisconsin
Chapter 11

Thomas Murry, PhD
Professor of Speech Pathology
College of Physicians and Surgeons
Clinical Director of the Voice and Swallowing
   Center
Columbia University
New York, New York
Chapters 1, 7, 16

Robert H. Ossoff, DMD, MD
Director, Vanderbilt Bill Wilkerson Center for
   Otolaryngology and Communication Sciences
Guy M. Maness Professor and Chairman
Department of Otolaryngology
Vanderbilt University Medical Center
Nashville, Tennessee
Chapter 23

Sharon L. Radionoff, PhD
Director, Sound Singing Institute
Singing Voice Specialist/Voice Technologist
Team Member—Singing Voice Specialist
Texas Voice Center
Houston, Texas
Consultant Singing Voice Specialist
University of Texas Health Science Center at
   San Antonio
Department of Otolaryngology-Head and Neck
   Surgery
Chapter 6

Josef Schlömicher-Thier, MD
Consulting Physician to the Salzburg Festival
Consulting ENT Surgeon Private, Clinic Wenle
   Salzburg
Chairman, Austrian Voice Institute
Salzburg, Austria
Chapter 13

Robert T. Sataloff, FACS, MD, DMA
Professor and Chairman
Department of Otolaryngology-HNS
Associate Dean for Clinical Academic
   Specialties
Drexel University College of Medicine
Professor, Department of Otolaryngology
Jefferson Medical College
Thomas Jefferson University
Chairman, Department of Otolaryngology–Head
   and Neck Surgery

The Graduate Hospital
Philadelphia, Pennsylvania
Chapters 24 and 25

Michael D. Seidman, MD, FACS
Henry Ford Health System
Director Division of Otologic/Neurotologic
  Surgery
Medical Director Center for Integrative Medicine
Detroit, Michigan
Chairman Committee for Complementary/
  Integrative Medicine for The American
  Academy of Otolaryngology-Head and
  Neck Surgery
Chapter 15

Rahul Shrivastav, PhD
Assistant Professor
Communication Sciences and Disorders
University of Florida
Gainesville, Florida
Chapter 10

Matthias Weikert, MD
Specialist in ORL, Voice and Speech Disorders,
  and Pediatric Audiology

Consultant Surgeon, Department of Head and
  Neck Surgery
St. Hedwig Hospital of the Catholic Hospital
Regensburg, Germany
Chapter 13

Judith Wingate, PhD
Clinical Assistant Professor
Communication Sciences and Disorders
University of Florida
Gainesville, Flordia
Chapter 10

Peak Woo, MD
Professor of Otolaryngology
Eugene Grabscheid, M.D., Voice Center
Mt. Sinai Medical School
New York, New York
Chapter 8

Gayle E. Woodson, MD, FACS
Professor, Department of Otolaryngology
Southern Illinois University School of
  Medicine
Springfield, Illinois
Chapter 2

This book is dedicated to our families;
Kathy, Ryan and Kaylin
Marie-Pierre and Nicholas

It is their love and support that has made this book possible and
our lives meaningful.

Part I

Overview

Chapter 1

INTRODUCTION

Michael S. Benninger
Thomas Murry

"Your voice is the mirror of your soul."

Our voices influence nearly every part of human interaction and culture. Until relatively recently in human history, the voice was the sole method of communication. Early human history and recording of events was exclusively through oral history. It is only in relatively recent history that communication has been both written and oral. Despite the information explosion in written, printed, and digitalized/computerized recordings, most people still use their voices as their primary means of communication. Even when people are alone, they will use their voices, to sing or to "speak to themselves."

Voice communication begins at birth. The birth cry is the first sign of life. The cry soon becomes the communication link between baby and mother. The voice of the mother soothes the crying voice. As the child develops, his or her voice plays a pivotal role in satisfying the needs of hunger, pain, and play. Some children develop pleasurable sounds while others use their voices strenuously and develop hoarseness or harshness. Still others find that humming or singing brings pleasure and reinforcement from family and friends. And, that is often how these children go on to bigger and more prominent acting and singing roles in primary school, high school, and beyond. For some adults, singing is an enjoyable hobby while for others it becomes their passion and finally their profession. Even for those who did not get the principal part in the high school musical, training and practice under watchful eyes and ears help to develop the voice for later success in a vocally demanding profession. Eventually, these individuals become the voice professionals.

Who are professional vocalists? Loosely defined, professional vocalists are individuals who rely on their voices to be the major part of their occupation. This includes teachers, salespeople, coaches, politicians, broadcasters, singers, orators, clergy, and numerous other professionals. The voice demands, the techniques and style of use, and the overall quantity of use may vary considerably among these groups. Similarly, the quality demands and the ability to maintain their professional value may differ. Newscasters must talk rapidly with clear articulation, teachers must talk for long periods of the day, and sports coaches must talk loudly. Ultimately, however, the need to maintain a strong, effective, and clear voice affects each of these professionals and contributes in some way to their success. Without their voices, these individuals can no longer perform the duties required.

One unique group of professional voice users is professional singers. Of all the voice professionals, singers are perhaps the most affected by problems with their voices, even subtle ones. There is a general expectation that a singer will always perform at his or her best, with a strong, pure, and clear voice with a broad range and unique character. Minor changes in quality are immediately scrutinized, far more so than minor hoarseness in other voice professionals. Because of these voice expectations, singers tend to also spend the most time of any voice professionals developing their voices through practice and training. They demand a higher quality for their own voices than even their audiences do. They are driven to perfection and will work diligently to crystallize their quality and refine their vocal style whether it is opera, gospel, or cabaret. This perfectionistic drive and focus on hard work and repetition is not only what leads to excellence but may increase the risk of injury. Any injury to the singer's voice has dramatic implications not only on their voices but also on their psyche and sense of self-worth.

> "First, I lost my voice, then I lost my figure and then I lost Onassis!"
> Maria Callas

What happens when a singer is injured and cannot perform at a level that either they or their audiences expect? That depends on many factors including the professional level of the singer, the magnitude of the injury, the importance of the performance, the experience of the singer, the type of music to be sung, and the expectations from the audience for the performance. It is a simplification to suggest that the expectations of the performance of an elite opera singer are greater than that of a rock singer. There are too many variables to think like this. The demands of the performance vary for each individual and for each performance. Even for the experienced, elite opera singer, there may be an important difference between a Metropolitan Opera premiere and a light-hearted recital at a hometown outdoor venue. The audition for entrance into a school of music is usually more critical to a developing young singer than the third performance of the weekend in the school play.

For some singers and for some performances, "the show must go on." But there is a danger in thinking like that. Singers usually injure their voices when they are sick, fatigued, or under strain. When the experienced singer feels that he or she cannot perform to a known level, he or she will cancel the rehearsal or the show. Canceling at the last minute, however, becomes more difficult for the lead singer at a small college in the Midwest where there is no one else to take over the role. The need to perform must always be balanced against the probability of vocal injury. When the singer cannot use his or her full voice, the decisions must be made with the singer's long-term career in mind. For some, it is simply of matter of rest and hydration; for others, their show cannot go on unless they seek treatment from knowledgeable individuals who understand the ramifications of voice care and vocal injury.

> *Madonna Cancels NJ Show*
> A sore throat forced Madonna to cancel the final NY area date of her Drowned World tour last night at the Meadowlands Arena.
> *New York Times*, August 2001

To treat singers, one has to be aware not only of the important principles of anatomy, physiology, and pathology of the voice, but also the critical interfaces between the voice, the sound produced, and the unique aspects of each individual singer. A comprehensive understanding of the differences in individual voice production, between musical styles and the more complex relationships the singer has with teachers, audiences, agents, and promoters, is necessary to comprehensively address the singer's voice needs. Each singer is different and each needs to be considered individually. Although there are a number of variables in the assessment and treatment process, the best rule to approach an injured singer is that there are no rules. Knowledge, education, compassion, and a thoughtful, deliberate approach bolstered by appropriate tools and equipment for evaluation and treatment are needed each time a singer comes to the clinic or studio with a voice problem.

One fortunate aspect of the treatment of singers is that the characteristics of hard work and drive that can lead to injury are usually also applied to assessment, treatment, and rehabilitation. Singers sing because they love it. They rehabilitate their injured voices to resume their profession. They respect a knowledgeable voice clinician and will often follow the advice and recommendations without hesitation. In a large sense singers are vocal athletes. Their bodies are the source of their vocation and like other athletes they base their careers on a somewhat fragile machine that is prone to injury.

And, like athletes, they will do what is necessary to return to performing. In doing so, they rely on the specialized voice practitioners, primarily otolaryngologists and speech-language pathologists who specialize in voice disorders, and colleagues in the music community to help them return to their careers at the same level as before their injury.

Actors and actresses also require exacting standards for their speaking voice. Projection, articulation, and endurance in the speaking voice range require training and practice. Injuries may occur in actors' voices that restrict use and therefore income. Medical care and rehabilitation of the injured actor's voice also falls to the otolaryngologist, speech-language pathologist, vocal pedagogist, and singing teacher.

The current approach to caring for the performer's voice is to use an interdisciplinary team of clinicians. The performer's voice care team is usually under the direction of an otolaryngologist or laryngologist. Laryngologists are otolaryngologists who specialize in diseases and disorders of the larynx. However, the performer's internist should always be kept apprised of changes in the performer's health status and of the prescribed medications.

Speech-language pathologists are an integral part of the performers' voice care team. Speech pathology encompasses many subspecialties of communication disorders. Relatively few have special training or intimate knowledge of the anatomy and physiology of the vocal mechanism or even an interest in the performing population. Most speech pathologists who routinely treat performers are closely aligned with an otolaryngologist and work together with the injured performer to achieve rapid and safe recovery of vocal injuries.

Phoniatrists, singing voice specialists, and vocal coaches are also involved in the care of the performer. Phoniatrists are specialists in European countries who are trained as physicians but not as surgeons. They may prescribe medicines and offer behavioral treatments. Singing voice specialists are usually singers who go on to study the medically related aspects of voice use.

They are usually affiliated with voice care teams and offer special singing-related information to the singer and the members of the voice care team.

There is a wealth of information available to the singer with a voice problem since the advent of modern voice care. Singers should be educated by their voice care team and team members owe it to the singers to share the most up-to-date practice methods that are available. It is important for the voice care team to communicate with the performer's other health care specialists, voice teachers, and others in the performing industry so that conservative and appropriate care is given when there is a voice injury.

This book is written to present the most current and comprehensive approach to the care of the singer's voice. The important anatomic, physiologic, and pedagogic principles of voice production for the singer will serve as the foundation for the care of the singer. The authors represent a wide array of people who have dedicated their careers to the prevention of voice injury, the diagnosis, treatment, and rehabilitation of the injured singer, and the education of others who continue to advance the science and art of voice care through education, research, and clinical practice. The diversity of the authors supports the important principles of the multidisciplinary approach to the care of the vocalist, particularly the singer.

This book serves as a concise reference for the otolaryngologist or speech-language (voice) pathologist who wishes to focus their practice on the evaluation and care of vocalists, particularly the professional singer. It also provides a strong foundation in the understanding of the singer's voice for singers, teachers of singing, pedagogues, and those who contract and produce vocal performances, and others who have already developed a foundation in voice and wish to become more familiar with the intricate principles of the performing voice. Ultimately, we hope that this book will continue to strengthen the fundamental foundations of voice care and will expand the multidisciplinary interests in the care and preventive treatment of the singer's voice.

Chapter 2

HISTORY OF PROFESSIONAL VOICE CARE

Gayle E. Woodson

It is generally considered that the specialty of laryngology was born when Manuel García, a singing teacher, introduced the technique of indirect laryngoscopy to the medical profession.[1] Vocal performance is an ancient art and performers have sought care for voice disorders throughout history. However, the treatment of hoarseness was empirical and traditional until the larynx could be examined, to accurately identify pathology. There are still mysteries and some unsolvable problems in voice care, but in the past century and a half we have made tremendous progress. Although the means to examine the living larynx was a major factor, advances in voice care have been fueled by developments in other realms as well (Table 2-1).

Table 2-1. Developments That Have Advanced Knowledge in Laryngology

Ability to Examine the Larynx
Surgical Technology
Advances in Knowledge of Structure and Function of the Vocal Tract
Pharmacology
Voice Therapy
Objective Voice Assessment

LARYNGEAL EXAMINATION

García's presentation to the Royal Society of Medicine in 1855 was a turning point in care of the voice. However, as noted by Bailey in a recent review, others, both before and after García, made significant contributions to the development of indirect laryngocopy.[2] In 1829, Babington presented a system of mirrors coupled to a tongue retractor that he had developed for examining the larynx, and published his report in *The London Medical Gazette*.[3] However, this device was cumbersome and was not widely accepted. M. Baumes in Lyons, France in 1838, and Liston, in Scotland in 1840, reported using mirrors to examine the larynx. García's report introduced the use a common, simple, and ancient instrument, the dental mirror, with reflected sunlight for illumination. After García's report, Turk, in Vienna, and Czermak, in Budapest, began to work with mirror laryngoscopy, and Czermak developed a very user- friendly system that employed artificial light. The ability to view the larynx during phonation was fascinating and allowed physicians to appreciate for the first time how the normal voice was produced, and how pathology supervened.[4] Many types of laryngeal pathologies were beautifully illustrated by physicians, who were also artists, who skillfully reproduced what they saw in their laryngeal mirrors. Figure 2-1 is a fanciful sketch by Dr FJ Knight, one of the founders of the

Figure 2–1. Drawing by Dr. F. J. Knight, circa 1885. (Reproduced with permission from the Historical Documents Collection of the American Laryngological Society, http://www.alahns.org/Historical_CD/pages/74_jpg.php)

American Laryngological Society. Laryngeal photography was also occasionally accomplished via the laryngeal mirror. Figure 2–2 depicts one of the earliest laryngeal photographs, from a patient with laryngeal paralysis.

Through the years, technologic advances have improved our ability to examine the larynx. Table 2–2 chronicles the developments in this area. High-speed cinematography and stroboscopy were used in research in the early 20th century, but slow-motion views of vocal fold motion were not applied clinically until the availability of improved optics in the latter 20th century.[5] Rod-lens telescopes provided vastly improved and magnified views of the larynx, with detail compa-

rable to that of operative microlaryngoscopy.[6] Flexible laryngoscopy permits laryngeal examination even in patients with unfavorable anatomy or prohibitive gag reflex.[7] Both mirror exam and telescopic exam are restricted to use in a narrow range of vocal behavior, and sometimes only during phonation of the vowel "ee." Flexible laryngoscopic examination can be performed throughout a wide spectrum of laryngeal behavior, including connected speech, breathing, cough, and Valsalva maneuver. The view through a flexible laryngoscope is only consistently obscured during a swallow, when the pharynx completely collapses. Optical technology has also allowed the larynx

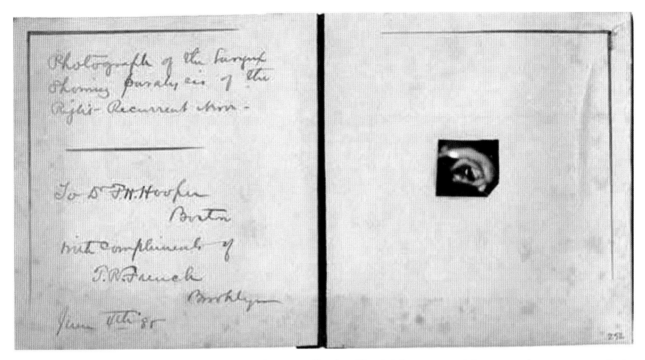

Figure 2–2. Photograph of the larynx in a patient with right recurrent laryngeal nerve paralysis. Photo taken by Dr. J. R. French of Brooklyn, and presented to Dr. J. H. Hooper on June 4, 1885. (Reproduced with permission from the Historical Documents Collection of the American Laryngological Association, http://www.alahns.org/Historical_CD/pages/3_22_jpg.php)

Table 2–2. Development of Laryngeal Examination

Transoral Laryngeal Surgery	1852
Mirror Laryngoscopy	1854
Direct Laryngoscopy	1896
Suspension Laryngoscopy	1916
High-Speed Motion Picture	1940
Operative Microlaryngoscopy	1950s
Stroboscopy—Research	1954
Telescopic Laryngoscopy	1974
Fiberoptic Laryngoscopy	1979
Videolaryngoscopy	1980+
Stroboscopy—Clinical	1980+
Chip Camera	2000+

to be examined with stroboscopic illumination. The addition of a camera provided a magnified view and the ability to record the examination for a more detailed review and a permanent record.[8] In the 21st century, the distal chip camera has further enhanced clinical laryngeal examination, providing large and clear images in nearly every patient.

SURGICAL TECHNOLOGY

Just as mirror laryngoscopy permitted the development of laryngeal diagnosis, direct laryngsocopy opened the doors to laryngeal surgery. Green reported transoral removal of laryngeal polyp in 1852.[9] However, a formal system for operative laryngoscopy, termed "autoscopy" was developed by Kirstein and first reported in American literature in 1896.[10] Chevalier Jackson popularized operative laryngoscopy in this country and refined the instrumentation.[11] The addition of a suspension arm stabilized the operative field and allowed the surgeons to use both hands. The operating microscope not only enhanced surgical precision, but allowed a more detailed examination of the larynx, with better identification of pathology. The concept was pioneered by Albrecht and refined and popularized by Kleinsasser.[12,13] Geza Jako developed a laryngoscope that permitted binocular visualization.[14] He also developed precision microsurgical instruments. Instrumentation is still evolving to provide precise and atraumatic tissue handling. The development of laser surgery allowed precision, no-touch surgery. This technology has also evolved, with various wavelengths, smaller spot size, and superpulse mode.

ADVANCES IN KNOWLEDGE OF STRUCTURE AND FUNCTION OF THE VOCAL TRACT

Both voice therapy and laryngeal surgery have benefitted tremendously from improved understanding of physiology and anatomy. As mentioned above, the advent of mirror laryngoscopy profoundly stimulated interest in laryngeal diseases, and in this country led to the establishment of the American Laryngological Society. This provided a forum for laryngologists to present new knowledge and greatly fostered advances in the field. However, in that early era, laryngology was not greatly concerned with voice care because of preoccupation with infectious and neoplastic problems. In addition, there was little or no collaboration between laryngologists and other voice professionals, such as singing teachers and speech-language pathologists. Frequently discussed topics at meetings of the American Laryngological Association included diphtheria, syphilis, and tuberculosis. However, there were some discussions of professional voice issues. One paper presented at the Fourth Annual meeting was entitled "On the Singing Voice, its Physiology, Pathology, and Treatment. (Figure 2-3).[15]

Despite some sporadic interest in professional voice care, little attention was devoted to it in the American medical literature. Dr. Hans von Leden has noted that, during the 1950s, the reputation of a laryngologist depended to a large degree on how many laryngectomies (total removal of the larynx due to cancer) he had performed.[16] Dr. Van Lawrence, an otolaryngologist who became physician to the Houston Grand Opera in the 1960s, found little available

information or guidance when he began caring for performers (personal communication, 1985). The field of American voice care benefitted significantly from phoniatrists who immigrated from Europe in midcentury. Hans von Leden has said,

> It is true that in the 1930s and 1940s a number of leading Phoniatricians including Froeschels, Brodnitz, Moses, Weiss and Arnold came to the United States as refugees. It is sad to report that most of these distinguished foreign leaders encountered considerable prejudice in addition to difficulties with the English language and with adjusting to totally different academic standards. Over a period of years, only a very few were able to adapt successfully. Paul Moses became the leading voice specialist in California, and his book on the *Voice and Neurosis* is still a valuable text. Dr. Friedrich Brodnitz became an authority on voice in the city of New York and in the American Academy of Otolaryngology (he became one of my mentors); Arnold was eventually successful in becoming the Chairman of a new Department of Otolaryngology in Jackson, Mississippi.[16]

One development that profoundly facilitated scientific advances in the field was the establishment of the Voice Foundation in 1969. This effort was spearheaded by Dr. Wilbur J Gould, and the transactions of those meetings were for years faithfully edited by Dr Van Lawrence. The yearly symposia sponsored by this organization have provided a forum for interdisciplinary collaboration and sharing of knowledge among physicians, speech pathologists, singing teachers, and basic scientists. The rich and varied programs provided a much needed stimulus to the field (http://www.voicefoundation.org).

One particularly significant example of the impact of knowledge on voice care is Hirano's description of the layered microarchitecture of the vibratory edges of the vocal fold.[17] Understanding of the importance of the intricate structure of the lamina propria has driven the development of the microsurgical principles of mucosal preservation, minimal touch. It also explains the profound implications of vocal fold scar, and we hope that current research into the biology of the lamina propria will enable us to rehabilitate the scarred larynx by restoring the submucosal tissues.

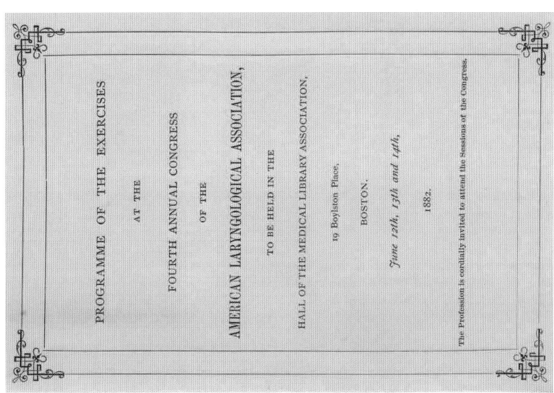

Figure 2–3. A page from the Program of the Fourth Annual Congress of the American Laryngological Society, held in Boston, June 12–14, 1882, listing a presentation by Dr. S. W. Langmaid, "On The Singing Voice: Its Physiology, Pathology and Treatment." (Reproduced with permission from the Historical Documents of the American Laryngological Association, http://www.alahns.org/ Historical_CD/pages/36B3_Jpg.php)

ADVANCES IN PHARMACOLOGY

Advances in pharamacology have profoundly benefitted voice care. Until the early 20th century, the available treatments for laryngeal inflammation were meager and lacked scientifically supported rationale. Various topical and inhaled therapies were recommended. Here is an example of a recommended therapy for acute laryngitis:

> The patient should then put a large bath-towel round his neck and shoulders and, taking hold of his tongue with one corner of the towel, pull well out whilst sitting so that the funnel of the spray is not more than two inches from his open mouth. He should then, while keeping the tongue well out, inhale the vapour deeply into his lungs for five or ten minutes at a time—including also the nose when there is catarrh of that organ—and then get back to bed and roll his head up in the shawl. This can be repeated three times a day.[18(p540)]

Another text recommends these measures for acute laryngitis: "correct the pathology in nose or pharynx, instruct patient in voice use, heroin or codeine for cough suppression, and strychnine as a general tonic and stimulant of vocal cords. It is stated that local treatment is of no avail, except for relief of pain."[19]

The value of rest and voice retraining were widely recognized as the best treatment for chronic laryngitis, but the details of voice retraining were often proprietary secrets held by recognized experts. One therapeutic textbook published in 1911 made this recommendation for the treatment of chronic laryngitis: "For those who can afford it—it is best to begin treatment by a course at Aix-les-Bains, Mont Dore Ems, or Salsomaggiore, where the local treatment is thoroughly carried out."[18(p541)]

We currently take for granted the availability of powerful antibiotics, antihistamines, decongestants, and acid-suppressive medication. These drugs provide profound relief, and their efficacy has illuminated the pathogenesis of voice disorders, fueling further progress. For example, the efficacy of proton pump inhibitor therapy provided supports for the use of fundoplication surgery in chronic laryngitis, which has proven to be quite effective.

VOICE THERAPY

Voice therapy has long been recognized as a vital component of voice care. One 1911 textbook notes that acute laryngitis is ". . . usually met with in males who have been indulging too freely in alcohol and tobacco, or overusing the voice."[18(p540)] The best treatment for recurrent laryngitis was voice retraining. The following treatment was recommended for chronic laryngitis: "In the writer's experience, the greatest good is obtained from skilful massage of the neck and larynx combined with vibration. . . . it is sometimes very difficult to get patients out of their old habits, which is so necessary in these cases before they can learn to produce their voice with a wide-open pharynx and, therefore, without 'pinching' or 'squeezing.' "[18(p541)] Despite the recognized importance of voice therapy and observed efficacy over many years, it is still not adequately reimbursed by third-party payers. This is difficult to comprehend, considering that one would not consider treatment of many orthopedic disorders without the inclusion of physical or occupational therapy. A major goal of clinical research should be the collection of data to identify and support the efficacy of the best approaches to voice therapy so that the benefits of voice therapy are more available to those who need them.

OBJECTIVE ASSESSMENT OF VOICE

Objective assessment of vocal function is vital for documenting response to treatment of voice disorders so that we can make progress in improving therapy. To a limited extent, acoustic analysis, standardized perceptual scores, aerodynamic measures, and validated questionnaires have allowed us to answer some important questions. However, despite a significant body of research, we still do not have testing for the voice that can compare to the diagnostic audiometric assessment of hearing. Several factors contribute to this. Acoustic analysis, although objective, is not usable in very severe voice disorders. Second, it has not been possible to objectively or quantitatively identify the qualitative parameters that we perceive in voices. Aerodynamic measures hold promise in describing physiologic parameters of voice production, but measurement to date is cumbersome and standard parameters have not been defined. However, the research efforts thus far have been quite effective in recognizing what cannot be done. Goals for the future include standardized protocols for the diagnosis and management of the voice based on large prospective research efforts.

SUMMARY

Advances in voice care have been sparked by breakthroughs in optical technology, fueled by curiosity about the vocal system, and ultimately driven by love and respect for the human voice. The greatest understanding of the voice and vocal disorders will result from continued interdisciplinary collaboration among all those who care for those who treasure their voices.

REFERENCES

1. García M: Observations on the human voice. *Proc Royal Soc Med.* 1855;7:399.
2. Bailey, B. Laryngoscopy and laryngoscopes—who's first?: the forefathers/ four fathers of laryngology. *Laryngoscope.* 1996;106:939-943.
3. Wells WA. Benjamin G. Babington—inventor of the laryngoscope. *Laryngoscope.* 1946;56:443-454.
4. Mackenzie M. *The Use of the Laryngoscope in Diseases of the Throat.* Philadelphia, Pa: Lindsay & Blakiston; 1865:9.
5. Moore GP. Vocal fold movement during vocalization. *Speech Monogr.* 1937;4:44-55.
6. Ward P, Berci GI, Calcaterra TC. Advances in endoscopic examination of the respiratory system. *Ann Otol Rhinol Laryngol.* 1974;83:754-760.
7. Sawashima M, Hirose H. New laryngoscopic technique by use of fiberoptics. *J Acoust Soc Am.* 1968;43:168-170.
8. Yanigasawa E, Casuccia A Jr, Suzuki M. Videolarlyngoscopy using a rigid telescope and video home system color camera: a useful office procedure. *Ann Otol Rhinol Laryngol.* 1981;90:346-350.
9. Green H. Morbid growths within the larynx. In: *On the Surgical Treatment of Polypi of the Larynx, and Oedema of the Glottis.* New York, NY: GP Putnam; 1852:56-65.
10. Scheppegrell W. A new communication upon autoscopy of the respiratory passages—examination of the larynx and trachea without a mirror. *Laryngoscope.* 1896;1:370.
11. Jackson C, Jackson CL. *Disease and Injuries of the Larynx.* New York, NY: Macmillan; 1942:330.
12. Albrecht R. Uber den Wert kolposkopischer Untershchungsmethoden bei Leukoplaken und Carcinomen des Mundes und Kehlkopfes. *Arch Ohrenheilk.* 1954;164:459-463.
13. Kleinsasser O. Mikrochirurgie im Kehlkopf. *Arch Ohrenheilk.* 1964;183:428-433.
14. Jako GJ. Laryngoscope for microscopic observation, surgery, and photography. *Arch Otolaryngol.* 1970;91:196-199.
15. Langmaid SW. On the singing voice, its physiology, pathology, and treatment: Transactions of the Fourth Annual Congress of the American Laryngological Association; June 14, 1882.
16. von Leden H. 100 Years of German phoniatry and pediatric audiology: a tribute to Professor Herman Gutzmann, Sr. XXIV Kongress der Union Eurpoäischen Phoniater; Berlin, Deutschland; September 16-18, 2005. Available from: http://www.phoniatrie 2005.com/gruss_leden.htm.
17. Hirano M. Phonosurgical anatomy of the larynx. In: Ford CN, Bless DM, eds. *Phonosurgery.* New York, NY: Raven Press; 1991.
18. Hutchinson R, Collier H. *An Index of Treatment by Various Writers.* New York, NY: William Wood; 1925:539-542.
19. Packard FR, Inflammatory conditions of the larynx. In: Packard FR, ed. *Diseases of the Nose, Throat, and Ear.* Philadelphia, Pa: Lippincott; 1909: 223-233.

Chapter 3

ANATOMY OF THE VOCAL MECHANISM: STRUCTURE OF THE VOICE

Nicolas E. Maragos

The mechanism that produces voice is, on the surface, a rather mundane structure that mostly is taken for granted. We know intuitively that everyone's voice is a little bit different, but even though we use the sound of someone's voice to figure out very quickly who is on the telephone, and whether or not they are sick or tired or worried or in a hurry, we still do not think much about it. For the singer, however, and for others who tend to stretch the vocal mechanism "to the limit," the voice and its health take on added importance. To understand the conditions that may do harm to the voice we must, therefore, understand what it is that produces the best sound over the course of a lifetime. Thus, the study of the anatomy of the vocal mechanism is paramount to understanding the basics of vocal health, hygiene, and preservation of our gift of voice.

VOCAL MECHANISM AS A WHOLE

Although the larynx ("voice box") generates the vocal sound, it is neither the beginning nor the end of the vocal mechanism. Before delving into the finer details of the larynx itself, we should spend some time understanding the anatomy of the remainder of the vocal

mechanism. Voice is produced when the lining tissue of the vocal folds, the mucosa, is put into oscillation and changes a steady stream of air into a rhythmically interrupted airstream.[1] The air, of course, has to come from the lungs, and the power pushing the air out of the lungs comes from the contraction of the abdominal and chest muscles, and the relaxation and recoil of the diaphragm. Normal exhalation takes place with a larger flow of air at the beginning of exhalation and a quickly decreasing flow thereafter. This pattern is fine for quiet breathing, but for a smooth, steady, and prolonged vocal output the airstream needs to be modified for a steadier flow. Thus, anything that hampers the normal action of the diaphragm, chest, or abdominal muscles may have a great impact on the voice.

The action of diaphragmatic contraction is mediated through the phrenic nerves on both sides. The phrenic nerves are a mix of motor nerves from the third through fifth cervical roots (C3–C5) in the neck and come directly out of the spinal cord through spaces between the vertebral bodies (spinal column).[2] Branches from roots C3 to C5 combine into a single nerve high in the neck on each side, travel downward in the neck to the posterior mediastinum between the lungs, and finally lie next to the heart before reaching the top surface of the diaphragm. Because the diaphragm is dome-shaped curving upward, contraction of the diaphragm through phrenic nerve stimulation leads to an increase in size of the chest cavity and inhalation.[3] Thus, if one or both phrenic nerves are injured or weakened the person is not able to breathe in to stay alive. The most recent well-known individual suffering from this was actor Christopher Reeve whose spinal cord was injured above C3, that is, above the formation of the phrenic nerves. He spent his last years on a portable respirator because of his total loss of diaphragmatic function.

The intercostal muscles of the chest and the abdominal muscles also receive their motor nerve supply through the spinal nerve roots exiting the spinal column farther down. The intercostals span the distance between adjacent ribs and pull the ribs together when they contract. The abdominal muscles surround the abdominal contents and squeeze everything inward during contraction. The balance of tension between the abdominals and intercostals on one hand (pushing air out) and the diaphragm on the other (pulling air in) is what voice professionals and, especially, singers spend years mastering. A deficit in this part of the vocal mechanism will, therefore, lead to a decrease in peak performance and a less than optimal vocal output.

VOCAL MECHANISM AT THE CENTER

"The living voice is that which sways the soul" (Pliny the Younger—*Letters*. Book ii. Letter iii. 9). Educators, writers, and philosophers from ancient civilizations understood well the meaning and essence of voice. From Pliny the Younger's quote from the first century AD to Longfellow's more recent quote that "the larynx is the voice of the soul," people knew there was something special about good vocal production. At the center of euphonia ("good sound") is the larynx, and it follows that a normal or near-normal laryngeal organ must be available for the voice user to produce the sounds that "sway the soul" of the listener.

The larynx is a composite structure situated in the midneck, or rather suspended in the neck from the skull above. Muscles connected to the larynx from both above and below act upon it to change its position in the neck and help it carry out its three vital functions: airway closure during swallowing, airway opening during breathing, and airway modulation during voicing. These outside (extrinsic) muscles are often those which the voice teacher, either consciously or unconsciously, tries to manipulate to improve the student's voice. Those muscles that raise the larynx in the neck are called elevators, and those that lower the larynx are named depressors. The hyoid bone at the top of the larynx is the primary point of attachment of these elevators and depressors. The names of these suprahyoid (above) and infrahyoid (below) muscles are not important to the student, but speech pathologists, voice therapists, and voice teachers need to be reminded of their existence and the great value (or harm) that may come to the student if these muscles are injured, too tense, or malfunctioning in any way.

VOCAL MECHANISM: EXTERNAL SUPPORT

The larynx by definition includes those bony, cartilaginous, and internal soft tissue structures spanning from the top of the hyoid bone to the bottom of the cricoid cartilage (Figure 3–1). The rigid external skeleton from superior to inferior includes the hyoid bone, thyroid cartilage, and cricoid cartilage. These structures form a semirigid tube that normally can be bent forward and shortened in a superior/inferior direction, but cannot be bent from side to side. This tube is also rigid when rotated making it possible to operate on the posterolateral larynx with this maneuver in the awake patient. All the internal cartilaginous and soft tissue structures are attached to the thyroid and cricoid cartilages or are supported by them through a system of muscles, ligaments, and membranous sheets of thicker fibrous tissue.

The thyroid cartilage is the largest cartilage of the larynx and is formed by two relatively flat and broad plates of cartilage fused anteriorly at the midline of the neck. It connects posteriorly to the hyoid bone above and the cricoid cartilage below through two pairs of horn-shaped projections, the superior and inferior cornua, respectively. The superior cornu attaches to the hyoid bone above through a ligament on each side, the lateral thyrohyoid ligament, as part of the suspensory system of the larynx mentioned earlier. The inferior cornu forms a joint with the cricoid cartilage on either side, the cricothyroid joint, which allows the forward flexing of the thyroid cartilage on the cricoid cartilage but not sideways flexing. The anterior angle of the two lamina of the thyroid cartilage are different in men (90°) than in women (120°), hence, the greater protrusion of the man's thyroid cartilage, which prompts the term, "Adam's apple." The cricothyroid joints, as we will learn in a later chapter, are important for the normal action of the cricothyroid muscles during vocal pitch modulation.

Two of the most important structures of the larynx are the paired cricoarytenoid joints (Figure 3-2). As their name implies, these joints connect the cricoid cartilage to the arytenoid cartilages. Located posteriorly and just below the level of the vocal folds, these joints support arytenoid movement including a gliding motion for adduction and abduction of the vocal folds,

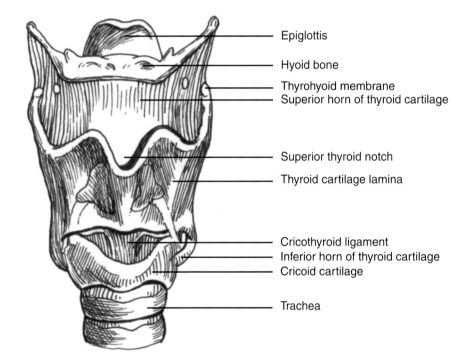

Figure 3-1. External structure of the larynx, anterior view.

Epiglottis

Hyoid bone

Thyrohyoid membrane
Superior horn of thyroid cartilage

Superior thyroid notch

Thyroid cartilage lamina

Cricothyroid ligament
Inferior horn of thyroid cartilage
Cricoid cartilage

Trachea

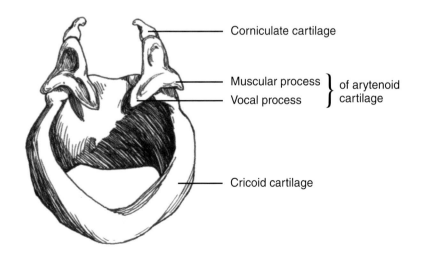

Figure 3-2. Cricoarytenoid joints, anterosuperior view.

Corniculate cartilage

Muscular process ⎫ of arytenoid
Vocal process ⎬ cartilage

Cricoid cartilage

tilting forward and backward to put the vocal processes in better vertical alignment during phonation, and a rotation around a vertical axis. The cricoarytenoid joint capsule and, in particular, the posterior cricoarytenoid ligament hold the arytenoid in place on top of the cricoid.[4] Without this support the arytenoid would fall into the larynx from its rather precarious perch atop the cricoid. Abnormalities of these joints (scarring, arthritis, etc) will impact laryngeal function by affecting vocal fold movement and position. Better treatment of these problems is one of the future directions in laryngeal surgery.

VOCAL MECHANISM: INTERNAL SUPPORT

The study of medicine and human anatomy may be daunting and, at times, confusing, but the language of medicine is actually very simple once one understands a few rules of the system.[5] So it is with the anatomy of the larynx and all the structures therein. For example, we can now use all the information given above regarding the laryngeal external support system to understand and remember the intricate and fascinating internal structures of the larynx. Thus, the muscle of the vocal fold itself, beginning at the thyroid cartilage anteriorly and ending at the arytenoid cartilage posteriorly, is named the *thyroarytenoid* muscle, not the "arytenothyroid" muscle, because its origin is at the thyroid cartilage.

The arytenoid cartilages are the heart of the larynx. The attachments to these cartilages include the muscles, ligaments, and fibrous tissue important in voice production. The arytenoid cartilages are mostly pyramidal in shape with three processes or points of attachment to other structures. These are the vocal process anteriorly, the muscular process laterally, and the superior process.[6] The vocal process protrudes from the anterior portion of the arytenoid body and attaches to the medial thyroarytenoid muscle and ligament (vocalis muscle and vocal ligament, Figure 3–3). Attached to the muscular processes are the lateral and posterior

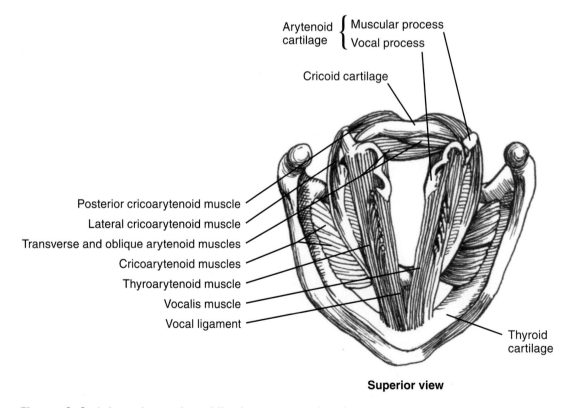

Arytenoid cartilage { Muscular process / Vocal process

Cricoid cartilage

Posterior cricoarytenoid muscle
Lateral cricoarytenoid muscle
Transverse and oblique arytenoid muscles
Cricoarytenoid muscles
Thyroarytenoid muscle
Vocalis muscle
Vocal ligament

Thyroid cartilage

Superior view

Figure 3–3. Internal muscles of the larynx, superior view.

cricoarytenoid muscles, and spanning the distance between the arytenoid cartilages posteriorly is the interarytenoid muscle. These latter muscles position the arytenoid cartilages in the airstream to facilitate breathing, swallowing, and voicing.

As mentioned above, the vocal folds are suspended between the thyroid cartilage anteriorly and the arytenoid cartilages posteriorly at the vocal processes of the arytenoids.[7] The thyroarytenoid muscle makes up most of the body of the vocal fold. As most muscles contract when stimulated by their motor nerve supply, the action of the thyroarytenoid is to pull the arytenoid toward the thyroid cartilage to both shorten the length of the vocal fold and bulk it up isometrically. The lateral cricoarytenoid muscle arises from the anterior and lateral cricoid cartilage and inserts onto the laterally placed muscular process of the arytenoid, whereas the posterior cricoarytenoid muscle arises from the posterior surface of the cricoid cartilage and also inserts onto the muscular process (Figure 3–4). Contraction of these muscles moves the arytenoid into its various positions so that the larynx may complete its normal functions. Finally, contraction of the interarytenoid muscle will pull the arytenoids closer to each other and fill the interarytenoid space with folds of overlying soft tissue and mucosa, thus effectively obliterating any opening between these cartilages.

All the above-mentioned muscles obtain their motor nerve supply from the recurrent laryngeal nerve.[6] The last muscle affecting the voice, the cricothyroid muscle, acts indirectly on the vocal fold. It is situated on both sides in the anterolateral space between the cricoid and thyroid cartilages. Its motor nerve supply is through the external branch of the superior laryngeal nerve. Cricothyroid muscle contraction changes the tension of the vocal fold by increasing the distance between the vocal process of the arytenoid and the anterior attachment of the vocal ligament and thyroarytenoid muscle to the thyroid cartilage. This is accomplished through the cricothyroid joint mentioned earlier, a joint that allows pivoting and anterior flexion of the thyroid cartilage upon the cricoid. Alterations in

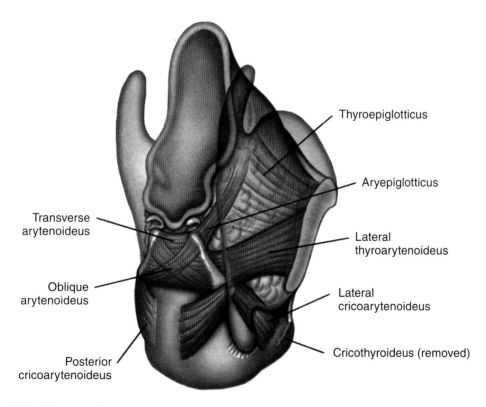

Figure 3–4. Intrinsic muscles of the larynx, posterior oblique view. (From Tucker HM. *The Larynx.* New York, NY: Thieme Medical Publishers, Inc; 1987:14 with permission).

cricothyroid muscle strength or imbalance of strength between the right and left sides is probably the most overlooked deficit of the vocal mechanism but one that is extremely important to singers and other voice users alike.

Some laryngeal structures are not directly responsible for vocal production. However, they do impact the resonating quality of the voice, especially if they "get in the way" of the outflow from the larynx. These are the epiglottic cartilage and the false cords. The epiglottis sits anteriorly and above the vocal folds and is attached by its petiole to the inside of the thyroid cartilage, and the false cords reside above and lateral to the vocal folds. The primary purpose of these supraglottic (above the vocal folds) structures is to help protect the airway during swallowing. However, they may partially or totally obstruct the vocal output in those patients with, for example, muscle tension dysphonia or spasmodic dysphonia. Without an easy passage through the larynx the voice will be impaired.

The medial thyroarytenoid muscle and the vocal ligament make up the body of the vocal fold over which the flexible mucosa of the vocal fold moves. Ultrastructural studies have shown a division of the submucosal fibrous tissue in this area, also called the lamina propria, into three distinct parts: superficial, middle, and deep layers (Figure 3–5). The superficial layer of the lamina propria is the most important of these layers for its sparse and pliable collagen binds this tissue loosely and allows the shearing force from the airstream out of the lungs to rhythmically open and close the airspace between the vocal folds during

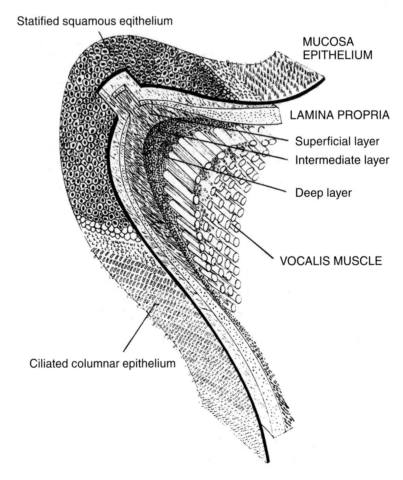

Figure 3–5. Ultrastructure of the vocal fold. (From Hirano M. Phonosurgery—Basic and Clinical Investigations. *Otologia (Fukuoka)*.1975;241 with permission).

normal phonation. Sound production without this movement leads to a dysphonic voice. The importance of the middle and deep layers of the lamina propria are its increased ability to produce thicker fibrous tissue (scarring) after injury, thus having a negative impact on the voice.

VOCAL MECHANISM: VASCULAR AND PHYSIOLOGIC SUPPORT

The arterial blood supply to the larynx comes mostly from the inferior thyroid artery through its inferior laryngeal branch.[6] After entering the larynx posterolaterally with the anterior branch of the recurrent laryngeal nerve just above the cricothyroid joint on both sides, this artery joins branches from both the cricothyroid artery anteriorly and the superior laryngeal artery superiorly to form a rich anastamosis inside the thyroid cartilage.[8] As these vessels further divide into smaller and smaller vessels, they finally reach the submucosal tissue and, in the vocal fold, they run parallel to the edge.

The capillary supply to the vocal folds and surrounding structures brings nutrients in and takes metabolic waste products away, but it also removes the heat generated in the mucosa from the energy expended during phonation (mechanical movement, muscle contraction). Increased capillary flow, however, is not the most efficient way to protect the vocal folds from harm. Mucous glands occupy the superior mucosa of the anterior vocal fold in the ventricle, and the mucus secreted here is used for cleaning, lubricating, and protecting the vocal folds. Thus, the anatomy of an area of the body and its physiologic function once again go hand in hand.

VOCAL MECHANISM: NEUROLOGIC SUPPORT

The peripheral motor nerve supply to the larynx is well known and has been mentioned already. The internal laryngeal muscles are supplied by the vagus nerve which gives off two branches to the larynx before it continues downward to supply the rest of the

gastrointestinal or GI tract.[9-11] These are the superior and inferior (recurrent) laryngeal nerves. The superior laryngeal nerve (SLN) further divides into an internal sensory branch and an external motor branch. The internal branch enters the larynx between the hyoid bone and thyroid cartilage and pierces the thyrohyoid membrane one centimeter in front of the superior cornu of the thyroid cartilage (Figure 3-6). It carries information from touch-sensitive receptors, heat-sensitive (thermal) receptors, and mucosal receptors sensitive to chemical changes back to the brainstem. In addition it picks up information from the internal muscles and joints of the larynx as well. Meanwhile the external branch of the SLN is dedicated to supplying motor innervation to the cricothyroid muscle but also picking up sensory information from the anterior subglottic mucosa.[12]

The inferior or recurrent laryngeal nerve (RLN) takes its name from its course through the neck and into the upper chest, and its subsequent looping

Figure 3-6. Innervation of the larynx, right lateral view.

around the aortic arch on the left and the subclavian artery on the right. It then "recurs" in the lower neck running in the groove between the trachea and the esophagus and traveling upward to finally reach the posterolateral larynx.[13] As the RLN reaches its target muscles it sends motor fibers in succession to the posterior cricoarytenoid muscle, the interarytenoid muscle, the lateral cricoarytenoid muscle, and the thyroarytenoid muscle. It also has sensory branches connecting to the subglottic mucosal sensory receptors and the internal laryngeal muscles. If the patient has a congenital anomaly of the right subclavian artery a "nonrecurrent" RLN will be present.[14] However, the RLN *always* enters the larynx just above the cricothyroid joint to gain access to the internal muscles it must innervate.

SUMMARY

The vocal mechanism is an intricate system of balances between the abdomen, chest, neck, and head. It is no wonder that physicians and philosophers throughout recorded time have marveled at the human ability to communicate vocally with other people. The voice is part of our individual identity, and to protect that part of our identity we must, therefore, understand how the voice works and how to maintain it throughout our lives. Learning vocal anatomy is the fundamental step in preserving our gift of voice, and one well worth taking.

REFERENCES

1. Tucker, HM. *The Larynx*. New York, NY: Thieme Medical Publishers, Inc; 1987:136-137.

2. Anson BJ, ed. *Morris' Human Anatomy*. 12th ed. New York, NY: McGraw-Hill Book Co; 1966:1059.

3. Anson BJ, ed. *Morris' Human Anatomy*. 12th ed. New York, NY:McGraw-Hill Book Co; 1966:30.

4. Sellars I, Sellars S. Cricoarytenoid joint structure and function. *J Laryngol Otol*. 1983;97:1027-1034.

5. International Anatomical Nomenclature Committee. *Nomina Anatomica*. 6th ed. Edinburgh, New York: Churchill Livingstone; 1989.

6. Anson BJ, ed. *Morris' Human Anatomy*. 12th ed. New York, NY: McGraw-Hill Book Co; 1966: 1409-1427.

7. Hirano M. Phonosurgery—basic and clinical investigations. *Otologia (Fukuoka)*. 1975;21:239-298.

8. Mihashi SK, Okada M, Kurita S, et al. Vascular network of the vocal cord. In: Stevens KN, Hirano M, eds. *Vocal Fold Physiology*. Tokyo:University of Tokyo Press; 1981:45-58.

9. Strong MS, Vaughan, CW. The morphology of the phonatory organs and their neural control. In: Stevens KN, Hirano M, eds. *Vocal Fold Physiology*. Tokyo:University of Tokyo Press; 1981:13-20.

10. Tyler HR. Neurology of the larynx. *Otolaryngol Clin North Am*. 1984;17:75-79.

11. Kambic V, Zargi M, Radsel Z. Topographic anatomy of the external branch of the superior laryngeal nerve: its importance in head and neck surgery. *J Laryngol Otol*. 1984;98:1121-1124.

12. Wallach JH, Rybicki KJ, Kaufman MP. Anatomical localization of the cells of origin of efferent fibers in the superior laryngeal and recurrent laryngeal nerves of dogs. *Brain Res*. 1983;261:307-311.

13. Caiot P, Bousquet V, Cabanie P, et al. The nerve loops crossing below the subclavian artery and their anatomical variations. *Anat Clin*. 1984;6: 209-213.

14. Saunders G, Uyeda RY, Karlan MS. Nonrecurrent inferior laryngeal nerves and their association with a recurrent branch. *Am J Surg*. 1983;146: 501-503.

Chapter 4

PHYSIOLOGY OF VOICE PRODUCTION: HOW DOES THE VOICE WORK?

Jack Jiang

The production of voice requires the interaction of many physiologic processes whether one sings an aria or simply has a conversation. Most commonly the word, "phonation," conjures images of vibrating vocal folds. The vocal folds serve as an energy transducer; they are responsible for converting aerodynamic power into acoustic power. There are many other contributors to speech, however. The aerodynamic power necessary for voice production is generated subglottally by the chest, thorax, and abdomen. Then, above the vocal folds, resonators modulate the sound into a human voice. This chapter looks more in depth at how these physiologic processes interact to create the voice and how singers can control and master their voices.

THEORIES OF PHONATION

Theories and models of vocal fold vibration have undergone considerable development over the past 150 years. As early as 1741, the vocal folds were demonstrated to be the source of sound production.[1] A model from the 1950s termed the neurochronaxic theory described each vibration as being controlled by individual nerve pulses.[2] The neurochronaxic theory

has now been rejected in favor of more empirically validated models, namely the myoelastic-aerodynamic theory and the body-cover theory.

Myoelastic-Aerodynamic Theory

Published in the late 1950s,[1] the myoelastic-aerodynamic theory is now one of the most widely accepted theories for how vocal fold vibration is initiated and maintained. This theory is most appropriately studied by breaking it into its two components.

Myoelastic refers to the gross neuromuscular control of vocal fold tension and elasticity during phonation. Regulation of elasticity in turn influences the vibration characteristics of the vocal folds. Muscular control over how close the vocal folds are held is also important. During normal exhalation, the vocal folds are about 60% apart, or abducted.[3] During phonation, the muscles are contracted to adduct (bring together) the vocal folds into the stream of airflow. By controlling the configuration of the glottal aperture (opening between the vocal folds), the body can influence pressure differences above and below the glottis. This helps drive the aerodynamic features of vocal fold vibration.

The aerodynamic component of this theory emphasizes the role of fluid dynamics during phonation, specifically the continuity law and Bernoulli's principle. The continuity law assumes an incompressible flow confined in a duct. At all points in the duct, flow must be equal; this is the proverbial "what goes in must come out." Airflow is equal to the cross-sectional area multiplied by the particle velocity. Therefore, if the duct narrows, the velocity must increase proportionally to maintain constant flow (Figure 4–1). In algebraic form:

$$v_1 A_1 = v_2 A_2 = constant,$$

where v is the particle velocity and A is the cross-sectional area at a given point.[4]

This leads to Bernoulli's principle, which deals with the conservation of energy of a flow confined in a pipe. At any point in the flow, the total energy of the fluid is composed of two components: the kinetic energy due to the particle flow and the potential energy due to the pressure on the walls of the pipe. Total energy in the fluid must be conserved. Thus, when the particle velocity increases at a constriction and the kinetic energy of the fluid increases, the potential energy of the fluid must decrease. This is observed by a reduction in pressure on the walls of the pipe. This is especially relevant during the opening and closing of the glottis during phonation; as air passes through the narrowed glottis, it increases in velocity and decreases the pressure exerted on the glottal walls.[4]

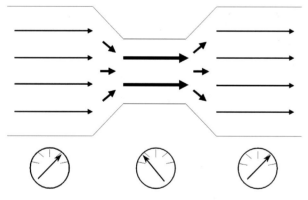

Figure 4-1. Bernoulli effect. As an incompressible flow enters a constriction, flow must remain constant. This is accomplished by increasing velocity, as represented by arrow width, proportionally to the reduction in area. The gauges beneath the diagram indicate relative pressure at each point in the tube.

At a simplistic level, Bernoulli's forces are credited for maintaining vocal fold oscillation. As air passes through the narrowed glottis, the particle velocity increases (continuity law) and the pressure subsequently drops (Bernoulli's law). This reduced pressure draws together and collapses the vocal folds. When subglottal pressure builds up, it reportedly blows the vocal folds apart and allows the cycle to repeat. This repetitive process goes on hundreds of times each second of phonation.

This explanation is inadequate, however. Bernoulli forces are present in the glottis without preference to whether it is opening or closing. Although these forces are effective for drawing the vocal folds together, they ultimately will lead to vocal fold damping. In other words, the Bernoulli forces are such that, instead of maintaining vibration, they will eventually lead the vocal folds to rest.

The additional input necessary to maintain vibration comes from the supraglottal air column. The air column has a degree of inertance, or resistance to change. When air passes through the glottis, it collides with the stagnant air particles already in the supraglottal air space. This creates an area of high pressure (a compression) that aids in driving the vocal folds together. Similarly, when the vocal folds collide with each other, they cut off airflow, but the air above the glottis continues moving forward. This creates an area of low pressure (a rarefaction) that aids vocal fold reopening.[4]

These forces can all be incorporated into an explanation of how vocal fold vibration takes place (Figure 4-2). To initiate phonation, the vocal folds are adducted so there is only a narrow channel between them. As expiratory pressure builds up from the lungs at the glottis, the air pressure pushes against the elasticity of the vocal folds. Eventually, the pressure reaches the minimum pressure needed to begin vibration, the air pushes the vocal fold tissue aside, and air flows through the vocal folds. The difference between the subglottal and supraglottal pressures combined with the deflection of the vocal fold mass creates a positive pressure which draws air up through the trachea. As described by Bernoulli's law, the airflow increases in velocity as it flows through the narrowed glottis.

As air escapes through the glottis from the subglottal reservoir, the subglottal pressure decreases, thus decreasing the force holding the vocal folds apart.

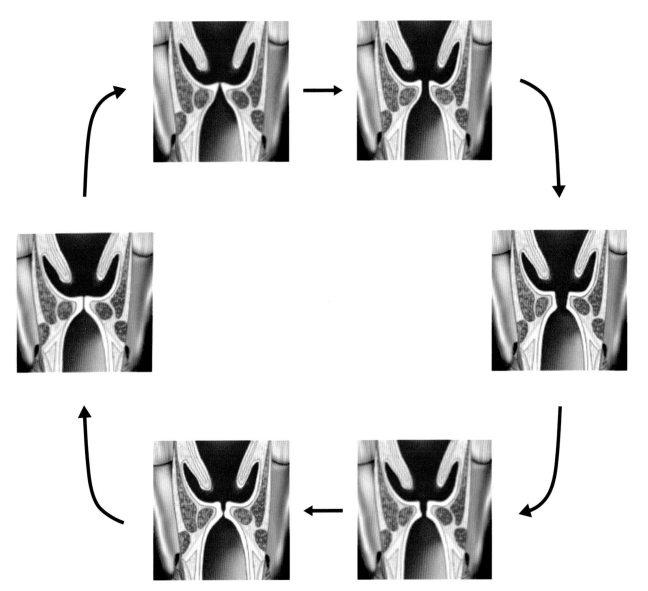

Figure 4–2. Vocal fold movement during one complete cycle. Beginning at the left, the vocal folds are adducted, followed by opening of the lower margins, opening of the upper margins, closure of the lower margins, and finally closure of the upper margins. (Adapted from *Vocal Parts*, 2001[24])

The Bernoulli effect generates a negative force, which pulls the vocal folds medially together again. Also, closure is aided by the passive recoiling (elasticity) of the vocal folds as they return to the position they were held in before being deformed by the transglottal pressure.[5]

When the vocal folds are drawn medially together, they once again obstruct the airflow, and the cycle repeats itself in what is termed the glottal cycle. The key point of the myoelastic-aerodynamic theory is that each glottal cycle is repeated without the need for repetitive muscular contraction after the vocal folds are initially brought together. Vibration is maintained through aerodynamic principles.

The number of times the vocal folds open and close each second is referred to as the frequency. The average frequency is 110 Hz in males and 200 Hz in females, but the human voice has a tremendous range and depends on many complex interactions.[5] The Bernoulli theory suggests that the effective mass and tension of the vocal folds, which are under neuro-muscular control, are the most important factors for controlling frequency.

Body-Cover Theory

The body-cover theory asserts that the five layers of the vocal folds can be classified into two groups to help account for vocal fold motion (Figure 4–3). The cover consists of the epithelium and the superficial and intermediate layers of the lamina propria. The cover is noted for being pliable and elastic but not muscular, and therefore not contractile. The deep layer of the lamina propria and the thyroarytenoid muscle fibers comprise the body. Active contractile properties of the body allow for adjustments of stiffness and concentration of mass.[6]

The morphologic structure of the vocal folds is important for controlling the tension of the vocal folds. The effective tension relies on the coupling of the vocal fold cover to the adjustable body. When the thyroarytenoid contracts, the body stiffens.[7] This contraction causes the distance between the arytenoids and the thyroid to shorten, so the cover becomes lax and pliable. The influence of the thyroarytenoid contraction on the fundamental frequency depends on the depth of vocal fold movement. If vibration is occurring primarily at the cover level, contraction of the thyro-arytenoid will make it more lax and thus lower the fundamental frequency. If vibration is deeper, however, and involves the body of the vocal folds, the increased tension for contraction of the thyroarytenoid will lead to an increase in fundamental frequency.[8]

The body-cover theory is used to account for the very large number of modes of vibration possible in the human vocal folds. Due to the loose coupling between the cover and the body, the cover can move independently of the body in an extremely variable ripple of tissue deformation.[6] This nonuniform tissue movement is characterized by normal modes of vibration, which detail the vibration patterns of the vocal folds. For instance, the lower margins of the vocal folds typically lead the upper margins in opening and closing of the vocal folds. This creates an alternation between convergent (closed at the top) and divergent (open at the top) shapes in the vocal folds whose asymmetry helps to sustain the oscillations.[4]

The more flexible the vocal folds are, the more potential there is for self-oscillation, and consequently, the more difficult it is to describe their movement. Current study of the vocal folds lacks consensus on the contribution of nonlinear dynamics to the vibration; multiple variables likely interact as either linear interactions of nonlinear systems or nonlinear interactions of linear systems.[5] Chaos theory (fractal analysis) has been employed to try to explain the complexity and redundancy of vibratory patterns.[9]

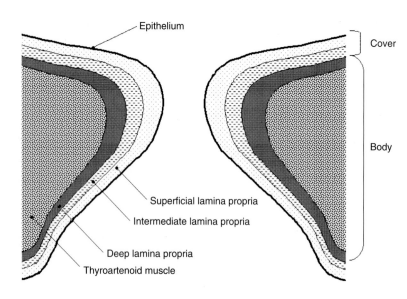

Figure 4–3. Layers of the vocal folds. The epithelium and superficial and intermediate layers of the lamina propria comprise the cover while the deep layer of the lamina propria and the thyroarytenoid muscle comprise the vocal fold body.

Mucosal Wave Movement

In addition to theories detailing how vibration is maintained, there is a clear model detailing how the vocal fold mucosa opens and closes in a wavelike pattern.[10] It is a common misconception that the sound produced by the vocal folds is a direct result of their vibration, much like a vibrating guitar string. On the contrary, the sound produced by the vocal folds is the result of small bursts of air that escape while the vocal folds vibrate. The vibration consists of an alternating sequence of medial (closing) and lateral (opening) movements. The asymmetry of these movements, which begin at the lower margins and travel to the upper margins of the vocal folds, helps to maintain oscillation. This movement is termed the mucosal wave because of its similarity to how waves travel in a fluid media.[5]

Canine larynges have been studied with videostroboscopy and other methods to show how different variables affect the mucosal waveform. Mucosal wave velocity has been shown to increase with vocal fold lengthening,[11,12] greater airflow,[11] greater subglottal pressure,[13] and laryngeal muscle contraction associated with higher fundamental frequency.[13]

PHONATORY INPUTS

The vocal folds are often thought of as the source of voice. Although they are essential in the conversion of aerodynamic power to acoustic power, the vocal folds do not act alone. Voice production requires contributions from subglottal pressure, the vocal folds, and supraglottal resonators.

Subglottal Pressure

Vocal fold vibration is powered by subglottal aerodynamic inputs. When intrathoracic pressure exceeds atmospheric pressure, there is a positive subglottal pressure. This subglottal pressure is primarily controlled by the lower respiratory airway, particularly the elastic properties of the chest walls and the active muscular contraction of the chest, diaphragm, and abdominal muscles. However, changes in the larynx

and upper airway can also influence subglottal pressure. These changes are dynamic and influence the phonation threshold pressure and glottal resistance. To respond to these changes, there must be complex and rapid feedback systems. Although not fully understood, feedback systems may include a combination of pressure sensors, proprioceptive sensors, muscle tension/stretch sensors, and auditory sensors.[5] This feedback helps the body to regulate the amount of subglottal pressure required to start phonation.

The phonation threshold pressure, the minimum subglottal pressure required to initiate and sustain vocal fold vibration, is very important in the study of phonation. A low phonation threshold pressure means that relatively little respiratory effort is required to drive vocal fold vibration. The phonation threshold pressure decreases when there is a decreased prephonatory glottal width (the vocal folds are closer together), the viscosity of the vocal folds is decreased,[14] the thickness of the vocal folds is increased, or when the pitch is lowered. Phonation threshold pressure is elevated in dehydrated vocal folds,[15] patients with vocal fold polyps,[16] and patients with Parkinson's disease.[17]

This necessary subglottal pressure cannot be generated without glottal resistance, which is the ratio of transglottal pressure to transglottal airflow. This ratio was originally constructed in an effort to define something invariant about the glottal region of the airway. However, it has been difficult to tabulate due to the large number of geometric factors that affect the ratio, including glottal width and shape.[4]

A more useful number to characterize flow through a constricted area, such as the glottis, is a measure called the Reynolds number. This number is defined as:

$$Re = (vd)/\mu,$$

where *Re* is Reynolds number, *v* is air particle velocity, *d* is the effective diameter of the constriction, and μ is the kinematic viscosity. When Reynold's number exceeds a certain critical value, the fluid exiting the constriction will exhibit turbulent flow, like raging whitewater. Below the critical value, fluid exiting the constriction will exhibit laminar or steady flow (Figure 4-4). Usually the flow resistance increases with turbulent flow because of the increased energy dissipation. This can be useful for phonating certain

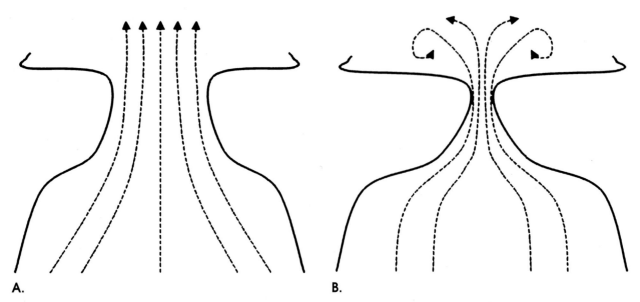

A.   **B.**

Figure 4–4. Reynolds number. **A.** If the speed of air is slow enough and the glottis wide enough, air exiting the glottis will exhibit laminar flow in parallel sheets. **B.** If these factors combine to give a Reynold's number above the threshold, turbulent flow will result.

sounds, like [h], but is not desirable for other sounds such as vowels.[4] It should be noted that most singers attempt to maintain laminar flow throughout phrases in the music.

Biomechanical Properties of Vocal Folds

Vibration of the vocal folds is a complex process whose characteristics are modulated by the biomechanical properties of the vocal folds. Specifically, the mass, stiffness, and viscosity of the vocal folds are important to regulating their vibration.

The fundamental frequency of vibration is inversely related to mass, as defined as the amount of vocal fold material that is effectively vibrating. While the actual mass of the vocal folds is fairly constant except in cases of edema or growths, the mass per unit length is easily modifiable. Longitudinal stretching of the vocal folds, as caused by contraction of the cricothyroid muscle, thins out the mass, modifies the cross-sectional shape of the vocal folds, and increases fundamental frequency. Contraction of other muscular fibers, namely, the thyroarytenoid, brings the arytenoid and thyroid closer together, thus increasing the

concentration of mass and decreasing fundamental frequency (Figure 4–5).

The second key biomechanical property of the vocal folds is stiffness, or the effective restoring force per unit of displacement. Stiffness is directly proportional to vocal fold tension and largely regulated by vocal fold length.[4] Contraction of the cricothyroid muscles increases the physical length of the tissues and thus increases the stretch tension. This is a passive state of tension because it occurs as a result of the tissue being spread over a greater area, much like a rubber band's tension increases as it is stretched. Contraction of the thyroarytenoid muscle fibers results in an active tensing of the vocal fold body. Although thyroarytenoid contraction increases the stiffness and tension in the muscular body, it reduces tension in the cover.[4] Optimum phonation requires a balance between the tension of the muscular body and the cover; the more closely the tensions of the body and cover are matched, the more efficient the conversion of aerodynamic to acoustic energy. This balance is not determined by the absolute level of contraction of each muscle but rather the differential control between them.[4]

Finally, viscosity is an important biomechanical property of the vocal folds. Viscosity is a measure of how resistant the vocal fold tissues are to change.[4]

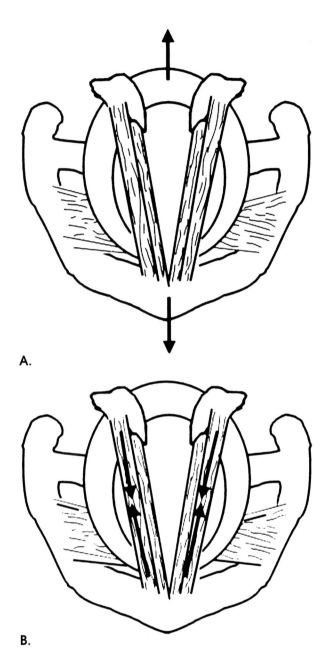

A.

B.

Figure 4–5. Muscular tuning of fundamental frequency. **A.** Contraction of the cricothyroid will elongate the vocal folds putting a passive stretch tension on the vocal fold cover. **B.** Contraction of the thyroarytenoid muscle results in an active tensing of the vocal folds.

Higher viscosity, such as results from dehydration of the vocal folds, translates to greater internal friction, greater energy loss in the form of heat, and a higher phonation threshold pressure. Viscosity is not independent of mass and tension; longitudinal tension increases viscosity, whereas the greater vocal fold thickness that results from contraction of mass reduces viscosity.

Supraglottal Resonance

The sound exiting the glottis consists of the fundamental frequency plus many harmonics, or overtones. The supraglottal vocal tract helps to shape those sounds from raw noise into a human voice. The filtering effects of the supraglottal vocal tract modulate the acoustic output of the glottis and regulate the acoustic power. The higher frequencies are more susceptible to energy loss because of the damping characteristics of the source spectrum of glottal vibration.[5]

When the waveforms reflect off other structures, resonance occurs. To appreciate resonance, we turn to the analogy of a bottle with a narrow neck. When one blows across the top of the neck, the air in the bottle resonates at a certain frequency. The resonant frequency is a characteristic of the bottle, not of the air being blown across it. Pouring liquid into or out of the bottle will change its resonant frequency by changing the air column's size and shape.

Similarly, air will resonate at a certain frequency in the supraglottal vocal tract. Each resonance in the vocal tract is called a formant. Changing the size and shape of the airway by moving the tongue, jaw, lips, and any other structures in the upper airway will change the resonant frequency. Lengthening the airways causes a decrease in formant frequencies, the energy regions of vowels. The resonance in the supraglottal air tract is responsible for the perceived differences in vowels. Each vowel is defined by the lowest two formants, which are a characteristic of the supraglottal vocal tract.[4] (See a more extensive discussion of formants in chapter 9.)

PHONATORY CONTROL MECHANISMS

Pitch

As described by the myoelastic-aerodynamic theory, two main factors interact to control pitch: tension and mass. The tension involves both the passive tension on the vocal fold cover and the active stiffness of the vocal fold body. Lengthening the vocal folds increases stretch tension on the vocal fold cover. Increasing the length also decreases the mass per unit length, which leads to an increase in frequency. The average person can control these changes to have an overall pitch range of about two octaves.

Raising the pitch primarily relies on contraction of the cricothyroid muscle. Contraction of the cricothyroid causes the vocal folds to lengthen and the medial edge to thin. Because the cricoarytenoid muscle limits the movement of the arytenoid cartilages, contraction of the cricothyroid also causes an increase in vocal tension. All of these factors can be fine-tuned to elevate the pitch. Breath pressure has also been shown to covary with pitch. This has been demonstrated in both excised larynges and computer models, but it is a complex relationship that is not yet completely understood.[18] Current evidence shows that while pitch and pressure are related, they do not have a causal link.

There are two mechanisms for lowering the pitch. From a higher pitch to a lower pitch, one simply relaxes the muscles in the larynx. The natural elasticity of the vocal folds returns them to the tension required to produce their normal pitch. Further lowering of the pitch requires contraction of the thyroarytenoid muscle. This draws the arytenoid and the thyroid cartilages together, thus increasing the concentration of mass and decreasing tension on the cover.[7] This rounds the medial edge of the vocal folds and allows for greater amplitude of vibration. Contraction of the thyroarytenoid can be used to lower the pitch below the normal pitch At high frequencies because there is little movement of the deep tissues, contraction of the thyroarytenoid is used to fine-tune the pitch.

Loudness

Loudness of voice is a measure of how we perceive pressure or power differences. The largest determinate of loudness is the intensity of sound, which is the physical measure of power or pressure ratios. Increased intensity requires the vocal folds to open and close with more vigor. Control of this is possible at the subglottal, glottal, and supraglottal levels. This control relies on the same basic mechanism that controls

frequency, so it is difficult to vary them separately. There are two contributors to subglottal regulation of vocal intensity: subglottal pressure and tracheal airflow.[19] At the level of glottal regulation, intensity is linked to the level of medial compression.[20] When the vocal folds are more tightly compressed, more force is required to blow them apart. They then are drawn together more forcefully and close more rapidly. Tightly compressed vocal folds stay closed longer and thus increase the intensity with which each burst of air escapes the vocal folds. This level of regulation is especially important at low pitches.[21]

Supraglottal factors can also affect vocal intensity. The size, shape, and placement of resonators are important. Trained speakers learn how to effectively control frequency and intensity independently. Trained singers can also increase vocal intensity with less respiratory and vocal effort by changing the shape and stiffness of the vocal tract to tune formants. It is well known that there is a major hump in the voice spectrum around 3000 Hz known as the "singers' formant" that allows the singer's voice to soar over the accompaniment.[4]

Voice Quality

One of the main ways to evaluate vocal quality is through vocal registers, which are perceptually distinguishable modes of phonation. The ideal phonation register is modal, or chest. This register is present in the middle frequency range. Because it is the most efficient mode of phonation, it is the mode used most commonly in daily conversation. Speech-language pathologists focus on teaching their clients to use this mode of phonation.

Below modal phonation is the pulse or glottal fry register. This low frequency of phonation (30–90 Hz) is distinguished by its crackly, "Strohbass" (straw bass) sound. It is important to note that it is not simply a lower frequency of phonation; it is a different mode of phonation that contains a secondary syncopated beat. During this syncopated vibration, two opening cycles occur in close succession followed by a prolonged closed phase that may last for up to 90% of the cycle. It requires only low subglottal pressure to maintain because the vibrating margin is flaccid and thick. The lack of tension allows air to slowly bubble through the vocal folds instead of pushing them into rapid vibration. To eliminate the crackly quality of this voice, one must increase the tension of the vocalis muscle.[22]

On the opposite end of the vocal spectrum is the high frequency (300–600 Hz and above) loft or falsetto register. The falsetto register is defined by a very short, or completely absent, closed phase with the vocal folds making contact only briefly. During this type of phonation, the vocal folds are thin and reedlike. The cricothyroid and thyroarytenoid muscles both exhibit heightened activity.[23] When the vocal folds reach the maximum possible contraction, they must use a different mode of increasing pitch. The posterior portion of the vocal folds is damped, and there is a reduced degree of movement.[22]

Two common variations on these modes of vibration are breathy and pressed voice. Breathy voice results when the vocal folds remain slightly abducted during vibration. This mode is inefficient because it causes air wastage and vocal fatigue, but it is not damaging to the phonatory mechanism. However, breathy phonation may be an indication of an underlying pathology, like vocal polyps, that is preventing complete closure of the vocal folds. On the other side of the spectrum, pressed phonation results from full glottal adduction. This variation on the voice is often viewed as strong and commanding but it is actually abusive to the vocal folds and can lead to damage.[5]

Nonregistered voice quality can be described based on its stability. Phonation with long-term modulation of intensity may be labeled as persistent, variable, or controlled; the terms traditionally given to these modulations in intensity are "tremulous" in pathologic voices, "nervous" in emotional voices, and "vibrato" in singing voices. Involuntary variations in stability are labeled "hoarse." Hoarseness may result from glottal incompetence in vocal fold paralysis, lesions that affect vocal fold mass, or vocal fold hyperfunction. For an objective evaluation of hoarseness, clinicians often refer to signal-to-noise ratio, or SNR.[5]

Overall voice quality, or timbre, is defined by the partial emphasis of different overtones. Essentially it is an evaluation of the qualities that make each voice unique and humanlike. Timbre is influenced by selective amplification by the walls of a series of resonators in the pharynx and mouth. Timbre is closely related to the skewing of the glottal volume velocity. This refers to the fact that the flow maximum occurs after the maximum glottal area. Skewing is linked to the iner-

tance, or resistance to change in airflow, of the airway. When phonation occurs, the stagnant air in the vocal tract must be pushed out. The resistance of the stagnant air increases supraglottal pressure and thus decreases translaryngeal pressure. Elongating the vocal tract with maneuvers such as lowering the larynx or protruding the lips can increase inertance. Greater inertance means greater skewing of the flow maximum, and the more the flow maximum is skewed, the more energy is in the higher harmonic frequencies of the voice.

SUMMARY

Overall, voice production involves the interaction of many physiological systems. It begins with the aerodynamic pressure generated by the chest, thorax, and abdomen. Muscles in the larynx can be used to control the width of the glottal opening and the tension in the vocal folds, which when combined with the pressure inputs, drive the vocal folds into a series of rhythmic vibrations. The result is a wave of air pressure changes sent to the upper vocal tract where it can be modulated by resonators and filters to produce the instrument known as the human voice.

REFERENCES

1. Van den Berg J. Myoelastic-aerodynamic theory of voice production. *J Speech Hear Res.* 1958;1:227–244.
2. Tucker HM. *The Larynx.* 2nd ed. New York, NY: Thieme Medical Publishers; 1993.
3. Stemple JC, Glaze L, Klaben BG. *Clinical Voice Pathology Theory and Management.* 3rd ed. San Diego, Calif: Singular Publishing Group; 2000.
4. Titze IR. *Principles of Voice Production.* Englewood Cliffs, NJ: Prentice Hall; 1994.
5. Jiang JJ, Lin E, Hanson DG. Vocal fold physiology. *Voice Dis Phonosurg J.* 2000;33:699–718.
6. Hirano M. Morphological structure of the vocal cord as a vibrator and its variations. *Folio Phoniatr.* 1974;26:89–94.
7. Titze IR, Luschei ES, Hirano M. Role of the thyroarytenoid muscle in regulation of fundamental frequency. *J Voice.* 1989;3:213–224.

8. Titze IR, Jiang J, Drucker DG. Preliminaries to the body-cover theory of pitch control. *J Voice.* 1988;1:314-319.

9. Baken RJ. Irregularity of vocal period and amplitude: a first approach to the fractal analysis of voice. *J Voice.* 1989;4:185-197.

10. Hertegård S, Gauffing J. Glottal area and vibratory patterns studied with simultaneous stroboscopy, flow glottography, and electroglottography. *J Speech Hear Res.* 1995;38:35-100.

11. Jiang JJ, Yumoto E, Lin SJ, Kadota Y, Kurokawa H, Hanson DG. Quantitative measurement of mucosal wave by high-speed photography in excised larynges. *Ann Otol Rhinol Laryngol.* 1998;107(2):98-103.

12. Titze IR, Jiang JJ, Hsiao T-Y. Measurement of mucosal wave propagation and vertical phase difference in vocal fold vibration. *Ann Otol Rhinol Laryngol.* 1993;102:58-63.

13. Nasri S, Sercarz JA, Berke GS. Noninvasive measurement of traveling wave velocity in the canine larynx. *Ann Otol Rhinol Laryngol.* 1994;103:758-766.

14. Finkelhor BK, Titze IR, Durham PL. The effect of viscosity changes in the vocal folds on the range of oscillation. *J Voice.* 1988;1:320-325.

15. Verdolini K, Titze IR, Fennell A. Dependence of phonatory effort on hydration level. *J Speech Hear Res.* 1994;37:1001-1007.

16. Jiang JJ, O'Mara T, Conley D, et al. Phonation threshold pressure measurements during phonation by airflow interruption. *Laryngoscope.* 1999;109:425-432.

17. Jiang J, Vlagos D, O'Mara TG, et al. Aerodynamic measurement of patients with Parkinson's disease. *J Voice.* 1991;13:583-591.

18. Shipp T, Doherty ET, Morrissey P. Predicting vocal frequency from selected physiologic measures. *J Acoust Soc Am.* 1979;66:678-684.

19. Holmberg EB, Hillman RE, Perkell JS. Glottal airflow and transglottal air pressure measurements for male and female speakers in soft, normal, and loud voice. *J Acoust Soc Am.* 1988;84:511-529.

20. Berke GS, Hanson DG, Gerratt BR, et al. The effect of airflow and medial adductory compression on vocal efficiency and glottal vibration. *Otolaryngol Head Neck Surg.* 1990;102:212-218.

21. Isshiki N. Regulatory mechanisms of voice intensity variation. *J Speech Hear Res.* 1964;7:17-29.

22. Seikel JA, King DW, Drumright DG. *Anatomy and Physiology for Speech, Language and Hearing.* 3rd ed. Clifton Park, NY: Thomson Delmar Learning; 2005.

23. Zemlin WR. *Speech and Hearing Science.* 4th ed. Needham Heights, Mass: Allyn and Bacon; 1998.

24. *Vocal Parts* [computer program]. Version 2.5. Lynnwood, Wash: Blue Tree Publishing Inc; 2001.

Chapter 5

NORMAL VOICE MATURATION: HORMONES AND AGE

Jean Abitbol

The life of the voice, its path, its challenges and limitations, its emotional impact through the existence is a journey. It will challenge us to understand how the cycle of life can leave its scars on the female and the male voice. The route is not the same. Voice matures primarily through its genetic inheritance, the DNA. There are many secondary reasons for maturation and aging of the voice. These are discussed in this chapter (see Figure 5–1).

We will come to understand the alchemy between mind, body, and hormones that create the voice and the impact of the passage of time. In the chaotic logic of the space and time continuum, this precious gift that is the voice is an emotional amplifier that we must protect.

Figure 5-1. Primary and secondary causes of aging.

HORMONES AND VOICE

A Complex Story of an Internal Clock

Why does puberty change the voice so much in men? Why a does a woman's voice change during her menstrual cycle? How can the vibrations change at menopause to result in breaking of the voice? How does a cyclic pathology appear on a vocal fold and is the voice injured after the hormonal "earthquake" around age 50?

So many questions, so many clues. If we are to solve this enquiry, we shall inevitably have to understand the hormones, their impact on the voice, and the scar of time. Between the cell and the larynx, the brain and language, hearing and vocalizing, the vocal landscape takes shape, but in all its forms, the voice is always a reflection of our personality.

What separates the infant's screams from that sexy female voice or from that male voice that charms us so? How does the hormonal revolution of adolescence transform the voice? How does our genetic mapping stamp the verbal expression of our thinking and our emotional universe?

Voice and hormones: two words that clash, meet, and harmonize. The voice is sexual. But is our voice's sex the same as our genetic sex? Is it determined by our XY, XX chromosomes, or by estrogen and progesterone hormones in women and androgens in men?

Our musical instrument, the larynx, is a hormonal target. At puberty, the larynx undergoes a host of changes. These transformations are determined by our genetic heritage, but more so by our hormones. Indeed, the castrato retains a child's voice, said to be feminine because he did not receive testosterone. This is proof enough of the unquestionable impact of male hormones on our vocal folds, and of their determining influence on our male genetic print.

Does voice have a sex? If it does, is its character hormonal or chromosomal? Our voice changes over the years, it changes with our life story, with our appearance, and with our physique. It also changes as a function of our emotional environment. Our fingerprint identifies a physical part of our anatomy specific and unique to us; it has no duplicate. Our voiceprint reveals our personality, our sensibility, and reveals our sexuality. Let's try to follow the trail of the sexual voice. Let's retrace the steps of this miracle of life, from the embryo through to the adult and the aged.

VOICE DEVELOPMENT: A HORMONAL TARGET

The infant's cries have no sex. In no way are some cries identifiable as feminine and others as masculine. By age 7 or 8, differences in the male and female pitch begin to occur. However, only at puberty will a sexual register impose itself on the children's voices.

The larynx is hormonally dependent and evolves with time and the sexual life of each individual.[1] When you hear people speaking on the radio or on the telephone, you can identify their sex from their voices within a few tenths of a second. The voice is a secondary sexual characteristic. Of course, sex hormones influence it, but so do others.

Time has an important influence on hormonal activity. This dimension plays a role not only in the evolution of life, but also in our day-to-day life. Certain hormones must be secreted at precise moments of our life: during our fetal development, at birth, or at puberty. Before those precise moments, it's too soon, after, it's too late.

This remarkable internal clock of ours isn't yet fully understood. The thyroid hormones are a case in point. If they don't do their work in the first years of our life, this brings on irreversible physical and intellectual anomalies that can lead to cretinism. Should one later try to palliate this hormonal deficiency with artificial substitutes, it would be to no avail, the damage will have been done. Nowadays, very early diagnoses enable appropriate treatment to be prescribed in good time.[2] But if the impact of our hormones dictates the need for a precise timetable, if they are to efficiently influence the evolution of our life, nowhere is this more evident than in a woman's menstrual cycle and our diurnal cycle. In our diurnal cycle, cortisone is naturally secreted by our body at the end of the day and in the early morning. These different secretions are controlled by an internal feedback system that avoids hormonal excess or insufficiencies through autoregulation.

The thyroid gland's role is to counter the aggressions of the outside world (the weather, cold, heat, stress). The thyroid hormones play a determining role in our vocal register. The thyroid gland at the base of our neck can become the seat of a goiter, basically a nodular increase in its volume, or conversely, it can become hyposecretive. The thyroid is indispensable to the evolution of the voice. It acts as do bellows on a fire, stimulating a majority of organs in our body and influencing our vocal timbre. In a serious case of hypothyroidism, the voice becomes harsh. The vocal folds present a slight edema and the vocal muscles become congested. This well-known pathology regresses as soon as thyroid extracts are administered. The voice recovers its normal register and its natural harmonics. However, the essential elements that modify the quality of our voice are our sex hormones: estrogen, progesterone, and androgen.

The role of our sex hormones is to enable our sexuality to adapt. Of all mammals, Man is the one with the greatest hormonal complexity—to such an extent that, if our hormonal secretion is upset, it can cause irreversible damage. If no substitutes are provided for certain glands when these are suppressed, the outcome can be fatal. Finally, the precarious balance between our hormones is what ensures the stability of the living being. Their action is key for the evolution of our adolescence. Our endocrine glands, the main ones being the pituitary gland, the ovaries, the testicles, the thyroid, and the adrenals, produce a hormone inside the gland and secrete it through an excretory canal into our blood vessels. The hormone stimulates a specific receptor organ, the organ that can facilitate the desired outcome: adrenaline accelerates the heart, testosterone increases our libido.

Only the ovaries secrete estrogen and progesterone, the female hormones, and then only if the ovaries have previously been stimulated by FSH and LH, the pituitary hormones.[1] Finally, estrogens and progesterone will, in turn, stimulate one of their main target organs, the genital organs, and bring on the menses in a woman, if she still has a uterus. If a woman has had a hysterectomy, she has no uterus, and therefore no menses; the target organ at the end of the line has been removed. The consequences of the menses are definitively gone, but not the consequences of the sex hormones' effects on her organism. Thus, other target organs like the vagina, the breasts, or the larynx retain their tonicity and their hormonal rhythm.

In certain respects, the hormone is like a cordless remote control, but its operating method is molecular rather than infrared. An infinitesimal amount suffices for a significant impact. Where vitamins are an indispensable element in our nutrition because the body does not produce them, hormones are produced by our cells, but are just as indispensable to our survival. They accelerate, stabilize, or slow down their target organ.

The Larynx as a Target Organ for Multiple Hormones

As a target organ, the larynx is warned by its specific receptors of the arrival of hormonal molecules. Our mighty hormonal factory gets into gear at puberty. Three masters manage it: the brain, the hypothalamus, and the pituitary gland. Their orders provoke hormonal secretions. The first intervenes: our neurologic center and emotional world pass information in the form of electrical impulses on to the hypothalamus at the base of the encephalon. The second takes over to pass this information on to the pituitary gland. The third now secretes substances and expedites them to the glands concerned. The informed gland then secretes its hormones and releases them into the bloodstream, where they will, on the one hand, migrate to the target organs and, on the other, inform the hypothalamus and the pituitary gland that all is well, that the secretion rate is satisfactory. This feedback is remarkably precise and maintains our hormonal balance just as it should be, neither too high nor too low. When hormonal secretions are excessive, the hypothalamus and pituitary glands jointly diminish the stimulation of the gland concerned. Hormones play an intermediary role between our brain and our various organs, notably the larynx.

Puberty, Vocal Metamorphosis: Male or Female, the Choice Is Made

Adolescence takes us down the path leading to sex-determined vocal frequencies. The adolescent, now virile, slim, and athletic, is ill-served by his shrill, unbearable falsetto voice. Meanwhile, the magic of evolution will have endowed others with the vocal vibration of a Caruso or a Callas, or simply the man-in-the-street, as much at home with his voice as he feels at home in his skin.

The Hormonal Revolution

At puberty, the threshold between childhood and adulthood, our secondary sexual characteristics develop and, with them, the physical and psychological transformations specific to each sex.[3] From the newborn to the old adult, chin- angle plays a role in vocal development and decline (Figure 5–2).

In the West, the average age of puberty is 10 to 13 years, in the East it is 9 to 12. The appearance of our sex hormones—estrogens and progesterone in girls and androgens in boys—triggers the development of the third layer of epithelium cells on the vocal folds (prior to this time, like the other mammals, we just have two layers). Thus, the harmonics of our voice become adult in part due to this third layer and in part due to the final development of the striated muscle of the vocal folds.[4] As a girl becomes a woman, she develops higher harmonics, as well as some lower ones that she previously lacked. In boys, the action of testosterone on the muscular and mucosal structure of the vocal cords favors the appearance of new low harmonics and the loss of some of the child's high harmonics. The hormonal revolution is more impressive in men. The shape and covering of the vocal cords changes, thickens, grows, acquires more volume, but the thoracic cage, lungs, stature, and brain are also evolving. In the West, men's left brain develops more than the right brain, whereas women maintain certain equilibrium between the rational brain and the emotional brain. The consequences of puberty for the voice may be more obvious in boys than in girls, but they exist in both sexes. It triggers emotional changes that are usually appropriate to the person's physical appearance. In women, the vocal pitch drops by a third of an octave compared to girls' voices; in men, the voice drops by an octave.

Puberty Can Take a Wrong Turn

Puberty can take an adolescent boy one to five years to acquire his adult voice. But puberty can take a wrong turn. A lack of harmony due to an imbalance between voicing and breathing produces a voice that "goes off the rails," like a Tyrolean melody. Compared to women, men have greater lung capacity, a more developed cardiovascular system, a higher level of hemoglobin and red blood cells, and more striated muscle mass.[5] In the boy turned man, a falsetto voice that can't stabilize itself must be treated. It produces an anachronism

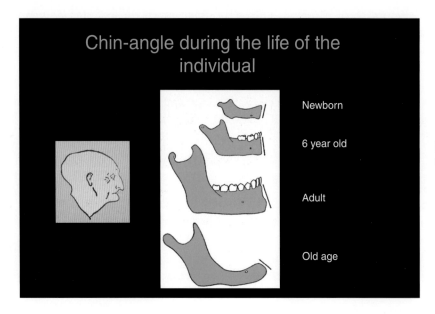

Figure 5–2. Changes in chin-angle over a lifetime.

between the apparent youth of the voice and the man's physical appearance. A difficult harmonization between voice and physical appearance is one of puberty's most delicate obstacles because the voice is seen to project its owner's personality. Therefore, one should definitely help adolescents to successfully complete this metamorphosis, should this be necessary. Voice therapy is the primary treatment to help an adolescent with this problem. Control of his exhalation during laryngeal voicing, and adapting his behavior to his sociocultural environment will help him discover his adult voice.

The Bend Has Been Successfully Negotiated: Male or Female, There's No Ambiguity

In male singers, a well-defined head voice and chest voice make their appearance after puberty. These two vocal techniques bring into play the ligaments and muscles located between the thyroid and the cricoid cartilages, which are more developed in men. They allow the larynx to rock, and the previous calcification of the Adam's apple greatly facilitates this. The significant lengthening of the vocal folds in men also makes it easier for them to sing in these two head and chest registers.

In women, the process of puberty is less eventful. It flows more smoothly. The thyroid cartilage and the cricothyroid membrane hardly change. The vocal cord lengthens slightly and increases its muscle mass. Despite the formation of the third epithelium layer, the vocal fold remains very supple, with a fine mucous membrane. Small glandular cells as depicted in Figure 5–3 keep the vocal folds lubricated and depend on feminine hormones (estrogens and progesterone).

The ovaries enter their active period of reproduction. The first menstrual cycles appear. They become progressively more regular. After a few months, the voice discovers new high-pitched and low-pitched harmonics. The periodicity of the female hormones' secretions gives rhythm to the adolescent girl's life cycles. The lunar cycle is orchestrated by the hypothalamopituitary axis due to the action of FSH and LH, two hormones that act directly on the ovaries to stimulate the secretion of estrogens and progesterone. Note that the menstrual cycle presents two distinct phases: a follicular phase between the first and the 14th day of the cycle, in which only estrogens are present—there's no progesterone—and a luteal phase between the 15th and the 28th day of the cycle, during which both estrogens and progesterone are secreted. In this context, ovulation occurs on the 14th day. The similarity between the follicular changes in the ovaries and the vocal folds is quite similar as shown in Figure 5–4.

Figure 5–3. Glandular cells depend on female hormones to keep the vocal folds lubricated.

Figure 5–4. Comparison of cervical and vocal fold smears during two stages of the female ovarian cycle.

All Is Sweetness and Light Between the Lunar Cycle and the Solar Cycle

In both men and women, the sex glands have two functions. The first is reproduction, through the formation of sperm in men and the preservation of the ovum in women. The second is synthesis of the sex hormones: androgens in men, estrogens, progesterone, and a hint of androgens in women. In girls, the number of ova is predetermined from birth. This is the number of follicles, which exist only in the ovaries. The ovum has 23 chromosomes, but they are all X chromosomes. Therefore, the sex of the baby will be determined by the spermatozoon, which can be X or Y. In men, the testicles ensure the regular production

of sperm almost until death. The male climacteric is delayed in some men until their 80s. Whereas men renew their sperm daily according to the solar cycle, women ovulate in tune with the "lunar cycle."

THE FEMALE VOICE

The Female Life Span: The Premenstrual Voice Syndrome

A Woman's Voice

The first menstrual cycle appears during adolescence. It is triggered by two hormones, FSH and LH, that launch the process of the life cycle. The lunar cycle harmonizes the next 40 years. The active phase of the genitals has begun. Each cycle is punctuated by a physical, mechanical, and ovarian impact, but equally by a molecular, hormonal, and chemical impact, with repercussions on the entire organism.[6] In this first part of the cycle, there is no progesterone, only estrogens are secreted. During the second period of the cycle, both estrogens and progesterone are secreted. But, and this is critical, the progesterone can only act if the estrogens have previously prepared the ground and informed the receptors of the target organs. The sudden drop in estrogens and progesterone production brings on the menses which is the first day of a new cycle.

Three Actors for Our Sex Life: Androgens, Estrogens, and Progesterone

Each molecule triggers a modification of the mucous membranes, muscles, and bony tissues; therefore, our laryngeal instrument, our voice, is also modified. It also influences the cerebral cortex, thereby influencing the brain.[7] This influence is primordial at puberty and persists for the rest of one's life.

The feminine voice has exerted its charms since millennia. In the Greek civilization, Apollo and Orpheus discussed the merits of the athlete's worship of the body and of the powers of a siren's voice to soothe emotions.

When estrogens are flowing, the vocal timbre is sharper. The estrogens secreted by the ovaries have different implications for the larynx. They result in a slight thickening of the cordal mucous membrane, which creates greater vibratory amplitude. The voice acquires a good timbre. The desquamation of superficial cells is reduced, accompanied by a decrease in the need to clear one's throat and in the amount of laryngeal mucous fluid. The lipid cells under the cordal mucous membrane are stimulated. The voice becomes more supple (in the menstrual cycle, this is called the maturation phase with a proliferate action).

The cells of the genital and the cordal mucous membrane: Are they different? By 1982, receptors for estrogen hormones had been identified on the vocal folds and in the uterus. These separate objective findings were confirmed by Abitbol et al. using comparative studies of smears taken from the vocal folds and the cervix of the uterus, during the same day of the menstrual cycle.[1] The results were amazing; in both cases, the cellular aspect was identical (see Figure 5-4). There was a perfect correspondence between the smears taken from the cervix of the uterus and those taken from the vocal folds. This correspondence had long been suspected. Given that both have the same type of mucous membrane, it is only logical that they should have the same cyclical impact. But now there was scientific, objective proof to support this. This is consistent with the observation that the voice can change with the menstrual cycle.

Estrogens also act on the mammary glands and their excretory canals to affect the growth of girls' breasts at puberty. Their action on the metabolism of calcium influences the bony and cartilaginous structures of our larynx. These structures increase or maintain global bone mass. Estrogens also improve the permeability of blood vessels and capillaries, which are very numerous in the vocal folds, thereby increasing oxygenation. They have no effect on striated muscle. They diminish the risk of Alzheimer's disease. They have an antagonist effect with androgens. Finally, for progesterone, the second, strictly female hormone, to be effective, the tissues must first have been impregnated with estrogens.

Progesterone appears exclusively in women: The voice is modified. Progesterone provokes a thickening of the vocal folds. Unlike estrogens, progesterone only exists in women, not men. As its name indicates, progesterone is a hormone that enables gestation to persist. It is secreted in the ovaries only during the active genital phase of a woman's life, from the age of 15 to approximately 55. It prepares the mucous membrane of the uterus for the nesting of the ovum. That is its primary role.

With respect to the vocal folds, progesterone causes cells on the surface of the mucous membrane to slough off (a process called desquamation). It thickens the secretions of the glands located below and above the vocal folds, causing dryness of the larynx, the need to clear one's throat, less agility when singing, and a narrow register during the four days preceding the menses. If the voice is strained during this phase, nodules may form (these are small supple swellings of the cordal mucous membrane).[8] Progesterone also brings on a slight decrease in the muscle tone of the vocal folds, and it diminishes, and may even inhibit, the permeability of capillaries. This causes the extravascular fluid, that is, fluid outside the blood vessels, to stagnate in the tissues of the vocal folds, bringing on edema of the vocal folds, which remain swollen during the week prior menses.

It is thanks to the estrogens that the intravascular fluid is transferred to the extravascular spaces in the surrounding tissues. Then, when progesterone is secreted, if the balance between the two hormones is satisfactory, the interstitial fluid will be well distributed. The edema of the vocal folds will be minimal. If, on the contrary, this is not the case, the progesterone will prevent the return of the interstitial fluid to the vessels, causing an edema to form. The progesterone in this instance closes the door of the capillaries and prevents them from draining the tissues.

Progesterone acts on the envelope of neurons.

Progesterone is secreted by the ovaries and was originally considered as a hormone involved only in reproductive functions. But Gago has demonstrated that it can be synthesized within the nervous system by neurons and glial cells.[2] The progesterone has promyelinating and neuroprotective effects. Moreover, it can be synthesized locally in the nervous system by neurons and glial cells and can, thus, be considered a "neurosteroid." It plays an astonishing role here. It activates the synthesis of the protective sheath of the neuron, the myelin sheath. The myelin sheath, a sort of protective sleeve that shields the nerve from all traumatic aggression and from differences in temperature, enables nervous impulses to be transmitted at a constant speed between the brain and its target organ. Nerves that have this myelin sheath conduct nervous impulses better and faster. The impact of the action of progesterone on the brain has led to a better understanding of therapeutic approaches to treating neurologic diseases, or certain myopathies that alter the myelin sheath and, therefore, nerve conduction, such as amyotrophic lateral sclerosis or multiple sclerosis. It seems that progesterone significantly slows the evolution of these afflictions.

Imbalance Between Estrogens and Progesterone

The imbalance between estrogens and progesterone causes a cyclical edema in the last week of the menstrual cycle, caused by the accumulation of interstitial fluid in the vocal folds. A similar process causes some women to have swollen legs before their menses.

The Voice Injured by Hormones and Premenstrual Phase

A violent pain, then no more voice. One autumn Friday around 5 PM, I received a phone call from the Bastille Opera, the diva S.L., an international lyrical soprano with a remarkable track record and an outstanding vocal technique, could no longer sing. Her voice was injured. I received her at 6:30 PM: "I'm dying, Doctor." Her impresario tells me what happened: "During the rehearsal, Mrs. S.L. felt tired. She has been feeling tired for the past few days. We just arrived this morning from Germany. But she insisted on attending rehearsals, to practice and to get to know the orchestra. All was going well. Today, I took her to the Opera House. She sang in a normal voice for a few minutes, without straining. But at one point she had to sustain a high-pitched note and she felt a violent pain on the right side, in her neck. I saw her grimace, but she carried on singing her lines. The tenor responded. During the forced rest of a few dozen seconds imposed by the tenor's verse, she was able to catch her breath. When she sang again, her voice had dropped, the high register was gone, and the B note and its pianissimo had evaporated. Impossible to do the vibrato! Her voice had gone! I asked if she could talk. 'Yes,' she answers, but softly. But she couldn't sing. We interrupted the rehearsal, and here we are." Worried, she bursts into tears and asks me: "Is my voice injured?" I examine her.

But first, I'd like to share with you a lesson I have learned from experience. Artists know their voice inside out. They know perfectly well if one fold is vibrating badly. Their knowledge of their laryngeal instrument is remarkable.

> *When artists complain of a vocal problem, most of the time they are right. If I can't detect pathology of the vocal cords, it doesn't mean that there isn't one, it simply means that I haven't found it.*

Consequently, I have to keep searching, dig deeper, carry out more technical examinations, and remain on the lookout for pathology. Who is guilty?

S.L. points to her larynx with her finger to indicate the exact place where she felt pain during her vocal effort. Her finger is indicating the right vocal fold. Palpation of her neck is normal. It reveals no particular sensitivity. The videoendoscopic examination shows a subepithelial hematoma on the right fold, but it vibrates. But it cannot lengthen and shorten. Its contour has changed. The precarious balance of this exceptional instrument has been damaged. What happened? How can a professional singer with perfect technical mastery and an irreproachable lifestyle be the victim of such a regrettable lesion?

The diva, S.L., in her 40s, is not on birth control. Her menses are normal. However, she informs me that those 4 to 5 days before she gets her period, her breasts are sore, her legs feel a little heavy, her pelvis is sore, and her voice alters slightly. I ask her to be more precise regarding the changes to her voice. She answers with exemplary precision. "I lose 10 to 15% of my voice, in order to be heard above the orchestra I have to control my breathing better and brace my pelvis more than usual on stage to counter the weakness of my vocal folds. My register is also affected. I lose a half-tone to a tone in the high notes, but my low tones are still great. My vocal control is also affected at this time; I often clear my throat and feel tired. By the end of the performance, my larynx feels sore. I am used to it, and usually, it goes pretty well." I ask her to explain what she means exactly by control: "By control, I mean sensing the timbre of my voice. In that phase of my cycle, prior to the menses, the color of my voice is a bit more metallic, the vibrato is a little harder to hold. But especially, I find it hard to do a pianissimo on certain frequencies. I have practically no problem in the forte. It's changing from one harmonic to another that bothers me, that's a problem. I find it hard to control my full voice." I ask her: "Mrs. S.L., what phase of your menstrual cycle are you in now and in how many days you think you'll get your period?" This was for me the crux of the matter. "In 2 or 3 days, doctor." I add: "Did you have time to warm your voice up properly before the rehearsal?" She thinks about this, and then confirms my intuition: "No, I was already late, and on top of that the air was dry because of the air conditioning, and I arrived this morning by plane . . . "

To all intents and purposes, the guilty party that had caused the hemorrhage of the vocal fold had now been flushed out.

This diva normally sings at 70% of her capabilities. In her premenstrual phase, just before her menses, she sings at 90% of her capabilities to produce a comparable timbre. But today, other elements perturbed her vocal musicality. The Opera House's air-conditioning had dried the atmosphere. She was feeling tired. She informs me that she had also slept badly the night before. She flew to Paris this morning. On examination with videolaryngostroboscopy, a large hematoma is found (Figure 5–5).

The reasons for the hematoma are getting clearer. The singer was suffering from a premenstrual vocal syndrome. The examination has revealed not only the hematoma on the right vocal fold, easily diagnosed, but microvaricose veins on the left vocal fold, sign of venous fragility. The singer doesn't suffer from them. The fold vibrates normally. The danger they present stems from their fragility. Her vocal power damaged the right vocal fold. That brought on the hematoma. Indeed, 4 days before the menses, the vessels are more fragile due to hormonal influence. The lubrication of the vocal folds was perturbed by the dryness of the atmosphere. The microvaricose veins burst, but only under the submucosal layer. They burst under pressure during the very powerful vocalizations of this lyrical soprano in a high register, the result being the submucosal hemorrhage.

Could she have avoided the misfortune, perchance? There was no way of predicting this accident. It was the first of her career. The reasons for it are simple. For years now, she's made it her practice to warm up her voice, to loosen her vocal folds, to oxygenate her laryngeal muscles. But today, around 2 PM she didn't have time to prepare her laryngeal instrument. It's just before her menses, and she's fragile. The reasons for the accident are now clear. To her fans' immense disappointment, her performances have to be cancelled. Her treatment begins. It's simple: strict vocal rest combined with sprays, phlebotonics, minerals, and anti-inflammatories medicine.

Two weeks later, all was back to normal. I recommend to the diva a cyclical treatment of 10 days each month, for a minimum of 2 years; also a regular stroboscopic examination, especially prior to her

2

Figure 5–5. Vocal fold hemorrhage in the premenstrual phase of the female ovarian cycle.

menses. The fragility of her blood vessels, the impact of the progesterone at the end of her menstrual cycle was partly responsible for her vocal predicament (Figure 5-6).

This type of problem must have been known in earlier times, because since the 19th century, any female singer performing at the Scala Opera House in Milan could during the five days preceding her menses and during her menses cancel her performance and still receive her fee. Back then, the influence of the hormonal cycle on women's voice was already known.

The Voice Changes During the Menstrual Cycle

A premenstrual cycle is evident in all women. But only a third of these present a more noticeable edema of the vocal folds and swollen breasts, symptomatic of the

Figure 5–6. Edema and microvarices of the vocal fold.

precarious balance of the sex hormones. Women on birth control can sometimes present these same symptoms if the pill is biphasic (one containing both estrogens and progesterone). What is going on? The case of Mrs. S.L., the diva, is a good illustration of the premenstrual vocal syndrome; however, she didn't present all the symptoms. The usual syndrome is an altered voice. This can be accompanied by a bout or recurrence of gastric reflux. But you'll recall that progesterone is already having a drying effect on the vocal folds. This causes a posterior laryngitis, as well as an edema of the cordal joint. But no pain will accompany this because neither the pharynx nor the larynx has been hurt. The dryness of the Opera House and, before that, the lack of humidity in the airplane had increased the risk of hematoma of the vocal folds.

The singer with a premenstrual vocal syndrome complains of tiredness, of a loss of pianissimo, of an alteration in certain harmonics in the higher registers, of a deficit in the power of the voice, and of a veiled voice. In some patients, I've also observed pharyngitis and cyclical sore throats, and halitosis, that required vaporization of the tonsils with the help of the laser in order to avoid a monthly intake of antibiotics and anti-inflammatories.

During this premenstrual period, the formation of an edema can create or aggravate the formation of nodules on the vocal folds. This causes a hoarse voice for the 6 days prior to the menses and for the first 2 days of the menses. If this cyclical, episodic dysphonia recurs too often or gets worse, the nodules also get worse. At first, they are soft and vibrate correctly. From one cycle to another, this simple nodule, the size of a small, supple button in the central third of the vocal fold, hardens. Now the hoarseness is permanent. This problem always requires voice therapy to enable the singer to rebalance the axis between her breathing and the vocal fold vibration. Sometimes, these voice therapy sessions carried out by the "clock makers" of physiotherapy, namely speech and language pathologists, are backed up by phonomicrosurgery. This intervention becomes necessary if the voice remains impaired between menses, as this can seriously handicap a singer's career. However, it's then more judicious to operate on these pathologic vocal cords well clear of the week preceding the menses, thus allowing the organism to spontaneously reabsorb the edema of the vocal cords just described, which normally disappears between the 3rd and the 20th day of the menstrual cycle.

The Voice and Pregnancy

A professional singer can sing remarkably well while 2 to 7 months pregnant. The vocal folds are then nicely plump and perfectly lubricated. The quality of the vibration is improved. The hormones that accompany a pregnancy confer a special warmth to the voice's harmonics. The voice is rounder, it carries well. It seems that pregnancy does beautify the voice. After the 7th month, the breathing support is impaired, which is only normal. The sole ailment that needs to be treated during a pregnancy is gastric reflux.

Menopause: With or Without Hormones?

Different Times, Different Problems

During the menopause, this cycle is progressively disrupted. But menopause, which today is of interest to us all, only relatively recently became topical. In the Greek civilization, 400 years BC, the menopausal woman didn't exist, or was an exception. The average life expectancy was 23 to 27 years. Menopause still didn't exist in the Middle Ages. Life expectancy was then 23 to 40 years. Only in the 20th century was menopause finally taken into consideration. Indeed, girls born in the 1980s can expect to live to the age of 92! Menopause now corresponds to practically half a woman's life. By the end of the 20th century, France accounted for nearly eight and a half million menopausal women. The importance of the voice, the development of verbal communication, and interpersonal relationships, all point to the essential problem that the voice and the menopause are now beginning to pose.

Why do these changes occur in a woman's voice around this period of her life? During the perimenopause, progesterone levels collapse. Very few estrogens remain. Equally, the secretion of male hormones also drops off considerably. But their presence, now that they are no longer counterbalanced by feminine hormones, can sometimes cause the voice to become more masculine. Thus, the ovary becomes a simple endocrine gland with no reproductive function.

The menopausal phase normally lasts from the age of 47 to the age of 55. The impact that the sex hormones had on their various target organs disappears, but not without consequences.

However, these days, the administration of substitute hormones enables the unpleasant consequences of this lack of sex hormones to be delayed to an increasingly later age, saving many women from a trying experience that is both mentally and physically hard to accept. In the 1950s, this perimenopause period was referred to as "the change of life," implying that an entire chapter in a woman's life was coming to a full stop. Our better understanding of the endocrinologic world has given the menopausal woman greater quality of life on a daily basis.

Hormonal substitutes may be contraindicated. They are not recommended in cases notably of breast cancer, a high-risk family background, cardiovascular pathologies, or cholesterol-related afflictions. For this reason, a medical checkup is a prerequisite for women in their 50s considering their options. Thereafter, a regular checkup should be performed.

The ovary becomes just an endocrine gland of estrogens and androgens. The receptors of sex hormones receive more androgens and become more receptive to them. As a result, the vocal cord mucous membrane thickens. This is accompanied by a lack of tonicity and a deficiency of its contours. The voice becomes deeper and more masculine.

Meanwhile, the 60-year-old woman may develop symptoms such as increased hairiness as an indirect consequence of androgens. A smear test of the cervix of the uterus indicates an atrophy of the epithelium. The same result is obtained from a smear test of the vocal folds: the parallelism is amazing.

Menopause and the Vagus Nerve

The larynx is controlled by the vagus nerve. At menopause, the brutal drop in progesterone results in a progressive slowing of nerve conduction that is barely noticeable. This slowdown is due to a relative lack of myelinization of peripheral nerves and induces slower nervous conduction from the brain to the larynx. As a result, vocal response slows down slightly, which can hamper rapid changes of frequencies when singing. Later, the vibrato (7 vibrations per second) cannot be maintained. The voice gradually gears down to the tremolo (4 vibrations per second).

The Modigliani Woman and the Rubens Woman

Observation of menopausal women has led us to categorize them into two vocal types. The voice doesn't necessarily become more masculine. Why is this? Put simply, one can distinguish two types of menopausal women. The first type, slim with very few fat cells, we will call the Modigliani type (as in Modigliani's paintings). The second, somewhat stouter, we'll call the Rubens type (as in Rubens' paintings).

Estrogen synthesis happens on three levels: at the level of the ovaries, when these are functional, at the level of the brain (hypothalamus, tonsils, and hippocampus), and finally at the level of fat cells. The latter cells are the ones that interest us here. They are particularly active during the menopause. For the past 30 years, we have known that, in both men and women, fat cells can turn androgens into estrogens. The relationship between obesity and a higher secretion of estrones (estrogen derivatives) is also age-related. It's higher in menopausal women. This is the work of a specific gene in our DNA (cytochrome 19 associated with P450 aromatase) that facilitates the transformation of androgen into estrogen in our adipose cells. Thus, the lower need for hormone substitutes of our Rubens-type woman is due to the fact that her fat cells will transform her androgens into estrones. Meanwhile, our slim Modigliani woman is more likely to need hormone substitute therapy, prescribed, of course, with due respect to contraindications.

Obese tenors have been found to have a higher level of estrogens and a slightly lower level of testosterone than those found in baritones and bass singers. Indeed, these slim, deep bass singers with their bony figures have a higher level of androgens. They have no fat cells that could help the organism to metabolize testosterone into estrogens.

With age, muscle mass diminishes; adipose mass increases; cells are redistributed differently about the body.[3,9,10] Corticosteroids encourage the increase of fat cells. Therefore, menopausal women need to be cautious about consuming them. A carefully considered hormone substitute therapy program, associated with vitamins and minerals, can bring considerable benefits to most female voice professionals if their body can tolerate it, which is far from being a given. I have noted that women thus treated are able to avoid developing a masculine voice as they age and are able to preserve a beautiful voice for significantly longer. I have been most impressed by certain sopranos who have kept the same tessitura until the age of 65.

Male Hormones: The Lower Frequencies Take the Voice Hostage

Women secrete androgens, the male hormone "par excellence," but in minute doses: on the one hand via the adrenal glands just above the kidneys, on the other hand via the internal theca, a very precise part of the ovaries themselves. Indeed, the female sex requires a touch of testosterone to ensure a satisfactory level of libido and enough low-pitched harmonics in her voice to distinguish it from a child's voice. But the level of testosterone must be around 150 µg/dl—if too low the libido disappears, if too high, masculinity sets in and excess pilosity or hirsutism can occur. This action is often irreversible. It is aggravated by steroids.

The consumption of androgens leaves indelible marks in women. That is why voice professionals should check their medication carefully for the presence of androgenic anabolic derivatives. These elements may also be present in certain progesterone preparations and their molecular derivatives.

THE MALE VOICE

The androgens secreted by the testicles have a direct effect on the voice. They certainly act on the bony tissues, but also on the brain. They increase aggressiveness. It is no accident that yelling is often an integral aspect of male expression in combat, both in men and in animals. This male hormone builds his laryngeal muscles, lends power to his call. The significant influence of androgens on his vocal print, on the power and frequencies of his call, without a doubt triggered the appearance of the secondary sexual attributes.

Androgens increase blood flow in the organism and improve oxygenation and muscle performance. Note that cortisone can have an androgenic effect and act as a euphoriant. This induces some voice professionals to overdose on it, hoping to be at their best vocally. But this is dangerous, because it can have a rebound effect. When you come off cortisone, muscle tone decreases abruptly and tiredness, possibly even a light depression, may set in.

THE AGING VOICE: DOES THE VOICE AGE?

Do Voices Wrinkle?

We age; it is a progressive alteration of the body's response in our life from maturity to death, a biological necessity for recycling of elements in nature. Our voice ages, as does our body.[2]

Aging is a natural, biological evolution. It is a consequence of stress, of age, of maturity, also of the state of our tissues, vessels, and brain. Different theories have tried to explain aging the free "oxygen" radical theory pretends that it weakens the proteins, the genetic heritage theory. Genes carry an innate blueprint of timetable for growth, repair, and death in every cell of our body. But we all have on chromosome 9 a gene for apoptosis. These genes are thought to be the "end-of-life" genes. They program our cellular death. Telomere length on the chromosome decides life span.

According to chromosomal research, the genetic heritage of *Homo sapiens* is capable of a life expectancy of 100 to 150 years. Aging is caused by life's vicissitudes. If we can't prevent the genetic inheritance, we may be able to avoid or to decrease the impact of accidents, infections, cardiovascular diseases, diabetes, mental stress, pollution, alcohol, tobacco, and drugs.[11] Lack of exercise is one of the factors as is diet. In France, in 1980, 9% of the population was over 65. By the year 2000, nearly 15% was over 65. In 2030, close to 25% is expected to be over 65.

The Voice Changes with the Passing Years: Why Does Presbyphonia Appear?

Thirty years ago, very little was known about the aging of the voice, or presbyphonia, which begins around the age of 80. A new medical field has opened up these past few years. As time goes by, the vocal folds lose their suppleness. The cord atrophies. There's a loss of hydration, a loss of collagen and elastin fibers. Remaining fibers are thicker; as a result, the laminar structure of the cordal tissue is less supple. Consequently, when you tighten your vocal cords, they arch and no longer make proper contact. They allow some air to slip through. If you speak for any length of time, you become breathless.

Many clinical signs are well known: (1) Intensity drops down due to vocal atrophy, (2) register narrows due to vocal elasticity, and (3) low pitch lowers due to vocal suppleness (fat cells substitute for muscular cells fibers).

- 1st formant and 2nd formant are low.
- Lost of suppleness of the resonators
- Lack of F_0 stability
- Vibrato becomes a tremolo.
- Presbyacoustic: feedback and importance of the audiophonatory loop weakens.
- Video laryngoscopy and stroboscopy are very useful to study the features. The following were found in older individuals.[1]
  1. Sulcus glottidis in 34%
  2. Bilateral amyotrophy with bowing vocal folds in 55.6%
  3. Arthrosis of the cricoarytenoid in 21.6% with hypomobility in 10%
  4. Superior laryngeal nerve paresis in 7.2%
  5. Lack of vibration in 71% (54 atrophy, 5 sulcus alone, and 10 bowing folds).

It May Be Mechanical

The larynx, the resonators, the feedback or the audio-phonatory loop may be altered (Figure 5–7). In addition, the oxygenation of brain area such as Broca's, and Wernicke's areas and the planum temporale will slow down the speaking and the singing voice.

There are multiple reasons why our voice changes as we get older. The first alteration is mechanical and anatomic in nature: the thyroid, cricoid, and arytenoid cartilages progressively harden, lose their suppleness, ossify, and calcify. The anterior part of the arytenoid cartilage, point of insertion for the vocal fold, and the epiglottic cartilage do not ossify, but they lose elasticity. As for the vocal fold joints, like any other joint they show signs of inflammation and arthritis. The crico-thyroid joint also shows signs of arthritis, causing increased difficulty in the head voice and a decrease in the agility and speed of the vocal folds when practicing musical scales. Joint suppleness is affected by a loss of collagen fibers and by a degeneration brought on by dehydration. The pharyngeal-laryngeal reflux is very common due to insufficiency of the cardia with elderly or obese people. This opens the road for arthritis of "the vocal folds" or more precisely of the cricoary-tenoid joint.

Figure 5–7. The audiophonatory loop.

Teeth and the Aging Voice

Our vocal instrument, the larynx, cannot shoulder all the blame. The buccodental point of articulation is part of the vocal aging process, yet is often ignored. Losing one's teeth causes the upper and lower lips to collapse, forming pinched lips. Our jaw is oddly designed. It is shaped like a horseshoe, with a very specific angle between the horizontal part and the two vertical parts. On the left and right sides, it articulates with the base of the cranium. This bony part is very strong. When the teeth fall out, it calcifies. The closed angle which normally forms an almost 90-degree angle between the horizontal section and the vertical section in adults opens wider in the toothless person.

With advancing age, lack of teeth causes the jaw to decalcify and erode; moreover, the angle between the horizontal and vertical parts becomes wider with an angle around 120° (usually it is around 90-95°), the horizontal part of the mandible becomes slimmer, the vertical part shorter, the profile of the face is changing. The mandible seems squashed under the cranium, the nose droops down to the level of the upper lip. Paradoxically, lack of teeth means the mouth is no longer able to open fully. The mandible joint, in other words the joint of the jaw, becomes less supple. This underscores the importance of maintaining an efficient set of teeth and resorting, when necessary, to dental implants, to ensure that the lips are able to rest against a satisfactory surface, thereby avoiding bone degeneration of the mandible: so much for the dental landscape of the voice.

Muscles and Neurons Must Keep Fit

The problem is simpler as regards muscles and ligaments. It is not only our vocal tract which may be impaired. The superficial and deep muscles of the head and neck are important as are the facial muscles. With age, but especially in case of insufficient physical exercise, the myofibrils of the striated muscles degenerate and turn into fibrosis and, secondarily, fat cells.[12] We know of exceptional singers who are 75 years old; we also know of teachers who, once retired, spend considerably less time speaking, as a result of which their cordal muscles atrophy. The internal biomechanical properties of the vocal fold are no longer stimulated. The neuromuscular junction is also normally solicited by phonatory activity. If it isn't, muscle activity decreases. Even our nerves undergo a reduction of the myelin sheath, which affects the speed at which messages are transmitted between the brain and the muscles: the elocution of these patients slows down. This combination of muscles and ligaments receives energy from the arteries and laryngeal capillaries feeding it. A decrease in physical and sports activity reduces the suppleness of the vessels, here and in the entire organism, and accelerates the onset of arteriosclerosis. It affects oxygenation and weakens the musculature: a vicious circle is triggered. The return to sports and voice activities should be very progressive and regular. The elderly need to be very patient in their renewed quest for fitness.

The Vocal Fold

By the age of 70, nearly 72% of patients who have stopped being vocally active present with atrophy of the vocal folds and epithelium that they didn't have prior to their 50s. Not only the synovial joints in the larynx but also those in the middle ear and the temporomandibular joint of the jaw are results of aging, as shown in Figure 5-8.

Gray has observed that the extracellular matrix sees its enzymes diminished, as a result the collagen fibers with collagen IV and VII decline. The interstitial matrix has less water and hyaluronic acid. There's a loss of elastic fibers, of the proteoglycans webbing. The lamina propria, an indispensable element under the cordal epithelium, becomes rigid and stiff. Triggering a vibration becomes more difficult. The viscosity increases and the gliding effect diminish. This suite of alterations, aggravated by deficient lubrication of the epithelium, often justifies supplementing the diet with substitute vitamins and with minerals that have a role to play in vocal activity.

- Before 50 years old: we don't observe atrophy (0%) of the vocal fold muscle. But there is 0.7% bowing vocal folds and 7% sulcus vocalis.
- After 70 years old: there is 72% atrophy, 8% bowing of the vocal folds and 64% sulcus vocalis.

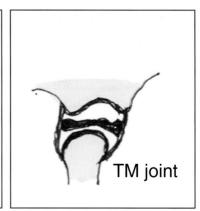

Figure 5–8. The synovial joints play an important role in the aging voice in the middle ear (*left*), cricoarytenoid joint in the larynx (*middle*), and temporomandibular joint in the jaw (*right*).

■ After 80 years of age: there is 81% fat with keratosis in the vocal muscle and ligament. There is an atrophy of the lamina propria. In males, the vocal ligaments shorten, the intermediate layer of the lamina propria (LP) is thinner (loss of the elastic fibers, atrophy of the deep layer of the LP, and loss of collagen fibers which leads to fibrosis). In females, the mucosal covering of the vocal fold becomes thicker, and there is also loss of elastic fibers.

Besides the vocal fold structure, the glandular cells located on the superior and subglottic epithelium atrophy as previously shown in Figure 5–3. So the lack of lubrication appears to also disturb the vibratory pattern.

The Breath: Power of the Voice

The energy of the voice is intimately connected with our breathing. Our lungs progressively weaken with age. In people who don't engage in physical activity, bronchial efficiency diminishes by almost 40% between the ages of 40 and 80 for a nonathlete population. That's a significant drop. Our lung capacity is affected by atrophy of the peribronchial muscles, a reduction in the number of alveoli in the lungs and in their elasticity. The thoracic cage loses its suppleness and there-fore its amplitude.[5] Asthma and asthmalike conditions are more frequent as are cardiopulmonary diseases. The stiffness of the thoracic vertebrae perturbs the elasticity of the thoracic cage. Physical activity is the antidote for this.

Thyroid Hormones

Besides these mechanical elements, the decrease in sex hormones plays a major role. With age, there's also a frequent drop in the secretion of thyroid hormones, hormones that generate energy for the muscles and that hydrate the organism. Hypothyroidism changes can be observed. The thyroid hormones should be controlled systematically in presbyphonia after menopause or andropause. Patients with a sluggish thyroid often require appropriate therapeutic treatment to get them out of their lethargy and feeling energetic again.

Man and Andropause

At the age of 70, andropause may appear. The blood analysis will diagnose the lack of androgens. If there is no contraindication such as cancer of the prostate, androgen treatment may be useful to recover the vocal folds' shape, the tonicity of the resonators, and consequently a powerful voice with a satisfactory register.

The Paradox of the Aging Voice

In Women

As the menopausal woman advances in age, her new hormonal balance, with its absence of estrogens and its very mild secretion of testosterone due to the atrophy of her ovaries, is no longer able to sustain the tonicity and strength of the vocal fold muscles. What are the consequences of this? The two vocal folds atrophy progressively. The mucous membrane covering them becomes thinner and dehydrates.

Initially, the voice displays a narrower register, the higher harmonics are lost, and the voice is less powerful and tires faster. But a paradoxic effect sets in. Because the vocal cord has diminished in thickness and becomes finer, the voice, which had become a little deeper, now becomes higher, more delicate, and sometimes even shrill. You often hear 80-year-olds speaking with a very high-pitched voice. One can thicken the vocal folds again by injecting a substance into them; this ensures reasonable timbre and vocal endurance.

In Men

After the age of 70, men can present these same vocal symptoms in the male climacteric. Yet the vocal structure in this case behaves like an athlete in all respects. As with women, hormone therapy is indicated in conjunction with specific nutrition hygiene, but vocalizations are indispensable. Androgenic hormonal therapy is rarely advisable because of its danger for an altered prostate. For men, vocal training is the best guarantee of keeping a young voice. An example I like to quote concerns of a professor of French at the Lycée Henri-IV, who also lectured at the Sorbonne and who was in the habit of speaking over 4 hours a day. I had known him for over 10 years. When he stopped his academic activities, he started writing his Memoirs and barely said a word for the next 6 months. He used to have an athlete's larynx. But when I saw him again a year later, I detected an impressive atrophy of his vocal folds. He was only 65 years old, yet he had the voice of an old man. The right treatment combined with intensive speech therapy enabled him to practically recover his normal voice. I advised him to carry on lecturing for a minimum of 3 hours a week. Our voice ages only if we isolate ourself from others. Regular practice and communication with others stimulates the voice and preserves its timbre.

Rejuvenating the Voice

This atrophy of the vocal folds can be corrected through voice and speech therapy and, on rare occasions, through phonosurgery (surgery of the voice). This phonosurgery consists of injecting a product into the shrunken cordal muscle to increase its volume to its previous state. The voice regains satisfactory power and tonality. The voice of these dysphonic, breathless patients once again becomes dynamic. This type of surgery is only practiced if the standard medical and speech therapy treatment has failed. This "voice lift" is often very successful. The key to preserving a youthful voice is to be serious about physical exercise, hydration, lubrication of the vocal folds, dental hygiene, muscular activity, nutrition, vitamin and mineral supplements, and possibly appropriate hormone therapy. Often, antireflux medication (to treat the acidity coming from the stomach to the larynx) is necessary.[13] If you take good care of the health of your voice, you can most certainly retain an efficient vocal tessitura and timbre.

Hormonal treatment may be used. A complete exploration of the thyroid gland often discovers a deficiency in thyroid hormones, which has to be treated. This appears more often in females. Other hormonal treatments in females and males is another story that we have developed above.

A Multifactor Treatment

More than 80% of patients undergo voice therapy for approximately 6 to 8 sessions. Some prefer to add singing lessons and join a choir, which is an excellent decision. They feel that they can improve their voice if they belong to a team and practice using it instead of being lonely and quiet.

Some may require an acute treatment for arthrosis (anti-inflammatory medicine or injection of steroid in the cricoarytenoid joint), reflux treatment (PPI), or injection of material in the bowing vocal fold. Alternative medicine with vitamins, minerals, and antioxidants such as omega-3 are now being added to the treatment regimen. An important point has to be made: we must not forget the lubrication of the vocal tract and eventually prescribe molecules such as, for example, acetyl-cysteine.

Dental care is critical; implants may be necessary; respiratory kinesitherapy is sometimes indispensable.

Prevention Is Possible

If you don't take proper care of yourself, the voice will age. Vocal registers will narrow, the voice will weaken, and the timbre will lose color and become metallic. This can be avoided by adopting a regular and constant healthy lifestyle, by taking antioxidants, vitamin C and vitamin E, minerals such as magnesium, and by keeping up physical and intellectual activities.

Unfortunately, the impact of passing years is sometimes less forgiving as regards our hearing. We have seen that listening and audiophonatory feedback are essential to the quality of the voice. All voice professionals should have their hearing checked regularly to test for partial deafness. If necessary, one should not hesitate to correct a hearing deficiency with a hearing aid. Nowadays, these hearing aids are very well tolerated and, in most cases, will help voice professionals to re-establish a correct balance between their vocal and auditory functions. A hearing aid keeps one in touch with the outside world. It is a safeguard against isolation; it stimulates the audiophonatory loop and contributes to a precise control of the voice while speaking and singing (see Figure 5-7).

The human voice is not immune to the effects of aging. Vocal quality and strength can be affected by a number of different conditions that increase in prevalence with age. The memory and the activity of the brain are indispensable to keeping a good voice.

Fortunately with appropriate diagnosis, environmental and hygienic interventions, specific medical treat-ments, and voice therapy, most people can maintain a functional, quality voice through all of their lives.[14]

REFERENCES

1. Abitbol J, Abitbol P, Abibol B. Sex hormones and the female voice. *J Voice.* 1999;13(3):424-446.
2. Gago N, Akwa I, Sananes N, et al. Progesterone and the oligodendroglial lineage: stage-dependent biosynthesis and metabolism. *Glia.* 2001;36(3): 295-308.
3. von Leden H, Alessi DM. The aging voice. In: Benninger MS, Jacobson BJ, Johnson AF. *Vocal Arts Medicine: The Care and Prevention of Professional Voice Disorders.* New York, NY: Thieme Medical Publishers; 1994:269-280.
4. Hammond TH, Gray SD, Butler JE. Age- and gender-related collagen distribution in human vocal folds. *Ann Otol Rhinol Laryngol.* 2000;109:913-920.
5. Scherer RC, Rubin JS. Laryngeal physiology: normal and disordered. In: Benninger MS, ed. *Benign Disorders of Voice.* Alexandria, Va: American Academy of Otolaryngology–Head and Neck Surgery; 2002:29-44.
6. Lee R. Hopkins V. *What Your Doctor May Not Tell You About Menopause.* Boston, Mass: Warner Books; 1996.
7. Kansaku K, Yamuara A, Kitazawa S. Sex differences in lateralization revealed in the posterior languages areas. *Cereb Cortex.* 2000;10 (9):866-872.
8. Benninger MS. Dysphonias secondary to neurologic disorders. *J Singing.* 1996;52:29-32.
9. Mueller PB. Senescence of the voice: morphology of excised male larynges. *Folia Phoniatr.* 1985;37: 134-138.
10. Hirano M. Aging of the vibratory tissue. *Acta Otolaryngol.* 1989;107:428-433.
11. Peres G. *Nutrition des Sportifs, Abrégé de Médecine du Sport.* 8th ed. Paris: Masson; 2002.
12. Malmgren LT, Jones CE, Bookman LM. Muscle fiber and satellite cell apoptosis in the aging human thyroarytenoid muscle: a stereological study with confocal laser scanning microscopy. *Otolaryngol Head Neck Surg.* 2001;125:34-39.
13. Kaufman JA, Amin MR, Aviv JE, et al. Laryngopharyngeal reflux (LPR). *Ear Nose Throat.* 2002; 81(9):1-32.
14. Abitbol J. *Odyssey of the Voice.* San Diego, Calif: Plural Publishing, Inc; 2006.

Chapter 6

ARTISTIC VOCAL STYLES AND TECHNIQUE

Sharon L. Radionoff

Voice professionals work in a wide range of disciplines and genres. The voice professional who is a singer may choose to use his or her vocal instrument as a singer/music educator, a singer/choral director, professional singer (opera; oratorio; musical theatre; clubs—pop/rock, jazz, country, mariachi, salsa), or as a professional actor/singer (theatre), to name a few. Each discipline demands peak vocal performance for longevity of career.[1]

In order to have a healthy singing voice, it is important to know how to: (1) Sing with healthy technique (ie, balancing airflow, phonation, resonance, articulation, agility), (2) sing in the correct voice category/range, (3) sing in the correct tessitura (pitch area where voice comfortably sits), (4) choose music that has a tessitura (pitch area) and range that matches one's own tessitura and range, and (5) sing the genre of music with the healthiest possible stylistic tools.[1]

In regard to vocal styles and stylistic tools, there are many vocal sounds that can be made but some sounds have the potential to be harmful. For example, "grit," "growling," and glottal onsets are stylistic effects found in rock, country, and pop music. These tools must be used with the least amount of tension needed to avert damage. Also, if used too often, a tension onset may become part of one's technique and no longer employed just as a stylistic tool.[2] These habits often creep into the speaking voice adding to the harmful effects. It is possible to create a desired vocal tool (ie, grit, growl) in more than one way. The key to longevity of career is finding and understanding the "system's balance" and alignment for singing before creating stylism. Balance must be attained before power, agility, or style. This analogy can be clearly seen in sports. For example, consider a gymnast. It makes sense that a gymnast stretches and finds his or her center of gravity first, whether it be on the balance beam or floor exercise, before doing any flips, turns, or difficult combinations. One might consider a gymnast foolhardy if he or she were to attempt difficult movements before balancing the body and mind. Singers, however, are notorious for ignoring balance and head immediately to agility, power, and style. They even attempt to "warm-up" by singing what they consider to be an easy song. There are so many variables to be aligned that it is critical for the voice professional to find his or her system's balance and alignment.

BALANCING

Sound: A Balancing Act

The act of singing can be compared to being on a teeter-totter or seesaw (Figure 6–1). The teeter-totter effect occurs as follows: a person sitting on the ground seat pushes with the legs and is propelled into the air.

Figure 6–1. Teeter-totter.

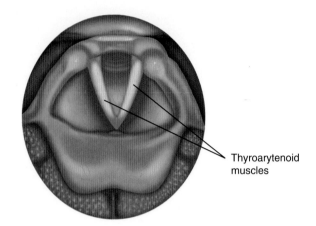

Thyroarytenoid muscles

Figure 6–2. The thyroarytenoid muscle makes up the body of the true vocal folds (vocal cords). (Courtesy of Blue Tree Publishing.)

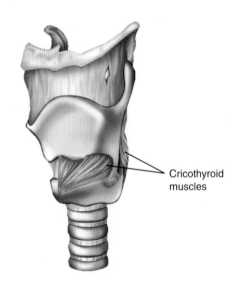

Cricothyroid muscles

Figure 6–3. The cricothyroid muscle runs between the cricoid and thyroid cartilages. (Courtesy of Blue Tree Publishing.)

Consequently, the opposite seat, which was in the air, goes down to the ground. Keeping the teeter-totter parallel to the ground requires a "balancing act."[3]

The shifting of power action in the teeter-totter example may be used as an analogy to singing. At different times, one muscle or muscle group is more active then another and a power shift takes place. Sometimes the shift is gradual and sometimes the shift is abrupt. The complex systems for sound production that interact and must be balanced are respiration (power source), phonation (the vocal folds = raw sound source/pitch source), and resonance (the supraglottic vocal tract = the quality shaper).[3]

Questions to keep in mind regarding balancing the vocal system are: (1) where does the work occur? (2) what does the work? and (3) how much work has to happen? These questions may be examined in terms of pitch, loudness, and articulation. There are a variety of muscles that work together to create pitch as previously discussed in chapter 4. This chapter discusses the two most important muscles. In the most simplistic terms, the thyroarytenoid (TA) muscle shortens, and thickens the vocal fold.[4] Therefore, when lower pitches are produced, the TA muscle (Figure 6–2) is active. When a higher pitch is produced, the cricothyroid muscle becomes more active (Figure 6–3). The cricothyroid (CT) muscle is the principal muscle for longitudinal tension. Contraction of the CT muscle lengthens the vocal folds and thins them, which allows for a higher pitch.[5] One does not have to vocally manipulate to make pitches change because this is intrinsically how the system works![3]

In regard to loudness, when the vocal folds vibrate with greater amplitude (are wider apart), there is more airflow passing through per vibration. Also, the impact or closure force of contact of the true vocal folds is greater thereby creating a louder sound. When the vocal folds vibrate closer together, there is less airflow

per vibration, which creates a softer sound. This is called amplitude variation and results in a change in intensity. This is perceived as a change in loudness.[4]

The questions asked above are especially pertinent to articulation. In order to have precise articulation, overwork may occur in terms of jaw clenching, chewing, tongue pressure, or excessive movement of the face and lips. For example, the consonant /n/ is created by the tongue tip moving up and touching the hard palate or, more specifically, the alveolar ridge.[6]

Figure 6-4. Sagittal (side) view of the resonance tract and articulators. (Courtesy of Blue Tree Publishing.)

Frequently the tongue posture for /n/ is produced with a closed or clenched jaw. This closing and/or clenching also is often true for the production of an /l/. The tongue is a powerful muscle, and a much larger structure than often perceived (Figure 6-4). Because the tongue has an attachment to the hyoid bone, tongue tension and excessive manipulation of the tongue may lead to vocal fatigue.[6]

No matter what the style of singing, balance is the key. If longevity of voice use is the desired outcome, then knowledge and excellent use of the vocal mechanism is critical. Therefore, singing and sound production are about balancing the systems necessary to achieve sound for a desired outcome in the healthiest way.[6]

BALANCING EXERCISES

Building Block Approach

Singing is like building a house. The foundation comes first, then the walls, and the roof follows before work begins on the inside. Likewise, as in building a house, there is a logical sequence when creating sound. Airflow management is the foundation (the respiratory system = power source), phonation (pitch source) is the walls, and resonance (sound shaper) is the roof. After you have layered these three systems then you can begin to work on agility, strength, and musicianship along with interpretation and style. An example of the building block approach would be the following: (1) begin with airflow on /sh/, /f/, or /s/; (2) next add phonation on a single note using /shu/, /fu/, or /su/; and (3) last add resonance by adding an /m/ to the previous phonation /shum/, /fum/, or /sum/ and repeat the pattern (shum-mum-mum). There is a direct link between the first step, airflow, to the second step, phonation. The same consonant and consonant combination for the respiratory mechanics of airflow begins both steps and then we add vocal fold vibration for the second step. Also, by adding the /m/ for resonance, the third step starts the same as the second but allows for frontal directionality for the resonance. As /m/ is the most frontal nasal consonant, it is not necessary to press or push air pressure forward. One simply closes the lips and the airflow travels forward. After the basic sound has been balanced, agility of vocal fold lengthening and shortening may be attempted. A desirable way to begin is by using small patterns so that one will not fight against oneself for control. The numbers used to define these patterns below are based on a major scale 1-2-3-4-5-6-7-8 (C-D-E-F-G-A-B-C). These patterns are 1-7-1 (C—down ½ step to B natural—back up to C), 1-2-1 (C—up a step to D—back down a step to C), and 3-2-1 (down the major scale E-D-C). Then these patterns may be added together to gradually increase the range of agility such as: 1-7-1-2-1, 1-2-1-7-1, 3-2-1-7-1, and so on.[7]

Stress Release Exercises

The voice can be misaligned for many reasons. It may simply be that one has just woken up and the brain and body are not awake enough to connect at the highest level. It may also be related to external or internal stress. A certain amount of stress is normal as one goes through the rigors of life, and stress can result from a variety of things. Just the pace of a busy day can induce the physical reaction of stress. This reaction will cause the body to tighten and the result will be less access to airflow. Less airflow means a diminished power source and the body and voice will feel pushed by the end of the day if one does not learn how to release body and mind tension. A good way to release stress and tension is to do a few repetitions of airflow management exercises—blowing air for a comfortable consistent length of time using /sh/, /wh/, /f/, or /s/ and after blowing, releasing the abdominal area, letting the body fill up with air and repeating.[8]

Vocal Tension Release Exercises

After airflow exercises, the next step would be "vocal tension release" exercises. These exercises consist of vocal slides using the phonemes /f/ and /v/ in combination (beginning with the unvoiced consonant and then moving down the slide on the voiced consonant) or /shu/. The main object of these exercises is to feel the air at the front of the mouth (f/v) with ease of sound, not listening for beautiful sound. It is important to do these exercises starting in a comfortable middle range and not in the high range. First, start on a comfortable middle range pitch and slide down to a comfortable low range pitch. It should be a moderately slow glide. Be sure that the upper teeth touch the bottom lip appropriately when using the f/v combination. Airflow should be felt behind the top teeth. The teeth should touch the bottom lip at the vermilion border. If one feels the airflow coming out between the teeth then one does not have the teeth touching the bottom lip enough or there is a gap between the teeth. This exercise may also be done by using an undulating wavy slide (Figure 6–5). Don't try to make exact pitch definition. Again, the important issue is a lot of air at the teeth and ease of sound. Another phoneme cluster to use is /shu/. Remember that when using /shu/ the tongue tip will not be behind the bottom teeth for the consonant cluster /sh/ but will then need to come behind the bottom teeth for the /u/ vowel. If you use the f/v combination then the tongue can be behind the bottom teeth the entire time.

Voice Balancing Exercise

The last exercise presented is called a voice balancing exercise. This consists of choosing a comfortable note in the speaking range. On a single note (eg, A3, Bb3, B3, or C4 for women—C4 = middle C) use the con-

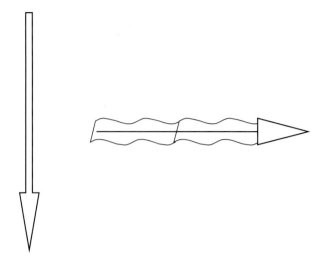

Figure 6–5. Descending and small wavy slides.

sonant vowel combination *"Bum" or **"Buhm." The object is to simply say easy repetitions of the combination of choice in slow and faster repetitions (bum-bum-bum-bum-bum). It is not necessary to push pressure forward into the /m/. Simply by choosing one of these combinations you will feel the sound move forward as /m/ is the most frontal nasalant consonant. All that one does is open and close the lips for the combination.[8]

Never forget that as a voice professional, the entire body is the instrument. What you do with your body will directly affect your voice. Also, because you only have one larynx, what you do with your voice when you are not singing will affect what you are able to do with your voice when you sing.[7]

BODY-MIND-SPIRIT CONNECTION

Another concept that warrants examination concerning vocal health is the understanding that each person is composed of body, mind, and spirit. One can put into practice all the appropriate exercises but the psyche can either hinder or help progress. When someone sings, all aspects of the persona are entwined. Our singing voice is our body, mind, and spirit. We cannot separate the influences of these elements.[9]

---

*International Phonetic Alphabet (IPA) used unless otherwise noted.
**Not IPA

Body

For healthy singing technique, the tongue and the neck are two common pitfalls to monitor. The tongue often gets us into trouble! The tongue is composed of 8 to 10 muscles that are interdigitated. In fact we can only see a small part of the tongue. We often try to control sound by controlling the position of the tongue (ie, pulling it back too far, pressing it down in the center) instead of having the most efficient "home resting place" for the tongue tip while we are producing different vowels. Of course the tongue will have to move for consonants and change shape for vowels, but we usually overwork with pressure and manipulation of the tongue rather than simply having the efficient position of the tongue for certain consonants.

Along with the tongue, the neck is often a source of control and manipulation. A stiff and stubborn neck is a sign of the inability to manage stress. Some singers often hold it stiff with extrinsic muscle tension to feel physical control for sound in the area of the larynx. This may be done in order to psychologically "feel" control.[10]

Mind

The impulse or idea for making sound begins in the cerebral cortex of the brain.[11] The brain is the control panel or central processing unit (CPU) of our body (Figure 6–6). It sends information to all the systems that have to balance in order to sing. The singing voice is trained by the concepts that we cultivate with various exercises. Please remember that practice makes permanent and not necessarily perfect! What we practice is what becomes a learned behavior. What we dwell on is what becomes part of us.

Manipulative control often happens with the tongue, jaw, neck, or torso to psychologically "feel" voice before it can leave out of the mouth. Learning efficient technique and the tools to sing facilitates healthy singing. However, as one learns efficient, healthy technique, one has to get out of the way, let go, and trust. Despite the overriding need to control, manipulate, and hold to make sound happen, one must consciously let go, trust, and believe that it will happen.[10]

Figure 6–6. Sagittal (side) view of the brain, nerves, and laryngeal skeleton. (Courtesy of Blue Tree Publishing.)

Spirit

What drives or motivates someone to sing? Is it a burning passion within or a desire to prove something? Is it the need for self-expression or applause? Does singing bring joy? Whatever the case may be, there is an internal reason why one chooses to sing. The essence or spirit of a person is expressed through music when they sing. If the technique is not at the level of the emotion or essence, then one will try to force singing to occur. In our vocal journey we can choose to approach singing by either "make my voice be" or "allow my voice to become." As stated above, efficient technique of course aids in healthy singing. Remember, however, that singing takes faith. We have to get out of the way, let go, and trust.

STYLES

Balance and alignment of the vocal instrument, comprising the body-mind-spirit connection, is just the beginning for the performer. If one knows where his or her center of balance is, then one can experiment with how far one may go from the central balance point for coloration and effect and still have integrity of technique. It really does not matter what style of music someone sings. What truly matters is the balance point of the voice. If a singer knows his or her balance point, then he or she will be able to experiment with breath, resonance (eg, nasalance), articulation, straight tone, and delayed vibrato (along with other aspects) for coloration and effect. It is no different than a painter having a palette with many colors to choose from to create nuance in his or her painting.

Broad Categories

Style is often discussed in terms of two broad categories: Classical music and commercial music. Vocal pedagogue Carolyn Binkley in Nashville defines classical and commercial music as the following: "Classical" is a term which represents many genres including opera, oratorio, art song, symphony, chamber music, and the manner of performance associated with those genres. "Commercial" can include the styles jazz, rock, country, pop, rhythm and blues, big band and swing, alternative, contemporary Christian, gospel, rap, hip-hop, and heavy metal but to name a few. These two terms are not descriptive of two areas, rather they are commonly used terms that are widely recognizable throughout the musical world (C. Binkley, personal communication, 1999). Although the acronym CCM is currently another reference to commercial music, one must be careful as the acronym has been used specifically to refer to the genre of Contemporary Christian Music for the past 25 years. There is a magazine called *CCM* devoted specifically to this genre of music as well (L. Poquette, personal communication, November 29, 2005). Furthermore, the term commercial music is well entrenched and used by colleges and universities to define a specific degree plan such as found at Belmont University in Nashville, Tennessee and Miami University in Miami, Florida.

Western

Classical music (as we know it) may be further categorized into "Western" classical music. A note is neces-

sary here about the term Western versus non-Western categories of classical music. Music historians often use this separation. However, noted ethnomusicologist Dr. Robert Trotter who taught "Music in World Cultures," preferred a more inclusive terminology (personal communication, 1987). This is especially relevant today given the culturally expanded nature of the world.

Non-Western

Non-Western music includes Latin styles such as Salsa, Cumbia, Merengue (which has its roots in the German polka and African drum beat), and a mixed style of music called Reggaeton (rap/hip-hop/Caribbean). There are also Hispanic styles such as Tejano and Mariachi music. In addition, the musical styles of Indian and Middle Eastern cultures vary significantly from what the Western ear is used to hearing. This list of non-Western music is by no means exhaustive. It is only meant to show that a plethora of diversity exists.

Choral

Another broad category subset is the choral tradition that exists in a variety of settings. Choral music exists in the school, community, and religious settings. In the school setting, ensembles may range from small chamber ensembles (12–20 voice, mixed chorus) to medium-size chorales (40+ voices, mixed chorus) to a larger oratorio chorus (150+ members, usually mixed). The larger choral works may include such diversity as "The Dream of Gerontius" by Edward Elgar to the well-known work the "Messiah" by Handel. In these large ensembles it can be difficult to hear oneself sing: Consequently, it is easy to "push" voice production to create more volume in order to hear oneself. Also, in the school setting there are show choirs with choreography and a live band as well as jazz ensembles with accompaniment ranging from a combo to a full jazz ensemble. Choreography and the different types of accompaniment both pose potential problems for healthy singing. If the singer pulls in the abdominal area when dancing then the breathing will be high and shallow. When there is a live band the singer will often push to hear him- or herself. This happens with and without monitors simply because of the sheer amount of sound from the instruments and prompts the singer to compete because of the inability to hear him- or herself.

In the community setting there are chorales, symphony choruses (often 250+ members), as well as Barbershop, Sweet Adelines, and Madrigals groups. The sound of the Barbershop/Sweet Adeline style is often described as a "laserlike" pinpoint sound. It is easy to get caught in a trap of using excessive pressure to create a frontal, laserlike sound if one is not careful.

In the religious setting there is a wide range of styles and service music. There is music for the traditional service versus the contemporary service (found in Catholic, Protestant, and nondenominational churches). Even within the contemporary service definition there is a wide diversity of style and definition. Some consider anything other than high-church music contemporary while others consider only current music contemporary. Two churches that have brought contemporary music to the forefront are the Brooklyn Tabernacle and Houston's Lakewood Church (choir roster of approximately 650 members). Cindy Cruse Ratcliff, Lakewood's Music Director, defines their style of contemporary music as "diverse and eclectic. It ranges from Rock to Pop to Rhythm and Blues (R & B) to Gospel and even Latin" (personal communication, October 15, 2005). She notes that the music often changes style within a song. A song may start as Pop-oriented while the bridge is in a Gospel or R & B style. A good example of mixed style would be "Gloria" from Lakewood's CD *We Speak to Nations* which has a Latin salsa feel but also incorporates a traditional "Gloria" from the carol "Angels We Have Heard on High."

In the contemporary tradition, amplification is used for the singers as well as for the instrumentalists. The volume of energy created by all this amplification can trick the singer into feeling like he or she needs to sing louder in order to be heard. This happens more when there are no monitors for the singers but can happen even with monitors (ear buds as well as wedge style). Many singers who use ear buds actually prefer to use only one in order to hear room sound and feel the audience energy. Also, when singers try to create the contemporary sound they frequently do this by using tension to stop vibrato (ie, straight tone) and sound more "pop" in style. To sing without vibrato actually takes more airflow, not less. This same issue of

inefficient production can be found in churches that ask sopranos to produce a young boylike sound in order to emulate the English Cathedral Choir sound.

Musical Theatre

In musical theatre, the performance practice "sound du jour" has historically gone through changes. In the book *The Complete Professional Audition* by Cohn and Perilstein, one can find songs and musicals in a variety of categories. Vocally, there is variation in singing style depending on when a musical was written. In the first chapter, Cohn[12] organizes shows into groups that encompass similar styles ranging from Country-Western influence (*Oklahoma*), Teens/Children (*Into the Woods*), Pop/Rock (*Jesus Christ Superstar*), and Outcasts/Underdogs (*Hairspray*) to name a few. In regard to different vocal sounds, there are musicals that are considered more classical in sound such as *Oklahoma* and *Phantom of the Opera*, while *Rent* and *Jesus Christ Superstar* use a contemporary pop/rock sound.

Those who perform the principal roles of a musical production are rarely asked to perform or play more than one character in an evening. However, *Jekyll and Hyde*, for example, demands two very different vocal productions from the male lead in every performance. It is very difficult to perform at the extremes of range and style every night and stay healthy. Other shows that have principals perform more than one character in an evening include: (1) *Into the Woods*, (2) *The Apple Tree*, and (3) *I Love You, You're Perfect, Now Change*. Also, in *Sunday in the Park with George* the cast plays different roles in the first and second act. Other difficulties include the use of character voices such as: (1) Little Bird (*Seussical*) and (2) Adelaide (*Guys and Dolls*). When creating a character voice, one has to be careful not to pass the point of healthy coloration and effect whether it is producing a cartoonlike voice or using nasalance. Each singer has a window of opportunity for coloration and effect and must experiment with how far he or she may go from the central balance point and still have integrity of technique. Another interesting twist is bringing Disney characters to life on the theatrical stage. It can be difficult to create an inanimate object such as a clock, teapot, or candle (*Beauty and the*

Beast) and keep integrity of body alignment (potential to adversely affect airflow).

Two terms that broadly categorize musical theatre are "legit" and "belt." Legit style includes such standards as *Oklahoma* and *Carousel*. Legit is defined by singing voice specialist Jeanette LoVetri (personal communication, November 8, 2005) as classically based vocal production generally using unmodified vowels. She further defines *belt* as chest register carried up above the traditional break, approximately E4–G4, at a loud volume (high intensity). The term belt is often treated as a dirty word. However, if done in a healthy manner, it can be a viable option. One can take pressure off the larynx by using more nasalance in this instance. Broadway belt includes shows as *Jekyll & Hyde* and *Wicked*. The advent of *Evita* however, brings about use of the mixed sound combining "belt" and head voice (P. House, personal communication, October 20, 2005).

In the August 2005 issue of *Opera News*,[13] Michael John Lachiusa (composer, lyricist, and librettist whose works include *Lady Suite, Hello Again,* and *The Wild Party*) discusses two other issues in regard to categorizing musicals. He defines what he calls the "faux" musical and the "jukebox" musical. He lists *The Producers* and *Hairspray* as two examples of the faux musical genre. He labels these musicals as "faux" because they are based on cult films, not original ideas. The other category of musical, referred to as "jukebox" musicals, is defined as such because they are basically a catalogue of songs by a group or solo singer. Examples of this include: *Good Vibrations* based on music by the Beach Boys and *Movin' Out* which is based on the music of Billy Joel. The musical that is given credit as being the first of this kind is *Mamma Mia*, which is based on the music of ABBA. Although these categories may have merit for organizational purposes, they do not detract from public interest in attending the performances.

There is potential for difficulty when music by well-known artists is used. It is possible that some of the listeners may be disappointed because they will compare the vocal sound of the performers in the current show to the original artists. Furthermore, a singer may be chosen to perform in these shows because he or she is able to mimic the sound of the original artist. However, if the vocal production is a manipulation for the singer, it has the potential to cause vocal problems after a period of time. If, for example, the lead singer in *Movin' Out* has to scoop his tongue in the center to press his larynx down to a lower than normal position to mimic the timbre (quality) of Billy Joel, then he has the potential of creating vocal distress in regard to his natural range and flexibility. Also, the lead singer(s) in the show may need a different key from the original. Hopefully, this will be taken into account. These same issues hold true for singers who primarily perform cover songs in clubs.

Currently, career marketability of young singers requires a broader ability than ever before in regard to genre. It is of note to mention that in 2002, an entire month's issue of *Opera News* (August)[14] was devoted to the crossover phenomenon between opera and the theatre. There has never been a time when being a crossover singer has been as important as now. Many opera and lyric opera companies include musicals in their programs. It behooves the singer to learn the elements of what makes a style a style.

SPEAKING VOICE

Theater Versus Musical Theater

In nonmusical theater, the actor may play one role throughout an evening's performance, or he or she may play several different characters. In Houston's Alley Theatre production of *The Devil's Disciple* by Bernard Shaw, one actor played both the British General Burgoyne and the commoner Uncle Titus; the comportment and voice of each were vastly different. The same actor, in the two-hander *Stone's in His Pocket* by Marie Jones, was required to use six different Irish dialects with a character age range from 6 to 78. Indeed, all the characters in this production were portrayed by only two actors. The virtuosity required to satisfy the textural and pitch demands in such instances is very taxing on the voice and can do damage without proper vocal technique (T. Waite, personal communication, September 28, 2005).

TOOLS VERSUS TECHNIQUES

The performer must remember that healthy technique must precede stylism and use of stylistic tools. It is also prudent to be reminded that there are some sounds that have the potential to be harmful. The examples outlined previously included "grit," "growling," and glottal onsets which can be found in rock, country, and pop music and must be used with the least amount of tension necessary in order to avert damage. There are also tools that are common in different styles of music. In Country music prominent stylisms also employed include yodeling, crying, and "riding" an "r." In Rock music screams are employed. In Jazz agility with scat singing and breathy voice are employed. In Alternative music, glottal tension and vocal fry are employed. In Musical Theatre we have "belt," "legit," and "pop" stylisms. Remember, if used too often, a tension onset may become part of one's technique and no longer employed just as a stylistic tool.[2]

SUMMARY

Learning to balance the voice and creating healthy phonation is an excellent foundation for a performance career. The balanced voice is like clay; you need to have it to be able to mold the sound into a shape (character/style/genre). Once you have the clay, then you will be able to shape it into a creation of your own choosing. The performers voice is the vehicle for expression. So, it is not about the person, but about being a communicator with the voice as the vessel or vehicle for communication.

Acknowledgments

Pictures for Figures 6-2, 6-3, 6-4, and 6-6 are courtesy of Blue Tree Publishing. The author thanks Inkwater Press for liberal use of content from the book *Faith and Voice* for the sections called Body, Mind, and Spirit. The author thanks *Texas Sings* for republication of material from several journal articles. The author thanks the following people for their support and editorial assistance: Leonard Radionoff, Jackie Gartner-Schmidt, Todd Waite, Cindy Cruse-Ratcliff, Lee Poquette, and Paul House.

REFERENCES

1. Garrett JD, Radionoff SL, Rodriguez M, Stasney CR. *Vocal Health*. Lynnwood, Wash: Blue Tree Publishing; 2003.
2. Radionoff SL, Binkley CK. *Commercial Singing for Classical Singers*. Professional workshop presented at The Voice Foundation's 25th Annual Symposium Care of the Professional Voice, Philadelphia, Pa; June 1996.
3. Radionoff SL. Sound: a balancing act. *Texas Sings*. 2005(Winter): 8-9.
4. Sataloff RT. *Professional Voice: The Science and Art of Clinical Care*. 2nd ed. San Diego, Calif: Singular Publishing Group; 1997:111-130.
5. Baken RJ. An overview of laryngeal function for voice production. In Sataloff RT, ed. *Vocal Health and Pedagogy*. San Diego, Calif: Singular Publishing Group; 1998:27-45.
6. Bunch M. *Dynamics of the Singing Voice*. New York, NY: Springer-Verlag Wien; 1993:113.
7. Radionoff SL. The music educator: a high-risk professional voice. In Stemple JC, ed. *Voice Therapy Clinical Studies*. 2nd ed. San Diego, Calif: Singular Publishing Group; 2000:397-409.
8. Radionoff SL. Choral directors vocal health and reviving the tired voice. *Texas Sings*. 2003(Fall): 4-5,11.
9. Radionoff SL. Sound: A balancing act—part II: body, mind, and spirit. *Texas Sings*. 2004(Winter): 13,19.
10. Radionoff SL. *Faith and Voice*. Portland, Ore: Inkwater Press; 2005:2-38.
11. Sataloff RT. The human voice. *Sci Am*. 1992(Dec): 108-115.
12. Cohn D, Perilstein, M. *The Complete Professional Audition: A Commonsense Guide to Auditioning for Musicals and Plays*. New York, NY: Back Stage Books; 2005.
13. Lachiusa J. *Opera News*. 2005(August).
14. Rauch RS (ed). *Opera News*. 2002(August).

Part II

Diagnostics

Chapter 7

CASE HISTORY, INTERVIEW, AND VOICE HANDICAP ASSESSMENT

Michael S. Benninger
Thomas Murry

THE CHIEF COMPLAINT

The most important step in the evaluation and assessment process of any person with a voice disorder is the elucidation of the history of the current complaint or concerns. The singer comes to a voice clinic because he or she has specific concerns about the quality of his or her voice. In some cases, the singer will give a very concise description of the problem, such as, "I fatigue after the first 4 or 5 songs" or "I am no longer able to reach the upper few notes of my range since I performed three weeks ago." At other times, it may be very difficult for them to articulate their concerns and it is incumbent on the practitioner to take extra time in this important step to clarify as specifically as possible the problems the singer is experiencing. A few extra minutes during the initial interview will allow the clinician to focus the evaluation on the singer's primary concerns and create a directed approach to specific treatment. It should be remembered that, despite a primary concern, there may be other factors that must be teased out slowly.

Care should be taken to elucidate the chief complaint as this will often play a major role in the ultimate diagnosis. Common chief complaints are shown in Table 7-1. We have found that the chief complaint can

Table 7-1. Chief Complaint and Probable Diagnosis.

Complaint	Probable Diagnosis
"Hoarseness"	Abnormality of the vocal fold (laryngitis, reflux, edema, masses)
Fatigue	Overuse of voice
Breathiness	Inability to approximate vocal folds (laryngitis, edema, masses)
Need for prolonged warm-up	(reflux)
Volume disturbances	Technique, intrinsic voice limitations, pathologic processes, age, neurologic disorders, hearing loss, endocrine dysfunction
Pain	URI or laryngitis, musculoskeletal strain, arthritis, reflux
Scratchy, itchy voice	Reflux, acute laryngitis, vocal abuse
Foreign body sensation, globus	Reflux, voice abuse

often serve as the primary mechanism for making the diagnosis. Table 7–2 lists some causes of overuse or improper use of the voice. The clinician should discuss each as multiple factors often occur over time to bring on the problem. Tables 7–3 and 7–4 list other considerations or conditions that may bring on the voice problem or contribute to changes in the voice of the singer.

A thorough history that focuses on the issues related to performance and postperformance voice changes along with a complete physical examination of the ears, nose, and throat will usually serve to crystallize the diagnosis. For example, a complaint of hoarseness might suggest a vocal mass, but examination is needed to confirm this diagnosis and identify the specific pathology.

The interviewer will be the most successful during the initial discussion with the singer if he or she engages the singer in aspects of lifestyle, rehearsal schedules, performances, and so forth. In this way, the singer will be more likely to discuss details about the onset of the problem. Other factors such as whether or not the singer is also a dancer, actor, or musician may also help the clinician to understand the reasons for seeking help.

As professional singers and actors are not the primary caseload of most otolaryngologists and speech-language pathologists, it is wise to have a prepared questionnaire. There are extensive ones such as that used by Sataloff[1] or shorter forms that are specifically for singers.[2] With a prepared questionnaire, the clinician is likely to identify issues that go beyond the current primary hoarseness or fatigue complaints.

The singer's initial interview may be aided by the presence of the singing voice specialist. He or she may offer the singer time to explain the details of the onset of the complaint, the feelings associated with the changes since its onset, and relay the concerns to the other clinicians. In any event, allowing extra time for the interview will put the performer at ease and demonstrate the clinician's interest in the details of the singer's problem.

Table 7–2. Common Causes of Vocal Overuse.

- Time and duration of practice
- Excessive performing
- Conducting and teaching
- Environment of performances
- Singing/talking excessively
- Singing/talking over noise
- Singing/talking under tension
- Social speaking
    Voice use different in speaking than in singing
    Expert training lost or ignored
- Noise volume—children, noisy backgrounds
- Telephone—sound amplified
- Airline travel—speaking over ambient background noise, dryness

Table 7–3. Additional Sources of Dysphonia in Singers.

- Inadequate preparation
    limited practice and rehearsals
    poor or inadequate training:
        in general
        singer's voice and level of training not suitable for the role
- Insufficient warm-up
- Poor environment for practice, rehearsing
- Working through injury
- Errors in technique
- Excessive muscle tension in tongue, neck, or larynx
- Excessive volume
- Poor or inadequate abdominal support

Table 7–4 Environmental Influences on Voice

- Humidity, dryness, mold
- Dust, dirt (set construction)
- Second-hand, primary smoke
- Smoke, fog machines
- Pollution
- Allergies
- Travel schedule
- Other vocal irritants

MEASURING QUALITY OF LIFE

Efforts to evaluate quality of life (QOL) in medicine have moved into voice clinical practice and research. The application of QOL to patients and the result of treatment or nontreatment are referred to as measuring outcomes. This section describes some general concepts of outcomes measures, the outcomes and quality of life research movements in medicine, and the present status of these movements as they relate to voice care, and the implications in determining treatment options for the voice patient.

ASSESSING THE SINGER'S QUALITY OF LIFE AND OUTCOMES

Health is a multidimensional concept that, according to the World Health Organization, incorporates physical, mental, and social states.[3] Handicap is defined as ". . . a social, economic, or environmental disadvantage resulting from an impairment or disability," and disability is defined as ". . . restriction or lack of ability manifested in the performance of daily tasks."[4] The degree of change in the parameters of physical, mental, or social status is considered an outcome. These outcomes, however, depend on a number of factors including the baseline level of function, other concomitant medical conditions, a person's perception of quality of life, and cultural or societal influences. In general, medical care strives to prevent and eliminate disease and thereby improve the quality of a patient's life. Traditionally, assessment of physical function was the only means of determining the impact of health or disease. This practice limits the clinician's ability to also assess the emotional or social impact of disease or its treatment. An acknowledgment of these limitations led to the development of a whole new way of looking at health and disease, and has been coined the "*outcomes*" movement.

Traditional assessment of outcomes in medicine has largely been through the perspective of the treating physician or clinician (ie, doctors, nurses, speech-language pathologists.) Therefore, an outcome was identified via changes in the physical examination, an improvement or change in symptoms and functions, or changes in laboratory tests or X-ray examinations. Clas-

sically the simplest two measurements of an outcome of treatment are the presence or absence of disease. In many ways, this distinction is very important, but it is often inadequate for assessing general life impact. For example, surgical treatment may be successful for a vocal fold polyp, yielding complete return of normal voice function. However, if the polyp and its treatment resulted in the singer missing an important performance, its effect on quality of life might be significantly different. Thus, when we consider the performer's voice, quality of life and outcome take on meanings that have fully yet to be understood.

The medical profession's early attempts to assess quality of life revolved around questionnaires that served to identify key issues that patients may have in relationship to their disease.[5] These questionnaires usually focused on questions that the physician or other person administrating the questionnaire felt were important, often not including factors that the person completing the questionnaire was most concerned about. Over time, following multiple revisions and adaptations, these questionnaires tended to address, to some degree, both these perspectives. Furthermore, questionnaires were not statistically validated, and, therefore, one could not be sure that they truly measured what was intended to be measured or that responses by individuals with the disease were different from those without the disease. It was also not clear whether or not the questionnaire maintained its validity over time so that a person who had no change in status would answer questions similarly at different times.

A realization that there are many critical issues related to the presence of a disease or the treatment of disease and efforts to measure the entire impact of health on individuals and society have driven the outcomes movement. Outcomes research attempts to observe patients in their typical clinical environment and uses patient-centered measures. In other words, they are measures of how the voice disorder affects function and quality of life.

Quality of life measurement instruments have been developed to try to measure the multidimensional nature of health with the questions and items within these tests usually clustering around broad health-related areas that can be measured in direct relationship to disease or response to treatment. Probably the most well-recognized and utilized quality of life measurement tool is the Medical Outcomes Study 36-Item

Short Form General-Health Survey, or "SF-36."[6-8] This instrument is self-administered and assesses 8 domains of health that are commonly affected by disease or its treatment: physical functioning, role functioning, social functioning, mental health, bodily pain, general health, vitality, and health transition.[6-8] Each of these subscales provides a score that is reliable and a valid measure of health for that particular dimension. The SF-36 has been used to evaluate a wide range of health issues and to compare quality of life as it relates to different disease processes.[9]

One of the disadvantages of using general health measurement tools to evaluate specific disorders is that they may not assess well the specific impact of the disease on an individual and how it may be affected by other medical conditions. This has led to an effort to develop disease-specific outcomes measurement tools.[8] The creation of these outcomes measurement tools requires a comprehensive, statistically validated assessment of reliability, predictability, reproducibility, responsiveness, and interpretability. In general, they should be easy to use (low burden) and should assist in the evaluation of the specific problem they were designed to assess.

MEASURING VOICE OUTCOMES AND QUALITY OF LIFE: STATE OF THE ART

Outcomes research is in its infancy as it relates to the care of people with voice disorders. Past attempts at trying to assess the impact of a voice problem on quality of life were limited by the types of tools that were available. Even with objective tests, there are often no generally agreed-upon gold standards of measurement. Furthermore, different objective tests have been designed for different measures of function, such as pitch, frequency range, airflow parameters, perturbation, or vocal fold vibration. Variation occurs among clinicians in the interpretation of these tests. These limitations have prevented valid comparisons between the impact of an intervention in different environments or in comparing two different interventions. Although it would be expected that improvements in objective tests would correlate with improvements in outcome, severity of disease as measured by these

tests does not necessarily measure its impact to an individual. Minimal variations in pitch for a performing vocalist would likely have a much greater impact than for a person who has minimal voice demands. A cured small laryngeal cancer may prevent a singer or other professional speaker from performing but would probably not limit the quality of life for a weekend volunteer choir singer. The impact on their quality of life would be expected to be significant and likely poorly represented by objective tests.

A recent study showed significant differences in perception of quality of life between patients with dysphonia and unaffected average people in the United States.[7] When evaluating the specific domains of the SF-36, we found significant differences in the domains of "emotion" and "physical" between individuals with dysphonia and normal speakers. These two domains deal with the ability to perform work and other daily tasks as a result of the physical or emotional impact of their disorder. As voice problems might be expected to have an impact on work and other daily activities, this finding is not unexpected. The "social functioning" score was also worse in patients with dysphonia. Because "physical functioning," "vitality," and "mental health" scores were also worse for dysphonic patients than for normals, it can be extrapolated that these disorders may affect a broader sense of well-being than would be expected from the types of problems people would generally be expected to have with a voice disorder. Objective tests of voice function or questionnaires would not be expected to measure these impacts on quality of life of dysphonia.

Traditionally, outcomes for patients with voice disorders have been measured with a clinical or biomedical frame of reference. The variables that are used to indicate a favorable or unfavorable treatment outcome do not rely on attitudinal input from the patients. In an effort to shift the focus from the clinicians' judgments to patients' self-perceptions of their voice disorders, we developed the Voice Handicap Index (VHI)[10] (Figure 7-1). The VHI consists of 30 statements that reflect the variety of experiences a patient with a voice disorder may encounter. Patients note a frequency of each experience on a 5-point, equal-appearing scale (0—never, 1—almost never, 2—sometimes, 3—almost always, 4—always), with the best score being 0 and the worst score 120.

VOICE HANDICAP INDEX (VHI)

Today's Date ☐☐ - ☐☐ - ☐☐

First Name ☐☐☐☐☐☐☐☐☐☐☐

Last Name ☐☐☐☐☐☐☐☐☐☐☐☐☐☐☐☐

MRN ☐☐☐☐☐☐☐☐

Birth Date ☐☐ - ☐☐ - ☐☐
Month   Day   Year

Age ☐☐   ○ Male   ○ Female

Provider ☐☐☐☐☐☐☐☐☐☐☐☐☐☐☐☐☐

Date of Operation ☐☐ - ☐☐ - ☐☐
Month   Day   Year

Type of Visit:
○ New Visit   ○ Pre-Treatment   ○ Pre-Surgical Treatment
○ Return Visit   ○ Post Medical Treatment   ○ Post Surgical Treatment

Diagnosis:
○ Functional Dysphonia
○ Spasmodic Dysphonia
○ Other Neurogenic Dysphonia
○ Bowing/Presbylarynges
○ Benign Masses (polyp/ nodule/ MRC)

○ Epidermoid Cyst/Sulcus
○ Vocal Fold Paralysis
  ○ a) unilateral
  ○ b) bilateral
  ○ c) SLN

○ Reflux Laryngitis
○ Leukoplakia
○ Benign Laryngeal Tumor
○ Malignant Laryngeal Tumor
○ Other (Describe)
_____

Instructions: These are statements that many people have used to describe their voices and the effects of their voices on their lives. Check the response that indicates how frequently you have the same experience.

	Never	Almost Never	Sometimes	Almost Always	Always
F1. My voice makes it difficult for people to hear me.	O	O	O	O	O
P2. I run out of air when I talk.	O	O	O	O	O
F3. People have difficulty understanding me in a noisy room.	O	O	O	O	O
P4. The sound of my voice varies throughout the day.	O	O	O	O	O
F5. My family has difficulty hearing me when I call them throughout the house.	O	O	O	O	O
F6. I use the phone less often than I would like.	O	O	O	O	O
E7. I'm tense when talking with others because of my voice.	O	O	O	O	O
F8. I tend to avoid groups of people because of my voice.	O	O	O	O	O
E9. People seem irritated with my voice.	O	O	O	O	O
P10. People ask "What's wrong with your voice?"	O	O	O	O	O
F11. I speak with friends, neighbors, or relatives less often because of my voice.	O	O	O	O	O
F12. People ask me to repeat myself when speaking face-to-face.	O	O	O	O	O
P13. My voice sounds creaky and dry.	O	O	O	O	O
P14. I feel as though I have to strain to produce voice.	O	O	O	O	O
E15. I find other people don't understand my voice problem.	O	O	O	O	O

Figure 7-1. The Voice Handicap Index (VHI) *(continues)*

7177008628

	Never	Almost Never	Sometimes	Almost Always	Always
F16. My voice difficulties restrict my personal and social life.	O	O	O	O	O
P17. The clarity of my voice is unpredictable.	O	O	O	O	O
P18. I try to change my voice to sound different.	O	O	O	O	O
F19. I feel left out of conversations because of my voice.	O	O	O	O	O
P20. I use a great deal of effort to speak.	O	O	O	O	O
P21. My voice is worse in the evening.	O	O	O	O	O
F22. My voice problem causes me to lose income.	O	O	O	O	O
E23. My voice problem upsets me.	O	O	O	O	O
E24. I am less outgoing because of my voice problem.	O	O	O	O	O
E25. My voice makes me handicapped.	O	O	O	O	O
P26. My voice "gives out" on me in the middle of speaking.	O	O	O	O	O
E27. I feel annoyed when people ask me to repeat.	O	O	O	O	O
E28. I feel embarrassed when people ask me to repeat.	O	O	O	O	O
E29. My voice makes me feel incompentent.	O	O	O	O	O
E30. I'm ashamed of my voice problem.	O	O	O	O	O

P Scale ☐☐

F Scale ☐☐

E Scale ☐☐

Total Scale ☐☐☐

Please circle the word that matches how you feel your voice is today.

Normal   Mild   Moderate   Severe

Figure 7-1. (continued)

Three subscales of the VHI measure the physical, emotional, and functional impacts of the voice disorder. The VHI, therefore, is able to measure not only the physical effects of a person's voice problem but also the functional and emotional aspects. Therefore it can serve as an independent, objective measure of the impact of voice dysfunction on the quality of life.

Two examples of how the VHI is used are shown in Figures 7-2 and 7-3. In Figure 7-2, the patient, a 32-year-old teacher who also sings with a club band on

Documentation:

Teacher/Singer

Figure 7-2. Use of the VHI in treatment of a 32-year-old teacher who also sings with a band on the weekend. The data show improvement but the VHI is above normal. She opted for surgical treatment.

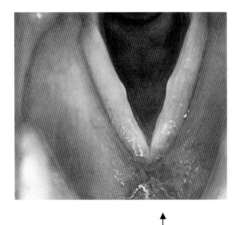

	VHI	F_0	F_0 Low	F_0 High	X flow	P.T.P.
Pretreatment	78	188	145	487	370 cc/s	5.2 cmH$_2$0
Posttreatment 6 sessions	47	201	140 Hz	600 Hz	295 cc/s	4.8 cmH$_2$0

Conclusion: Repeat examimation, consider surgery

Figure 7-3. A 28-year-old actress diagnosed with vocal fold nodules. Note that her VHI reduced to a near-normal value, Her nodules appear to have resolved at her examination 9 weeks later, as seen on the right.

Vocal nodules: Virtually all patients improve or return to normal vocal function.

Pretreatment VHI = 39
Posttreatment VHI = 19

After 9 weeks of treatment

weekends, presented with a lesion on the right vocal fold. Her initial VHI was 78, indicating a severe voice handicap in her estimation. She was given 6 sessions of voice therapy and returned for re-evaluation. Her VHI decreased to 47 and her acoustic and aerodynamic measures also decreased. However, her VHI was still significantly above normal and she opted for surgical treatment.

Figure 7-3 shows a 28-year-old actress who was seen shortly after performing in an outdoor theater during the summer. She was diagnosed with vocal nodules. Following a period of voice therapy (6 sessions over 9 weeks), her voice improved, her VHI decreased, and the vocal nodules were no longer present on follow-up stroboscopic examination. Her VHI went from 39, a moderately high score, to 19, a reduction of 20 points and a range considered to be normal.[10]

Our studies also show that the impact of dysphonia on quality of life is substantial even when compared to other chronic diseases such as angina, sciatica, chronic sinusitis, or back pain, particularly in the areas of social functioning and role-playing.[10] Overall, however, other chronic diseases tend to produce worse scores than dysphonia. As the SF-36 is scaled only relating to the individual domains and not for a total score, direct overall total comparisons cannot be made. Nonetheless, by evaluating the individual domains, a comparison of their impact on quality of life can be made between such disorders.

When attempting to correlate the VHI with the SF-36, strong correlations were found between the total VHI scores and the individual subscales of the SF-36 domains of social functioning, role functioning (emotional and physical), and mental health. The greatest disability of patients with swallowing disorders is in the functional areas, as validated by this study and the relationship of the VHI to the SF-36.[9] As patients with voice disorders generally do not have significant changes in bodily pain, general health, vitality, and general physical functioning, the VHI would not be expected to be very sensitive to changes in these domains of the SF-36.

Patients with vocal fold paralysis had worse scores in many of the domains of the SF-36 than patients with dysphonia from other causes, particularly in the domains of role-playing, physical, and physical functioning.[9] This is likely due to the impact of vocal fold paralysis on lifting and straining and other daily activities. In general, paralysis patients appear to be more disabled and have poorer overall quality of life than the other categories of patients with dysphonia as measured by both the SF-36 and VHI. When evaluated with the VHI, the group with vocal fold edema, which is not uncommon in singers, had better scores for the total, functional, and physical scores than the patients with vocal fold masses (eg, nodules or polyps). Individuals with vocal fold paralysis in general had worse

scores than other individuals with voice disorders on the VHI.[9] We have found the VHI to be an excellent tool when used to measure the success of either medical or surgical treatment in vocalists.[13]

Recently, Rosen and others offered a short form of the VHI, known as the VHI-10. The VHI-10 is a valid and reliable scale of a person's handicap. The VHI-10 was validated against the original VHI. It has been shown to be reliable in a group of 100 subjects. Its value in clinical situations is that it takes very little time to complete and offers a patient's self-estimate of his or her voice handicap. It has not been applied specifically to singers; therefore, its use with singers suggests the same caveat as the original VHI, namely, that singers tend to underestimate the speaking handicap as this questionnaire does not specify the singing voice in its statements. The VHI-10 is shown in Figure 7–4.

Published reports of the use of the SF-36 in evaluating performing vocalists or singers have not been presented to date, although we and other investigators are beginning use of the VHI to assess the level of disability and response to treatment.

As the VHI was developed from a group of patients with a broad range of voice problems, it may not be sensitive to subtle changes that may affect a performer. The broad measurement of emotional and social aspects may well represent the overall general life impacts of performing voice disorders.

> Singers, actors, and voiceover performers represent unique groups and when they present with voice problems; general questions or statements about the voice may not reflect specific problems that relate clarity, loudness effort, or emotional problems that develop as a result of voice injury.

All voice problems in singers may be interpreted as serious by the singer even though quality, loudness, or endurance issues may be minimal. However, as the vocal demands increase, the singer with a minor injury may require more time off, resulting in increasing loss of income.

Evidence of the continuing need to explore singers' voice problems and singers' perception of severity

The VHI-10

1. My voice makes it difficult for people to hear me. 0 1 2 3 4

2. People have difficulty understanding me in a noisy room. 0 1 2 3 4

3. My voice difficulties restrict personal and social life. 0 1 2 3 4

4. I feel left out of conversations because of my voice. 0 1 2 3 4

5. My voice problem causes me to lose income. 0 1 2 3 4

6. I feel as though I have to strain to produce voice. 0 1 2 3 4

7. The clarity of my voice is unpredictable. 0 1 2 3 4

8. My voice problem upsets me. 0 1 2 3 4

9. My voice makes me feel handicapped. 0 1 2 3 4

10. People ask, "What's wrong with your voice?" 0 1 2 3 4

Figure 7-4. The VHI-10[13] consists of 10 statements derived from the original VHI and has been validated against the VHI.

was offered by Rosen and Murry.[12] They found that singers' scores on the VHI are significantly lower than nonsingers. Moreover, they also reported that professional singers had lower VHI scores than recreational singers or those who have income from other professions. Reasons for the low scores on the VHI for singers may relate to the lack of specific questions related to the singing voice or the fact that professional singers come in for consultation soon after they detect a change in their voice. Although the VHI provides an estimate of the patient's perception of severity, it may underestimate their concerns. Nonetheless, the VHI provides an estimate of severity that cannot be obtained by other objective measures or subjective observations.

SUMMARY

The future challenges related to outcomes research in voice, particularly for singers, will revolve on the application of these types of instruments to allow identification of factors important to the patient. The first challenge is to determine the severity of a patient's handicap or disability from a particular disorder. This will influence the aggressiveness of treatment or, in some cases, whether or not to treat. The second challenge is to utilize outcomes research to identify the best treatment. This may also be used to develop new treatments that take the singer's response to treatment into consideration. Finally, voice outcomes research should focus on how improvement of a specific disorder will affect the global quality of life for the singer and his or her family.

The future in outcomes research in voice is bright. There is much effort directed at improvement of quality of life and measurement. These efforts in combination with traditional voice evaluations, basic voice research science, and prospective, randomized clinical trials should have a dramatic impact on voice care in the future. The application of objective outcomes tools such as the VHI and the SF-36 to performing vocalists will ensure that the global impact on quality of life is measured.

REFERENCES

1. Sataloff RT. *Treatment of Voice Disorders*. San Diego, Calif: Plural Publishing Inc; 2005:365–372.

2. Greene MCL, Mathieson L. The *Voice and Its Disorders*. 5th ed. San Diego, Calif: Singular Publishing Group;1991:77–81.

3. World Health Organization. The economics of health and disease. *WHO Chronicle*. 1971;25:20–24.

4. World Health Organization. *International Classification of Impairments, Disabilities and Handicaps: A Manual of Classification Relating to the Consequences of Disease*. Geneva, Switzerland: Author; 1980.

5. Benninger MS, Gardner GM, Jacobson BH. New dimensions in measuring voice treatment outcomes. In Sataloff RT. *Professional Voice: The Science and Art of Clinical Care*. 3rd ed. San Diego, Calif: Singular Publishing Group; 2006:471–478.

6. Ware JE, Sherbourne CD. The MOS 36-Item Short Form Health Survey (SF-36). I. Conceptual framework and item selection. *Med Care*. 1972;30:473–483.

7. McHorney CA, Ware JE, Raczek AE. The MOS 36-item Short Form Health Survey (SF-36). II. Psycho-metric and clinical tests of validity in measuring physical and mental health constructs. *Med Care*. 1993;31:247–263.

8. McHorney CA, Ware JE, Lu JF, Sherbourne CD. The MOS 36-Item Short Form Health Survey (SF-36). III. Tests of data quality, scaling, assumptions and reliability across diverse patient groups. *Med Care*. 1994;32:40–66.

9. Benninger MS, Ahuja AS, Gardner G, Grywalski C. Assessing outcomes for dysphonic patients. *J Voice*. 1998;12:540–550.

10. Jacobson BH, Johnson A, Grywalski C, Silbergleit AK, Jacobson GP, Benninger MS. The Voice Handicap Index (VHI): development and validation. *J Speech Lang Pathol*. 1997;6:66–70.

11. Benninger MS, Gardner G, Grywalski C. The outcomes of botulinum toxin treatment for spasmodic dysphonia. *Arch Otolaryngol Head Neck Surg*. 2001;127;770–773.

12. Rosen, CA, Murry T. Voice Handicap Index in singers. *J Voice*. 2000;14(3):370–377.

13. Rosen CA, Lee AS, Osbourne J, Zullo T, Murry T. Development and validation of the Voice Handicap Index-10. *Laryngoscope*. 2004;114: 1549–1556.

Chapter 8

LARYNGEAL EXAMINATIONS AND VISUALIZATIONS

Peak Woo

SINGERS AS PATIENTS: WHY ARE THEY DIFFERENT?

Some physicians and health professionals see singers' complaints as being dominated by psychogenic issues. It is true that singers want to see doctors earlier and more frequently than other voice professionals such as teachers and reporters. Thus, singers with their complaints often earn the undeserved reputation as psychosomatic in their complaints. Were it the only issue, most of us would be happy to send singers to psychologists and educate them on coping issues. But it is true that even well-educated, well-adjusted, and well-tempered singers experience transient voice loss and voice difficulties in a lifetime of productive singing; they may need help from a health professional when they have voice loss.[1]

Psychological issues particular to the singer's world may bring the singer to an otolaryngologist. Anthony Blunt said it best in his treatise on the singer's and actor's throat.[2]

Fame, wealth and realization of artistic ambition apart, the life of a leading international singer is not to be envied. These artists become unsettled by constant change of scene and climate, by uncomfortable traveling from airport to airport and from hotel to hotel, and also by the lack of "roots" with a home, family and close friends. Young singers, especially, suffer from insecurity and disruption of personal attachment. It is not unusual for a consultation to start on the theme of "laryngitis" and end with tears and the story of a broken engagement.

For singers who depend on their voices for a living, their voice is the instrument that expresses their individuality and their character. Singers depend on the fine-tuning of their instrument for their livelihood. This investment in time and energy may well merit the extra attention given to their instrument when it is not behaving correctly. Such concern, however, would not explain the fear, anxiety, and mental anguish that accompany some calls from singers to explain their voice difficulties. After all, trial lawyers, stockbrokers, and auctioneers all fall into similar professional voice categories. The identity of a singer is defined by his or her voice quality not by what is said or expressed in content. Thus, its potential loss is magnified to a much greater extent than for other voice professionals. For a singer, there is no greater nightmare than waking up without a voice, with the uncertainty of return of voice. This fear may seem incredible to a rational person and may indeed even seem irrational to the singer. But the relationship that a singer develops over time with his or her "voice" is unique. Often, the singer's voice has a separate identity which must be treated well, managed carefully, and coaxed into action by the singer. As if the voice "coexists" within the singer in a symbiotic fashion, it has good and bad days. The treating professional should not trivialize these feelings.

Singers are labile, sometimes emotionally fragile, and often prone to emotional extravagance. But would the public want a singer in any other way? Singers sing by tactile sensation, not by sound feedback. They sing by feeling sensations developed over many lessons and hours of practice. Sensory kinesthetic abnormalities are common when swelling, edema, dryness, phlegm, or lubrication problems of the throat become an issue. Singers feel it in the effort required for singing. They feel it in the ease in which one note melds into another. They feel abnormal when the singing gesture needed for expression is accompanied by tactile sensations at odds with those that they know are "perfect." Such need to explain the abnormal sensations are common symptoms that will bring a singer to the doctor's office before there is an audible problem in the singer's voice. This helps to explain why singers will tend to present to the doctor earlier than other voice professionals.[3]

LISTEN TO THE COMPLAINT

In the previous chapter, the common reasons for seeing an otolaryngologist (voice doctor) were presented. In addition, singers may seek an otolaryngologist simply to "bless the instrument" prior to going on with an important endeavor. The instrument, once verified to be true and healthy, can then be used with freedom and in a worry free state.[2] The singer may present with acute voice breakdown before a performance. Voice breakdown may be due to acute illness, real or imagined, or due to nonmedical causes.[1,3,4] Singers also present for a nonurgent evaluation for voice deterioration or vocal deficit due to spiraling or progressive voice loss surrounding body and life span changes.[5] Sometimes singers' failure to progress with a singing teacher or a singing technique will prompt a consultation to evaluate the vocal apparatus. Westerman Gregg has suggested that posture, respiratory support, change in hydration, phonatory hyperfunction, speaking pitch too high or low, lack of resonance, tongue tension affecting resonance and voicing are some of the factors to be explored.[6] Life span changes such as puberty, menopause, and senescence may be accompanied by voice changes that are difficult to decipher. These changes may prompt the referral for consultation.[7,8]

LISTENING TO THE VOICE

The history and the general examination have been discussed in previous chapters. Several important points should be reiterated. The history should especially inquire as to the menses in the adult female singer.[5] Prior to examination of the patient by instrumentation, it is important to note the quality of the voice. The GRBAS scale is a good scale for determining what instrument and what visualization tests to perform. The GRBAS scale rates the voice based on perceptual qualities of grade, roughness, breathiness, asthenia, and strain. Some singers will have a normal speaking voice but have specific singing difficulties. Patients with vocal strain, voice breaks, and specific voice range issues are examined by flexible laryngoscopy.[9] If the patient is complaining of a difficulty with passagio, excessive tremolo, wobble, or pain with singing, flexible laryngoscopy will be necessary. The inherent advantage of a flexible scope for evaluation of the singing apparatus without holding the tongue should be obvious.

As part of the general examination of the singer's speaking and singing voice, perceptual evaluation of their voice quality should be done beyond the GRBAS quality as discussed in chapter 10.

As part of the examination prior to instrumentation, ask the patient to sing some simple notes. The purpose of this is not to ask the singer to demonstrate his or her singing prowess but to systematically but simply test the voice. A five-tone ascending scale in the vowel "ee" or "oo" is easily modeled by the examiner and can be followed by the patient even if he or she has no prior training. The singer is then asked to progress up the scale until an audible voice break or a problem is detected. A simple tool to use is a pitch pipe, which is available at music stores for nominal cost (Figure 8–1). At the point of voice breakdown, the patient is then asked to sustain the voice at that note and the frequency is noted either by ear or by using a frequency analyzer on the stroboscope. The patient is asked to place the stethoscope of the stroboscope on the neck to pick up the fundamental frequency. Starting in the patient's most comfortable speaking voice will do. For males we start at C2, 125 Hz, for females we start at middle C, C4 or 250 Hz. The singers will then progress to approximately two octaves higher using the ascending five-tone scale. At the area of difficulty, the singer may be switched from a five-tone discrete vowel production to a voice glide. To facilitate discussion of musical notes and singing range difficulties, a musical chart of piano keys and their frequency is also useful (Figure 8–2).

In general, singers with voice problems will reveal the vocal difficulties in specific areas of their singing. These areas include:

1. High soft notes will be difficult.
2. Transition notes from chest voice to mixed or head voice will be noticeable by a break or a lack of ease during their production.
3. There will be difficulty with a fast staccato production.
4. Pitch glides may show distinct voice breaks with lack of smoothness.

Figure 8–1. Pitch pipe used for accurate modeling of singing pitch. Available in music supplies stores.

Figure 8–2. Keyboard with corresponding musical notation and frequency noted. This helps the examiner to test the frequency most troublesome to the singer.

PALPATION OF THE LARYNX AND NECK

In the examination of the neck and larynx, palpation should be done before visual inspection. Palpation of the larynx feels for evidence of appropriate laryngeal position, softness of the larynx during phonation, and confirms the presence of an easy posture without excessive tension. The common sites of excessive tension that may be elicited by palpation are:

1. Base of tongue and suprahyoid muscle tension. Figure 8-3 demonstrate the base of tongue palpation that elicits excessive tension with phonation.
2. Short thyrohyoid distance with contracted, tight thyrohyoid distance (Figure 8-4). The thyroid to hyoid distance is shortened with a barely palpable thyrohyoid membrane. This corresponds to a tight squeezed voice with a high larynx position.
3. Cricothyroid (CT) lock. Some patients have poor relaxation of the cricothyroid membrane. They have a locked distance at the CT membrane. Thus, pitch glides in the patient with fixed CT distance are associated with a higher pitch but with a strained quality. There is no closure of the crico- thyroid membrane with pitch elevation and there is a lack of opening of the cricothyroid membrane with low phonation.
4. Lack of freedom of movement of the larynx with phonation.

5. Figures 8-3 through 8-7 are photographs of the different sites of palpation done as part of the examination. Palpation of the base of the lesser horn of the hyoid bone and the superior cornu of the thyroid cartilage are used to elicit extrinsic laryngeal muscle tension. The cricothyroid mem- brane is palpated with pitch glides to feel for ade- quacy of laryngeal movement.

On palpation, the larynx should be supple. With rocking, the larynx should give easily and show the normal laryngeal crepitance. Consistent finding of iso- lated muscle tenderness after singing is not normal. The most common findings are tenderness of the

Figure 8-4. Palpation of the thyrohyoid distance and freedom during singing.

Figure 8-3. Palpation of the base of tongue for base of tongue tension.

Figure 8-5. Palpation of the hyoid horn for ten- derness and symmetry.

Figure 8–6. Palpation of the superior thyroid cornu for tenderness and motion.

Figure 8–7. Palpation of the cricothyroid membrane during a pitch glide.

suprahyoid muscles.[10] Over-activation of the stylohyoid muscles, the sternohyoid muscles, and the laryngeal elevators will result in tenderness of the greater hyoid cornu and the superior horn of the thyroid cartilage. Laryngeal isometric tension may involve either the extrinsic laryngeal muscles or the intrinsic laryngeal muscles or both. This muscle tension results in protracted tenderness to palpation. It is usually associated with a throaty voice with other vocal faults such as low-tone focus and lack of appropriate resonance.[11]

INSTRUMENTATION OF THE SINGER'S THROAT

There are no standardized examinations that will fit all singers. Some singers need a simple rigid examination that takes as little as a few minutes; others may need extensive examinations that require both the flexible laryngoscope and the stroboscope. With the video recording systems that are available, both flexible and rigid endoscopy can be recorded and analyzed.

Specific singing problems cannot be readily diagnosed by rigid stroboscopy alone and therefore flexible endoscopy with or without stroboscopic light should always be entertained in an initial examination. Examination of the biomechanics of the singing voice is best done by fiberoptic examination.[9] Once the diagnosis is clearly related to a vocal fold edge abnormality, follow-

up examinations may be shortened to include only the rigid or the flexible endoscope alone.

To efficiently conduct the examination of the singer, I prefer to start the examination in most patients with a rigid telescope. This examination is excellent for estimation of mucosal health, detection of lesions on the vibratory margins, and detection of gross movement abnormalities of the vocal folds. In the event that the vocal folds appear normal, a flexible examination of the vocal fold function is in order. Flexible laryngoscopy is the preferred imaging modality in patients with asthenic voice, vocal tremor, and vocal strain. Patients suspected of functional voice disorders and neurogenic voice disorders such as dystonia, Parkinson's disease, and dysarthria should also have a flexible laryngoscopy as the primary examination.

Fiberoptic Laryngoscopy

Fiberoptic laryngoscopy should be routinely used in singers presenting with specific problems in areas of their singing. Pitch elevation is associated with specific changes in the pharynx, base of tongue, and laryngeal position.[12] Whether these are adaptive, maladaptive, or normal depends on the clinical scenario. One may need the helpful eye of a singing teacher during such an examination. For example, if the singer is complaining of a difficulty with excessive tremolo or wobble in the vibrato, a flexible laryngoscopy of pharyngeal and laryngeal adjustments during singing will yield more valid observations than a rigid telescopic examination. Similarly, if the complaint is about difficulty during the passage or a problem in a specific note, the singing difficulty is best explored with a thin fiberscope with the singing teacher present to help with the accuracy of the sound production to be tested.

Prior to the instrumentation, the examiner may wish to ask the singer to produce the abnormal voice so that the test may focus on the problem. In patients with suspected spasmodic dysphonia or muscle tension dysphonia, the difficulties may not be during sustained vowels but may occur only with rapid onset and offset of the voice. Thus, the examiner must ask for speech and singing tokens laden with voice gestures most likely to reveal the abnormality.

The fiberoptic testing protocol is divided into three key areas. These three key areas are: (1) anatomy and mucosal health, (2) laryngeal movement evaluation with vegetative gestures, and (3) voicing gestures. Table 8–1 outlines the testing protocol.

Table 8-1. Test Protocol with Fiberoptic Laryngoscopy

A. Laryngeal anatomy and mucosal health

B. Laryngeal movement, vegetative, nonvoicing gestures
   1. cough
   2. eee . . . sniff
   3. whistle
   4. laugh
   5. deep inspiration
   6. rapid diadochokinesis evaluation with throat clearing

C. Voice testing
   1. sustained phonation and speaking
      a. pitch and loudness range testing
      b. register transition
      c. speaking sentences
   2. singing
      a. five-tone scale, steady vowel
      b. glissando
      c. messa de voce
      d. staccato
      e. singing in pianissimo
      f. singing a song the patient knows

The fiberscope should be introduced with a minimum of nasal anesthesia so as not to change the sensation of the singer and cause excessive secretion. The tip of the scope should be placed at the level of the uvula and not deeper lest it cause gagging and choking. The scope should be placed into the side opposite the vocal side suspected of the lesion. Thus, a patient with a left-side vocal fold lesions or paralysis should be examined through the right nostril. This takes the advantage of the fiberscope ability to be turned to slightly look to the side, revealing more information than from the top-down view. A panoramic view of the larynx and pharynx is used to evaluate the anatomy and the function. The anatomy of the larynx and pharynx is evaluated as to symmetry and motion. Some simple questions remind the examiner to systematically inspect the structures beside the vocal folds during flexible laryngoscopy:

- Is the base of tongue forward enough to see the larynx?
- Is there lingual tonsil and pharyngeal tonsil tissue?
- Are the pharynx and larynx hydrated and without excessive mucus?
- Is there pharyngeal pooling?

After the anatomy and mucosal hygiene are evaluated, laryngeal movement is checked. The "ee-sniff" gesture is used to check for adduction and abduction. Symmetry of arytenoid cartilage motion, and symmetry of pharyngeal constriction are important to evaluate for pharyngeal or laryngeal paresis. Patients with vocal fold paresis may show excellent adduction and abduction but subtle abnormalities may be revealed with gestures that require rapid diadochokinesis of the vocal folds. Thus, whistle, laughter, and cough are used to evaluate the symmetry of motion of the vocal folds. Asymmetric vocal fold motion should raise the suspicion of vocal fold motion abnormality such as paresis or ankylosis.

Examination of the vocal folds during voice production will evaluate steady voice production in different pitch and loudness modes. The voice system is then stressed to look at voicing during rapid voice transitions such as singing in staccato voice, full voice, and with common singing maneuvers. Singers with classical voice training background will understand the request for a five-tone steady scale in ascending or descending pattern, singing through their passage, singing with a glide (glissando), and singing from soft to loud in a steady pitch (messa di voce). Sometimes asking the singer to sing in supported full voice and nonsupported voice will show differences in laryngeal and pharyngeal movement. Some singers will also readily produce the voice in their singing that is problematic. These gestures then may be recorded and analyzed.

Some common abnormal patterns readily identifiable by flexible laryngoscopy have been identified. Several authors have addressed the laryngeal gesture changes accompanied by excessive muscle tension dysphonia.[9,13] Hyperfunctional voice disorders may result in excessive base of tongue tension, excessive false vocal fold adduction, and anterior/posterior arytenoid squeeze.

Clinical diagnosis of vocal fold motion impairment suggestive of paresis may be made by flexible laryngosocpy.[14] Vocal fold paresis may be on the basis of superior laryngeal nerve injury,[15] recurrent laryngeal nerve injury, or combined nerve injury. Paresis differs from paralysis in that there is preserved adduction and abduction in paresis but not in paralysis. The degree of paresis may be variable and office fiberoptic laryngoscopy testing is the best way to elicit more subtle cases. The criterion for the clinical diagnosis of paresis is based on findings of asymmetry of vocal fold movement compared to the contralateral vocal fold. The asymmetry may be obvious in differences in degree of abduction and adduction during phonation or respiration[15] or it may only be elicited by systematic testing.[16] Patients with vocal paresis may show asymmetry in pharyngeal squeezing during phonation, or lag of the affected vocal fold during laryngeal movements that require rapid movement such as in a whistle or laughter. Superior laryngeal nerve paresis may be elicited as an axis shift of the larynx during a pitch glide and/or the presence of vocal fold bowing of the affected vocal fold.

Muscle tension dysphonia (MTD) comes in many forms.[17] Observation of the patient and laryngoscopic examination may show evidence of MTD.[18] Extrinsic laryngeal muscles such as the suprahyoid muscles and strap muscles will tend to elevate the larynx and squeeze the pharynx. Base of tongue tension will push the epiglottis posteriorly and retroflex the epiglottis, making the view of the vocal folds difficult due to

epiglottis hooding. Thus, the finding of an elevated larynx during pitch glides, with retroflexion of the epiglottis would suggest the presence of excessive extralaryngeal neck muscle tension. Intrinsic muscles of the larynx may also be postured in a maladaptive way. There are typical laryngeal configurations due to intrinsic muscle tension dysphonia. Some of these are: (a) prephonatory ventricular adduction and constriction with release on phonation, (b) short thick vocal folds that fail to lengthen on pitch glide, (c) isometric tension with fixed vocal folds and a large posterior chink, and (d) false vocal fold phonation. Muscle tension dysphonia patterns have not been well studied by laryngeal EMG or laryngeal kinesthetic studies but are believed to be so on the basis of muscle imbalance during phonation. Some postulated abnormal patterns are (a) thyroarytenoid muscle hyperfunction (TA predominance pattern), (b) lack of engagement of the cricothyroid muscle (cricothyroid lock), or (c) isometric muscle tension pattern (posterior chink). Additional laryngeal research is needed to separate the different patterns.

The presence of muscle tension is indicative of adaptive or maladaptive functional compensation for the production of voice. The presence of MTD does not differentiate the problem of a primary MTD pattern from that of a compensatory MTD pattern. An example of secondary MTD is patterns of muscle hyperfunction due to reflux laryngitis.[19] Primary MTD is the presence of MTD without organic disease or injury. Thus, a singer who has spent too long during practice or lessons may show evidence of MTD after a long session. Compensation by MTD may be a consequence of adaptation after injury to the vocal folds by scar, hemorrhage, inflammation, or trauma. Therefore, a patient with an intubation injury to the larynx resulting in glottal incompetence may phonate with an MTD pattern that is adaptive to a need to generate greater subglottic pressure to drive the vocal folds in vibration. A singer with chronic reflux laryngitis may sing in a maladaptive way with MTD in response to edematous inflamed vocal folds and not as a consequence of poor singing techniques. After the examiner has identified the presence of MTD, the determination of its primary cause, be it primary or compensatory MTD, is a challenge to the diagnostician.

Chronic laryngitis (laryngeal edema) is one of the causes that promote MTD. Chronic laryngitis causes a mass effect by the edema of the vocal folds that raises phonation thresholds. In addition, chronic laryngitis affects the viscoelastic properties of the mucosal layer of the vocal folds. Inflamed vocal folds have thicker mucus making each vibratory cycle more labored. Early chronic laryngitis or laryngeal edema is one of the most difficult problems to identify. While classic posterior laryngitis resulting in gross arytenoiditis, contact granuloma, and pachyderma laryngitis is easily identified, subtle edema may show only erythema of the vocal folds with excessive mucus. Mucosal health may seem abnormal due to the thickening of the posterior pharynx and the presence of dry thick mucus throughout the upper airway. Fiberoptic laryngoscopy may give some clues as to laryngeal edema and inflammation but stroboscopy and evaluation of the vocal folds in vibration will give better details.

Rigid Videostrobolaryngoscopy (VSL)

The goal of videostrobolaryngoscopy (VSL) examination in the singer is twofold.[20] The clearest indication for VSL examination of the vocal folds is for vocal fold pathology such as cysts, polyps, nodules, and inflammation. The second and sometimes as important indication is the evaluation of laryngeal phonatory gestures that accompany the sound production.[18] VSL examination will open a new world for understanding of dysphonia. Errors and pitfalls that can be avoided by such evaluation may help to detect: (a) organic lesions previously attributed to functional etiology, (b) scarring and vocal fold injury that was not recognized, (c) unilateral polyps previously mistaken as nodules and vice versa. Clinical errors such as failure to consider multiple sources for inflammation, failure to try conservative medical or voice therapy, and recommendation for speech therapy for voice disorders when there is no evidence are far too common. Accurate stroboscopy evaluation can help to avoid such errors.

Not all patients with voice disorders should have a VSL examination. Some pediatric patients cannot be examined.[21] Good candidates for examination by VSL are based on the fact that the principle of stroboscopy is based on Talbot's law, which states that there is retention of image on the retina of 200 milliseconds after exposure. This optical illusion of apparent motion from a series of images presented with rapid succession is the basis for motion films. Thus, by exposing rapid microsecond flashes of light on a quasiperiodic vibratory source such as oscillating vocal folds, the image may be frozen. When the flashes of light are synchronized just off the fundamental frequency of vibration, the vocal folds may be seen to oscillate at 1.5 to 3 times per second. This multiple image from VSL recordings of vocal folds oscillating in slow motion is made up of hundreds of glottal cycles and is a montage of glottal vibration. Thus, based on the principle of stroboscopy, the best patients chosen for VSL examination should be those with a vibratory source that is quasiperiodic. The professional voice user, the singer with subtle dysphonia noticeable as a qualitative abnormality in the voice, the veiled husky voice, the voice with intermittent abnormalities, are considered ideal candidates for VSL. Low gag reflex and phonation time of greater than 5 seconds are desirable but not mandatory. Ideally the VSL patient should have enough insight and cooperation to produce phonation tasks directed by the examiner at sustained pitch and loudness.

For practical VSL recording in the office, four parameters are typically recorded. These parameters and the approximate frequency ranges for singers are shown in Table 8–2.

A. Modal phonation at habitual pitch and loudness;
B. High-pitched phonation at habitual loudness;
C. Low-pitched phonation at habitual loudness; and
D. Loud phonation at modal-pitch frequency.

These are guidelines that are easily achievable by most patients. Although VSL does not evaluate the true vocal range in frequency and amplitude of vocal phonatory function, it does test the larynx and its function by using different subglottic pressures and laryngeal muscles. By adding specific tasks such as pitch glides and loudness variation, different modes of phonation such as chest, falsetto, and flute register can be examined during the examination.

A cooperative patient can have the simple protocol examination done in one to two minutes. The playback can be reviewed with the patient and interpretation and report generation based on oscillatory patterns of the vocal folds may be made from examination of the recorded examination.

Table 8–2. Four Parameters Typically Recorded During VSL and the Frequency of Phonation That They Typically Represent

Parameters	Females	Males
A. Modal phonation at habitual pitch and loudness	225 Hz 70–75 dB	125 Hz 70–75 dB
B. High-pitched phonation at habitual loudness	300 Hz 70–75 dB	200 Hz 70–75 dB
C. Low-pitched phonation at habitual loudness	190 Hz 70–75 dB	100 Hz 70–75 dB
D. Loud phonation at modal-pitch frequency	250 Hz 80–85 dB	140 Hz 80–85 dB

Interpreting the Stroboscopic Examination

As the VSL is viewed at regular speed and in slow motion, several features of vocal fold anatomy will be rated relative to normal vocal fold anatomy and physiology. After the VSL is reviewed, the clinician should be able to decide on the primary diagnosis of the phonatory disorder, make a functional assessment of vocal fold vibratory function, and based on these make therapeutic decisions as to treatment. Great variations can occur in the normal larynx. For example, the presence of a small posterior chink that permits air leakage in females is normal. Elias and Sataloff investigated strobovideolaryngoscopic findings in normal professional singers without voice complaints. "Abnormal" strobovideolaryngoscopic findings occur in this asymptomatic population of "volunteers" with great frequency. These abnormalities might have been misinterpreted as causing dysphonia.[22] Therefore, it is a good rule to review any prior videos or prints of the singer's larynx before a new diagnosis of nodule or edema or scar is made. A great deal of variation of normal occurs in the normal larynx and by inference in the normal singing larynx. A great deal of latitude must be taken prior to a clinical interpretation of a specific laryngeal gesture as abnormal.

If the examiner sees the frequency of phonation to be consistently too high or too low during the examination from that experienced without the scope in place, the examiner should have the patient practice the desired token by asking for the sound "Heeeee . . . " without the scope in place. Once the patient has a consistent ability to produce the sustained vowel, then the patient can be examined with the scope in place. It does little good to examine the vocal fold vibratory patterns in too soft, too loud, or too high a pitch.

Glottal configuration is the overall shape of vocal fold closure during sustained modal phonation. Vocal folds are judged at their most closed phase. The common patterns are: (a) complete, when the vocal folds are in complete contact from the front to the back, (b) posterior chink, when there is complete closure in the anterior aspect of the vocal folds but there is a gap between the vocal processes, (c) midfold gap, when there is good closure in the front and back but there is bowing in the midthird with incomplete closure in the midmembranous portion of the vocal folds, (d) anterior gap, when there is a gap anterior to the posterior two-thirds of the vocal folds, (d) hourglass or midfold contact, when there is contact only in the midmembranous portion of the vocal folds, (e) irregular, when there is irregular edge making contact, and (e) incomplete, when there is a lack of contact. Figure 8–8 is a montage of a singer with a small nodular swelling and a large posterior glottic chink.

Next to be rated is the phase of vibration. Normal glottal vibratory cycle at modal pitch and loudness will spend approximately 60% of the glottal cycle in the opening or closing phase and 40% in the closed phase. Edema, mass, and tension abnormalities will change this pattern to too much in either the too-open phase

Figure 8-8. Stroboscopic video montage of a singer with nodular diathesis and excessive phlegm. Note the long opening phase and nodular swelling of the vocal margin.

pattern or too-closed phase pattern. Both soft phonation and vocal fold nodules will result in vocal folds vibrating with a long opening and closing phase. Pressed phonation or phonation in vocal fry will result in a prolonged closed phase. The rating of normal versus abnormal phase closure should have wide latitude. The ratings are simply divided into open-phase predominates, normal, or closed-phase predominates. Open-phase predominates is when greater than two thirds of the frames of the glottal cycle are in the open position. Normal is when vocal folds are in contact with about half the glottal cycle open and half closed. Closed phase predominates is when greater than two-thirds of the frames of the glottal cycle are in the closed position.

Vibratory amplitude of the individual vocal folds is rated next. The amplitude of the lateral excursion during vibration of a vocal fold during modal phonation should be about half the thickness of the visible vocal folds. Therefore, amplitude is normal if one-half to two-thirds of each vocal fold moves aside during each glottal cycle. The extent of lateral movement is rated as normal, decreased, zero, or increased. Normal vibratory amplitude is when one-half to two-thirds of the vocal fold lateralizes during each glottal cycle. Decreased amplitude is when there is reduction in the expected lateral movement (stiff vocal folds). Zero is when there is no visible movement of the vocal fold during each glottal cycle. Increased amplitude is seen when there is a large lateral excursion with each glottal cycle (ie, in patient with presbyphonia or vocal fold paralysis).

Mucosal wave is the traveling wave which crosses from below the folds to the superior surface. The mucosal wave travels on the surface of the vocal fold and is distinctly different from the vibratory amplitude. A normal mucosal wave should be visible across the superior surface and coincides with the opening of the upper lip of the vocal folds during each glottal cycle. More than the vibratory amplitude, the smoothness of the propagation of the mucosal wave is an indication of the intact nature of the superficial layer of the lamina propria. Its presence indicates the pliability of the Reinke's layer. The mucosal wave is larger when the vocal folds are shorter and are driven with large subglottic pressure. The mucosal wave is also larger in males than females. Mucosal wave is less distinct at higher pitch and soft phonation. Therefore, great care must be given to obtain consistent pitch and loudness recordings when one recording is to be compared to another. When there is scar or inflammation, the mucosal wave will usually become affected either locally at the site of scar or globally when there is diffuse inflammation or edema. The mucosal wave is rated as normal, absent, or reduced. Absent mucosal wave is a lack of visible traveling wave across a part or whole area of the vocal fold. Reduced mucosal wave is wave limited to the medial edge. Although reduced mucosal wave is usually associated with reduced amplitude, the mucosal wave abnormalities occur earlier and may be disturbed without an amplitude abnormality.

Asymmetry of vocal fold vibration is one of the easier pickups as the abnormal vocal folds will vibrate with a lack of symmetry compared to the normal side. Asymmetry of vocal vibration can be compared to the opposite side for abnormal edge, closure, vibratory amplitude, or mucosal wave.

Vocal folds should vibrate in phase relative to each other. When they fail to oscillate in phase, these phase differences contribute to dysphonia. Normal is when both vocal folds open and close together. Out-of-phase vibration is when one vocal fold is in the open phase while the other is in the closing or closed phase. Phase shifts can occur in the lateral/medial plane, resulting in a snake dance side-to-side undulation. Phase shift may occur in an anterior-to-posterior direction as the vocal folds peel open from the back to the front or the front to the back.

Because there are many possible variations in vocal fold oscillation, some seemingly abnormal vibratory patterns are actual normal variations. In the singer, it is especially important to recognize these normal variations lest they be a cause of undue anxiety.

The posterior glottal chink is a normal variation in many males and females. The female singer and speaker have a higher incidence of a small posterior chink. The chink is small and usually posterior to the vocal process. A small gap between the vocal processes may also be present. There is, however, rarely any extension of the posterior gap anterior to the vocal process and any gap that is present into the membranous vocal folds that is more than 25% of the length of the vocal folds should be considered abnormal. Such finding is indicative of muscle tension dysphonia, early vocal nodules, or other pathologic conditions.

Vocal swelling at the site of maximum vocal fold contact is a common finding. Nodular swelling at the midmembranous vocal folds may be present in many female singers and has been observed even in male singers. It may be present without vocal complaints. The pattern of vibration is unaffected despite the presence of soft vocal fold nodules. These findings should be labeled as soft vocal fold nodules without pathologic consequence or judgment.

Phlegm and mucous coating on the vocal folds can vary greatly. It depends on the hydration status of the patient, whether the patient has undergone vocal warm-up before the examination, the time of day, and when the last performance was finished. There should be great leeway in avoiding a diagnosis of reflux due to the presence of phlegm alone.

COMMON PATHOLOGIC CONDITIONS AND THEIR MANAGEMENT IN SINGERS

We now discuss some common findings in singers and their management.

Laryngitis

The red larynx and traumatic laryngitis are one of the most common findings in singers after loud or prolonged singing. The etiology may be due to quality or quantity of singing. After prolonged loud reading of a single passage, no significant changes were noted in trained singers but there were differences in vibratory amplitude noted in untrained speakers.[23] Prolonged voice use results are difficult to quantify but clinically they have a typical history and physical finding. The voice is characterized by early vocal fatigue. The singer has to push harder to make the desired sound. Singing in high and especially soft phonation becomes difficult and may be broken by unexpected breaks. Examination can suggest the presence of vocal fold swelling by asking the singer to sing in legato voice through the passage. Another way to test the voice is to ask the singer to glide the voice from low to high voice (glissando). During the singing passage, the examiner listens for unexpected breathiness before the sound is produced or hoarse, rough quality at the soft notes that can only be compensated by a hard glottal attack (coup de glotte). Stroboscopic examination will often show symmetrically swollen vocal folds that have either a large posterior chink or an hourglass appearance. The vocal folds during phonation may not thin out as the frequency of vibration is increased, resulting in short thick vocal folds. Vibratory examination will show a prolonged open or closed phase during the glottal cycle (hypo- vs hyperfunction). The vocal folds will have reduced vibratory amplitude with a mucosal wave that is difficult to see. Sluggishness of the mucosal wave is typical. The surface of the vocal folds may have a paucity of thin mucus with pale whitish phlegm at the nodal point.[24]

Treatment for traumatic laryngitis is vocal rest and voice re-education with a view toward injury prevention. If the situation is temporary, a brief course of steroid may be useful to allow the singer to sing through the disability. Hydration and use of mucolytics will make the viscoelastic properties of the vocal folds favorable to oscillation at a lower phonation threshold and may be enough to tide the singer through the singing engagement.

Dehydration and Lubrication

Dehydration and lubrication problems are such common issues in the singer that they warrant mention as a separate problem. Sympathetic discharge before a performance, poor hydration, and self-medication with agents that are drying are some of the common reasons singers may sing with a dry throat. Singing with a dry throat may sound like acute laryngitis or edema but it has different stroboscopic findings. Dry vocal folds differ from red vocal folds in the lack of capillary dilation. The surface of the vocal folds of dehydration and laryngitis sicca will often be uneven with a "salt and pepper" appearance due to air drying. The mucus is often thick and the vocal folds will stick together during the opening phase of vocal fold vibration. The condition is readily managed by bland nebulization of saline or water. A hydroscopic agent added to the bland nebulization such as 5% glycerine will help to wet the vocal folds and allow them to vibrate with greater ease.

Chronically dry throat due to steroid inhalers, medication negative side effects, and Sjögren's syndrome may cause a low-grade mucositis, which mimics laryngitis sicca. Laryngitis sicca results in keratinization of the vocal fold margin, thickening of the vocal fold edge with stiffness, and a mass effect of the vocal folds. The interarytenoid area is often thickened, resulting in pachyderma laryngis. The condition is difficult to differentiate from reflux laryngitis except in the diffuseness of the involvement of the larynx. Treatment of chronic laryngitis sicca depends on a careful search for medical causes of dry throat and review of past and present medications.

Reflux Laryngitis

Reflux laryngitis is common and may present with hoarseness, chronic throat clearing, excessive phlegm, or pain with singing as described in chapter 11. If left untreated, reflux laryngitis may progress to loss in vocal range, permanent voice changes, and development of mucosal abnormalities. Scar and vocal fold damage due to submucosal fibrosis may promote fibrovascular lesions that go on to scar and sulcus formation. Acute and chronic reflux laryngitis may be serving as inflammatory cofactors that act in concert with vocal overuse and abuse to produce unwanted lesions of the vocal folds.

The stroboscopic appearance of reflux laryngitis is characterized by sluggish swollen vocal folds with reduced fundamental frequency. Vocal fold edge may be irregular but is uniformly edematous or erythematous. Figure 8-9 is an example of chronic laryngitis associated with vocal abuse resulting in an ulcerated vocal fold edge. Vocal folds vibrating with open phase

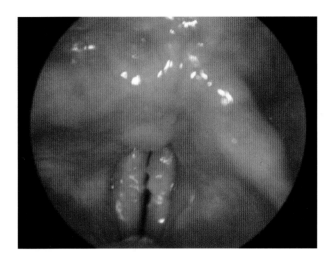

Figure 8-9. Reflux laryngitis.

predominating, and reduced mucosal wave and amplitude are other findings. There is frequently mucus collection swirling on the surface of the vocal folds. Treatment is by aggressive management of nutrition and careful mucosal hygiene. Empirical treatment by acid suppression by use of proton pump inhibition (PPI) is indicated.

Pathologic findings in singers beyond acute and chronic inflammation lie largely in the finding of benign mucosal lesions. These include varix, vocal fold nodules, pseudocysts, polyps, and cysts. Rarer problems may include sulcus vocalis, scar, and mucosal bridges. Careful differentiations between the lesions are necessary to allow the clinician to proceed with the most effective treatment. Keratosis and epithelial changes are usually of prolonged duration and are more of interest when they do not resolve as they may have implications for atypia or neoplasia.

Vocal Fold Nodules

Vocal fold nodules are the most feared lesions in singers. Nodules are difficult to diagnose accurately without stroboscopy. Nodules are symmetric swellings of the vocal fold at the margin of the membranous vocal fold experiencing maximal phonotrauma.[25] Fear of loss of the voice, income, and of permanent disability cloud the ability of the singer to judge rationally the implication of the diagnosis of nodules. This fear is not

to be trivialized. Thus, the use of the term nodules is frequently avoided.

Stroboscopic examination can differentiate between the various diagnoses that can simulate nodules. In the differential diagnosis, the following should be considered: fusiform polyps, laryngeal medina, pseudocyst, laryngeal papilloma. Some of the lesions mistaken for nodules are easily differentiated by the stroboscopy. A good VSL will readily differentiate symmetric lesions such as vocal nodules from asymmetric lesions such as laryngeal polyps. Furthermore, laryngeal nodules can be differentiated as to their stiffness. This is valuable for prognosis. Stiff vocal nodule versus soft vocal nodule can mean the difference between taking a day off versus prolonged voice rehabilitation. Cysts and pseudocysts will show abnormality on one side compared to the other. Figure 8-10 is an intraoperative photograph of a vocal fold mucous cyst. Figure 8-11 is an endoscopic photograph of a pseudocyst. Both are in singers. The pseudocyst does not have a capsule and is truly a fusiform polyp. The side with the cyst will appear to be larger and more massive. The reduction in mucosal wave will also be apparent. Vocal nodules will have a vocal fold configuration simulating an hourglass

Figure 8-10. Vocal fold cyst, mucous type.

Figure 8–11. Pseudocyst or fusiform polyp on a singing teacher.

Figure 8–12. Keratosis of the vocal fold edge in a patient with mature vocal nodules.

appearance. There will be midfold contact. The contact area may be keratotic or thickened. In some patients the thick keratotic edge may not soften and surgery may be needed despite their cause from phonotrauma has been moderated. Figure 8–12 is such an example of keratosis going on to surgery due to stiffness noted on stroboscopy. The mode of vibration will show a predominantly open-phase vibration. There may be a posterior chink. In early vocal nodules, the mucosal wave will be slightly diminished but the vibratory amplitude will be good. Testing the voice at different pitch and loudness combinations will show relative stiffness as the voice is put under more strain with increasing amplitude and subglottic pressure.

The importance to diagnostically differentiate cysts, pseudocysts, and polyps from nodules is in their subsequent treatment.[26] Surgical treatment is rarely indicated in the patient with vocal nodules. Vocal nodules require vocal retraining and a consultation with a qualified speech-language pathologist (voice therapist). Pseudocyst, polyps, and vascular lesions should be treated differently. Although these asymmetric lesions are often responsive to therapy such as steroid treatment, they do not uniformly respond to voice therapy. Surgical management of these benign mucosal lesions should be considered.

Pseudocysts

Pseudocysts differ from vocal polyps in the following way: pseudocyst is an excess of mucosa due to the shearing force from a harsh phonation. Polyps, on the other hand, come from submucosal hemorrhage leaking into the submucosa or lamina propria. The site of pathology in vocal polyps and pseudocyst also differ. Vocal nodules are primarily a dysfunction of the epithelium and the basement membrane. Pseudocyst is caused by redundancy of the squamous epithelium. Laryngeal polyps are due to an increase in the protein layer in the superficial layer of the lamina propria. Mass effect on the affected vocal fold will result in the heavier vocal fold vibrating asynchronously from the thinner, more pliable vocal fold.

Pseudocysts are more common in female singers. More often, this is an affliction of females undergoing classical singing training. It appears to affect singers with a higher tessitura. The onset of this condition is usually quite distinct. Sometimes, it is preceded by laryngitis or a cold. Occasionally, it is a combination of heavy singing surrounding a brief period of illness. After the illness is gone, the loss in the voice persists and does not completely resolve. The voice quality is often described as veiled with airiness to it. If the patient has had a prior examination, the patient often has been diagnosed to have laryngitis. Only videostroboscopy will show evidence of asymmetry and redundancy of mucosal membrane.

Vascular Ectasias

Vascular ectasia and varixes can form on the vocal fold margin. Their etiology is obscure but may be related to microtrauma as they form usually at the striking zone of the vocal fold margin.[27] The vessels may be on the superior or the inferior surface of the vocal fold margin. They cause difficulties by swelling during prolonged phonotrauma and may swell excessively during menses. The presence of dilated vessels on the superior surface of the vocal fold should prompt the examiner to seek additional vessels on the under-surface of the vocal folds. The undersurface of the vocal folds can best be examined by asking the singer to sustain a loud chest voice. This will maximize the phase difference between the upper and the lower lip of the vocal folds during stroboscopic examination. This gesture will allow the examiner to visualize the under-surface of the vocal folds, an area that is otherwise difficult to evaluate except under general anesthesia. Occasionally, small vessels will show a blush or frank vocal hemorrhage. Such an early vocal hemorrhage in a singer is shown on Figure 8–13.

Vocal Polyps

A vocal polyp is the most common type of lesion seen in males. It is a result of the vocal fold injury and may be related to a mucosal vessel hemorrhage. An evidence of a vascular ectasia may precede laryngeal polyps. Laryngeal polyps cause asymmetric vibratory patterns by reduction of amplitude and mucosal wave. Sometimes vocal cord polyps have a mass effect while at other times they may have a stiffness effect on the affected vocal fold. The vocal fold may lag behind the more pliable vocal fold. The mass effect from the polyp may result in a rocking motion on VSL that has its own frequency. Pedunculated vocal fold polyps are usually treated by surgery. An example is shown in Figure 8–14.

Figure 8–13. Early vocal fold hemorrhage with vascular blush on the left vocal fold.

Figure 8–14. Pedunculated vocal fold polyp, intraoperative view.

Vocal Fold Cysts

Vocal fold cysts may be of keratin or mucinous type. The keratin cysts are white with usually a visible feeding vessel. The mucinous type may arise on the under-surface of the vocal fold and may mimic a nodule or a vocal polyp. The mucinous cysts are yellow to brown in color and when small can be difficult to identify by constant light endoscopy. Stroboscopy is able to identify the lesion easily as the side with the intracordal mass will oscillate with markedly reduced vibratory amplitude and mucosal wave. The vocal fold may have a visible mass within the vocal fold. Such a mass may resemble an "egg" lying within the vocal fold.

Fibrovascular deposit lesions may resemble a cyst of the vocal fold. Yet they differ from cysts in that histologically there is mass, fibrin, fibrosis, and hyaline protein but there is no cell wall to suggest a true cyst.

Sulcus Vocalis

Sulcus vocalis and mucosal bridge are difficult to identify by office endoscopy or by stroboscopy. Sometimes the sulcus is readily visible as a vocal fold duplication or striae on the edge of the vocal fold. More often, a sulcus will present with a spindle-shaped glottic closure with markedly reduced vibratory amplitude and wave on the side of the sulcus. Asymmetric loss with loss of amplitude and wave on the side of sulcus in a patient without mass or edge abnormalities should make the examiner suspicious of a sulcus condition. In these patients, recording the voice in an aspirated voice may exaggerate the sulcus and show the lesion. If the sulcus cannot be identified by office endoscopy, surgical exploration may be necessary.

Some changes seen on stroboscopy are consistently found in patients with dysphonia associated with organic tissue change. These findings are: asymmetric amplitude, decreased amplitude, short closed phase, prolonged open phase, and failure of mucosal wave propagation on the side of pathology. With successive medical, rehabilitative treatment, improved vibration will result in improved vocal fold edge, better vocal contact, greater vibratory amplitude and mucosal wave. Less important findings that correlate to an improved voice are the degree of ventricular adduction and the perceived effort necessary for sustained phonation.

SUMMARY

Singers have special needs that bring them to the physician. Although not all problems before a performance are related to vocal fold dysfunction, otolaryngologists will nevertheless be called on to perform an examination and counsel the patient. A standardized examination protocol with some rudimentary knowledge of the singing process will go a long way toward establishing communication and efficacy in the management of this group of patients.

REFERENCES

1. Sataloff RT. Professional singers: the science and art of clinical care. *Am J Otolaryngol.* 1981;2(3):251-266.
2. Punt NA. Vocal disabilities of singers. Applied laryngology—singers and actors. *Proc R Soc Med.* 1968;61(11 part 1):1152-1155.
3. Mishra S, Rosen CA, Murry T. 24 hours prior to curtain. *J Voice.* 2000;14(1):92-98.
4. Mishra S, Rosen CA, Murry T. Acute management of the performing voice. *Otolaryngol Clin North Am.* 2000;33(5):957-966.
5. Davis CB, Davis ML. The effects of premenstrual syndrome (PMS) on the female singer. *J Voice.* 1993;7(4):337-353.
6. Westerman Gregg J. The singing/acting mature adult—singing instruction perspective. *J Voice.* 1997;11(2):165-170.
7. Boltezar IH, Burger ZR, Zargi M. Instability of voice in adolescence: pathologic condition or normal developmental variation? *J Pediatr.* 1997;30(2):185-190.
8. Woo P, Casper J, Colton R, Brewer, DI. Dysphonia in the aging: physiology versus disease. *Laryngoscope.* 1992;102(2):139-144.
9. Koufman JA, Radomski TA, Joharji GM, Russell GB, Pillsbury DC. Laryngeal biomechanics of the singing voice. *Otolaryngol Head Neck Surg.* 1996;115(6):527-537.
10. Morrison MD, Rammage LA. Muscle misuse voice disorders: description and classification. *Acta Otolaryngol Stockh.* 1993;113(3):428-434.
11. Morrison M. Pattern recognition in muscle misuse voice disorders: how I do it. *J Voice.* 1997;11(1):108-114.
12. Yanagisawa E, Estill J, Mambrino L, Talkin D. Supraglottic contributions to pitch raising. Videoendoscopic study with spectroanalysis. *Ann Otol Rhinol Laryngol.* 1991;100(1):19-30.
13. Morrison MD, Nichol H, Rammage LA. Diagnostic criteria in functional dysphonia. *Laryngoscope.* 1986;96(1):1-8.

14. Ellis SF, Pollack AC, Hanson DG, Jiang JJ. Video-laryngoscopic evaluation of laryngeal intubation injury: incidence and predictive factors. *Otolaryngol Head Neck Surg.* 1996;114(6):729–731.

15. Dursun G, Sataloff RT, Spiegel JR, et al. Superior laryngeal nerve paresis and paralysis. *J Voice.* 1996; 10(2):206–211.

16. Fleischer S, Schade G, Hess MM. Office-based laryngoscopic observations of recurrent laryngeal nerve paresis and paralysis. *Ann Otol Rhinol Laryngol.* 2005;114(6):488–493.

17. Belafsky PC, Postma GN, Reulbach TR, Holland BW, Koufman JA. Muscle tension dysphonia as a sign of underlying glottal insufficiency. *Otolaryngol Head Neck Surg.* 2002;127(5):448–451.

18. Behrman A. Common practices of voice therapists in the evaluation of patients. *J Voice.* 2005;19(3): 454–469.

19. Koufman JA, Amin MR, Panetti M. Prevalence of reflux in 113 consecutive patients with laryngeal and voice disorders. *Otolaryngol Head Neck Surg.* 2000;123(4):385–388.

20. Alberti PW. The diagnostic role of laryngeal stroboscopy. *Otolaryngol Clin North Am,* 1978;11(2): 347–354.

21. Hartnick CJ, Zeitels SM. Pediatric video laryngostroboscopy. *Int J Pediatr Otorhinolaryngol.* 2005; 69(2):215–219.

22. Elias ME, Sataloff RT, Rosen DC, Heuer RJ, Spiegel JR. Normal strobovideolaryngoscopy: variability in healthy singers. *J Voice.* 1997;11(1):104–107.

23. Gelfer MP, Andrews ML, Schmidt CP. Documenting laryngeal change following prolonged loud reading. A videostroboscopic study. *J Voice.* 1996;10(4): 368–377.

24. Mann EA, McClean MD, Gurevich-Uvena J, et al. The effects of excessive vocalization on acoustic and videostroboscopic measures of vocal fold condition. *J Voice.* 1999;13(2):294–302.

25. Lancer JM, Fisch U. Vocal cord nodules: a review. *Clin Otolaryngol.* 1988;13(1):43–51.

26. Milutinovic Z., Bojic P. Functional trauma of the vocal folds: classification and management strategies. *Folia Phoniatr Logop.* 1996;48(2):78–85.

27. Hochman I, Zeitels SM, Heaton JT. Ectasias and varices of the vocal fold: clearing the striking zone. *Ann Otol Rhinol Laryngol.*1999;108(1):10–16.

Chapter 9

AERODYNAMIC AND ACOUSTIC VOICE MEASUREMENTS

Philippe H. DeJonckere

Within the framework of voice education or training in singing, documentation provided by the acoustic and aerodynamic measures can be used by the singer as biofeedback to get a better control on voice production, to make relevant comparisons, or to monitor changes over time.[1]

In the case of singing voice disorders, acoustic and aerodynamic measurements provide a functional diagnosis and offer information concerning the characteristics, limitations, and possibilities for change of voice production. The main advantage of both approaches is noninvasiveness. If the singer has voice complaints or problems, acoustic and aerodynamic analysis make the dialogue between clinician and patient (singer) less abstract and more reality based. The clinician's and the singer's expectation is that the voice laboratory provides objective documentation of the condition of the voice. This concept of objective documentation is of major importance, although objective data sometimes may be interpreted subjectively. In addition, limitations remain with regard to standardization of procedures and normative values among laboratories.

Nevertheless, acoustics and psychoacoustics remain two distinct worlds. In case of vibrato for instance, it has been shown that perception of the singer's vibrato does not always agree with acoustic measurements.[2]

AERODYNAMICS

Aerodynamic analysis of voice production includes measurement of airflow, air pressure, and their relationships during phonation. Furthermore, a number of derived measurements can provide information regarding vocal efficiency.

Phonation Airflow

The simplest aerodynamic parameter of voicing is the maximum phonation time (MPT) in seconds. It consists of the prolongation of /a:/ for as long as possible after maximal inspiration and at spontaneous, comfortable pitch and loudness. It is one of the most widely used clinical measures in voice assessment, worldwide.[3] A prior demonstration is necessary, and three trials are required, the longest being selected for comparison to norm.[4] It has been shown to be very sensitive to learning and fatigue effects. Furthermore, in good voices, the duration of apnea, rather than the available air, can become the limiting factor. Children show significant lower values of MPT, as their lung volume is smaller.[5] A reduction of possible bias—for example, supportive respiratory capabilities compensating for poor membranous vocal fold closure—is possible by computing the ratio:

Averaged phonation airflow or

Phonation Quotient (PQ) = Vital Capacity (ml) / MPT (s).

Vital capacity (VC) is defined as "the volume change at the mouth between the position of full inspiration and complete expiration." It can be measured in a reliable way by using a hand-held spirometer.[6] VC depends, in normal subjects, on anthropometric factors, and is quite strongly correlated with height.[7] It is also sensitive to lung disease, especially for patients with carcinoma. As VC is not directly related to voice quality, it is meaningful to take it in account, certainly if children are investigated.

The mean airflow rate can also be measured by using a pneumotachograph. This device provides a direct measurement of the mean airflow rate (ml/s) for sustained phonation over a comfortable duration, usually 2 to 3 seconds, at the habitual pitch and loudness level, and following habitual inspiration. A pneumotachograph consists of a hand-held mouth tube (possibly connected to a mask) within which is placed a fine-mesh wire screen in order to create a (small) resistance to airflow. This resistance results in a pressure difference across the screen that can be measured with a differential pressure transducer; the pressure difference increases with the flow. Pathophysiologic backgrounds and normative values have been reported by Hirano,[3,8] Verdolini,[9] Colton and Casper,[10] and Woo et al. [11,12]

The variation of averaged phonation airflow varies considerably among normal subjects and there is a large overlapping range of values in normal and dysphonic subjects. This limits the value for diagnostic purposes.[13] Nevertheless, when comparing glottal function before and after surgical intervention or non-surgical voice training techniques, airflow measurement may be useful in monitoring therapeutic effects,[14] such as in cases of paralytic dysphonia[15,16,17] or when microlaryngeal phonosurgery is performed.[12] The method is especially useful for demonstrating changes in a single test subject over time.

For comparisons (pre- and post-treatment), it is recommended to use the same kind of technique (PQ or mean airflow rate measured by pneumotachography).

Example of Specific Application in Singers

In healthy students in singing, measures of flow rate and MPT demonstrated significant improvement after regularly practiced isometric-isotonic vocal function exercises for 4 weeks. This suggests an increase in glottal efficiency.[18]

Flow Glottography

Flow glottography (FLOG) consists of an inverse filtering of the oral airflow waveform. The basic tool is a high-frequency pressure transducer incorporated within an airtight Rothenberg mask.[19] The inverse filtering procedure removes the resonant effects of the vocal tract and produces an estimate of the waveform produced at the vocal folds. The special advantage of this technique is that it differentiates and, after calibration, quantifies the leakage airflow (the DC component of the airflow) and the pulsated (AC) airflow. Leakage airflow is an important concept: it assumes that there is an opening somewhere along the total length of the vocal folds through which air escapes. Calibration is critical for reliable measurements. Flow glottography can also be used to analyze the voice onset (Figure 9–1). Glottal airflow waveforms can be used for computing open, closing, and speed quotients, which are related to sound pressure level of the voice.[20] Such quotients demonstrate significant differences between normal subjects with and without vocal training.[21]

Example of Specific Application in Singers

Sundberg et al showed that the perceived phonatory pressed voice quality in the singing voice could largely be accounted for by variations in the normalized amplitude quotient (NAQ) of the flow glottogram: that is, the ratio between the peak-to-peak amplitude of the flow pulse and the negative peak amplitude of the differentiated flow glottogram and normalized with respect to period time.[22] This NAQ has been shown to be related to glottal adduction, which in turn affects mode of phonation and, hence, perceived phonatory pressed quality.

A. Soft onset

Time (sec)

Figure 9-1. Investigation of voice onset type by means of flow glottography (FLOG) with the Rothenberg mask. **A.** Physiologic, soft onset with transglottal airflow before the oscillation of vocal folds starts. **B.** Hard attack where vibration starts with a closed glottis. One vertical division corresponds to 100 ml.

B. Hard onset

Time (sec)

Subglottal Air Pressure

Measurements of subglottal air pressure made using esophageal balloons or pressure transducers, transglottal catheters, or by tracheal puncture are semi-invasive or invasive and limited to research situations. An accurate estimation of subglottal pressure can be obtained by measuring the intraoral air pressure produced during the repeated pronunciation of /pVp/ syllables (ie, a vowel between two plosive consonants). A thin catheter is introduced in the mouth through the labial commissure, sealed by the lips, and not occluded by the tongue. If there is no closure of the vocal folds, the intraoral air pressure should be similar to the pressure elsewhere in the respiratory tract. During the production of a voiceless consonant, the vocal folds are abducted and should not impose any significant obstruction to the airflow from the lungs. Thus, the pressure behind the lips is the same everywhere and reflects the pressure available to drive the vocal folds if they were to vibrate.[23,24] Pressure is usually reported in pascal units: 1 Pa is equal to 1 newton/m^2. 1 kPa is 10 cm of H_2O. This technique also allows measurement of the phonation threshold pressure (PTP), the minimum pressure required to initiate phonation.[25,26] Jiang et al used an airtight mask over the mouth and nose, with interruptions of the airflow.[26] PTP is related to sound pressure level: In normal subjects, the measured mean PTP is 2.38 ($\pm$ 1.27 = standard deviation) cm H_2O at 75 dB, 2.67 ($\pm$ 1.88) cm H_2O at 80 dB, and 2.98 ($\pm$ 2.23) cm H_2O at 85 dB. In case of pathology these values are significantly higher.

Efficiency of Phonation

Together with airflow and vocal intensity, subglottal air pressure can be used to estimate the efficiency of phonation. Obviously, reduced efficiency is expected to induce voice fatigue. Vocal efficiency is defined as the ratio of the acoustic power to the aerodynamic power and can be estimated by dividing the acoustic intensity of the utterance by the product of the air pressure and the airflow used to produce the utterance.[27]

ACOUSTICS

As with aerodynamic measures, acoustic measures reflect the status of vocal function and do not relate specifically to various voice disorders because basic biomechanical changes resulting in acoustic features can be induced by various types of lesions or dysfunctions.

Acoustic measures provide an objective and non-invasive method to obtain information about vocal function. Increasingly, these measures have become available at affordable cost, and appear to accurately monitor changes in voice quality across time especially before, during, and after treatment.

Visible Speech

Acoustic analysis can be used to make the voice and speech visible, in "spectrograms"[24] also sometimes called "sonagrams" (Figure 9-2). This visual representation may be a considerable aid to the perception and description of the voice characteristics.

Spectrograms are also useful for comparing normal phonation with phonation characterized by excessive noise. Commercially available software packages provide synchronized displays of the microphone signal and the spectrogram, showing the frequency distribution of acoustical energy over time. A choice can be made between narrowband filtering (frequency resolution, mainly demonstrating fundamental frequency, harmonics, interharmonic and high-frequency noise, subharmonics) and broadband filtering (temporal resolution, mainly demonstrating periodicity, but also formant location). Voice characteristics such as sound pressure level, fundamental frequency, and formant central frequency can also be displayed over time for analysis of singing voice. Modern technology allows a display of the spectrogram practically in real time; this type of feedback can be extremely useful in singing pedagogy.

Spectrograms, particularly when focused on higher harmonics, are very well fitted for demonstrating vibrato characteristics, as rate, extent, and regularity. Vibrato has been found to be one of the two most consistent acoustical differences between professionally trained and untrained voices, respectively.[28] Vibrato samples perceptually judged as good are the most periodic ones (Figure 9-3A and 9-3B).[29]

Power Spectrum

The power spectrum is a visualization of a fast Fourier transform (FFT) analysis. It shows the distribution of the acoustic energy, fundamental frequency, harmonics and harmonic emergence, and formants. The singer's formant—a strong spectral peak near 2.8 kHz—is typical for classic Western operatic style of singing. It results

Figure 9–2. Visible speech (or spectrogram, or sonagram), as displayed by the Computerized Speech Lab (Kay Elemetrics Corp., Lincoln Park, NJ). (*Top*) Microphone signal and spectrogram with frequency display (0–4000 Hz) over time (about 0.8 s; narrow band with frequency resolution). (*Bottom*) Microphone signal and spectrogram with frequency display (0–4000 Hz) over time (about 0.6s;broadband filtering with time resolution). This display provides qualitative information about noise components, regularity of glottal pulses, F_0-shifts, subharmonics, voice onsets, formant location, and formant shifts.

A.

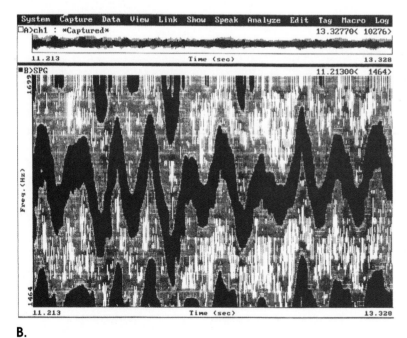

B.

Figure 9–3. A. Selected portion of a spectrogram (frequency range: 1523 to 1757 Hz) showing a rather regular pulsation of the higher harmonic, corresponding to a vibrato perceptually rated as esthetic. **B.** Another portion of the same spectrogram (frequency range here is 1464 to 1699 Hz), showing an irregular pulsation of the higher harmonic, corresponding to a vibrato perceptually rated as inesthetic.

from a "fusion" of the third, fourth, and fifth formants, and provides extra power (necessary when singing with an orchestra) as well as a specific color to the timbre ("ring of the voice").[30,31] Country singing is not characterized by a singer's formant.[32] The most consistent acoustical difference between professionally trained and untrained voices is the presence or absence—besides vibrato—of the singer's formant in the singers versus the nonsingers, respectively (Figure 9–4).[28]

Omori et al proposed an easy computation derived from the power spectrum of a sung /a:/ and based on the concept of singer's formant for objec-

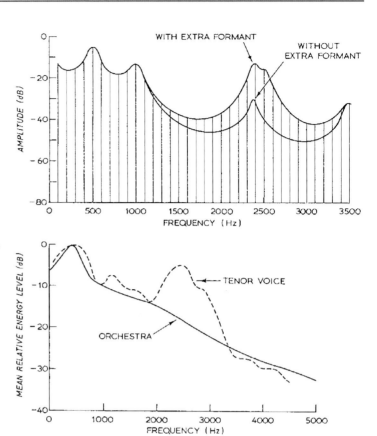

Figure 9-4. Top: Schematic power spectrum of a normal voice with and without singing formant. **Bottom**: Long-term average spectra for the sound of a symphony orchestra with and without a singer soloist (*solid and dashed curves*). The "singer's formant" constitutes the major difference between the orchestra with and without the singer soloist.[37]

tively evaluating singing voice quality.[33] The "singing power ratio" (SPR) is defined as the ratio of the greatest harmonics peak between 2 and 4 kHz and the greatest harmonics peak between 0 and 2 kHz (Figure 9-5). The SPR of a sung /a:/ was found to be significantly greater in singers than in nonsingers, and in singers, the SPR of a sung /a:/ was significantly greater than that of a spoken /a:/. Furthermore the SPR had a significant relationship with the perceptual scores of "ringing" quality of the voice. Power spectra can be averaged over a long time (long-time average spectra: LTAS), such as that shown in Figure 9-4, bottom.

Acoustic Parameters

Acoustic analysis can also provide precise numerical values for many voice parameters, from averaged fundamental frequency to sophisticated calculations for noise components or tremor features.

Factor analysis allows the large number of acoustical parameters to be reduced to a limited number of clusters[34]:

1. Short-term fundamental frequency perturbation
2. Short- or medium-term amplitude perturbation and voiceless segments
3. Harmonics-to-noise ratio
4. Long-term frequency and amplitude modulation
5. Very long-term amplitude variation
6. Subharmonics
7. Tremor

Perturbation measures (in period and amplitude) as well as the harmonics-to-noise computations on a sustained vowel (/a:/) at comfortable frequency and intensity, appear as the most robust measures and seem to determine the basic perceptual elements of voice quality: grade, roughness, and breathiness. Nevertheless, correlations with perceptual data remain usually moderate.[35,36] Jitter is computed as the mean difference

A.

B.

Figure 9–5. A. Power spectrum 0–4 KHz. Normal male voice, sustained sung /a:/, without vibrato. The vertical arrow indicates the strongest harmonic between 0 and 2 kHz, for computing the Singing Power Ratio. **B.** Power spectrum 0–4 kHz. Normal male voice, sustained sung /a:/, without vibrato. The vertical arrow indicates the strongest harmonic between 2 and 4 kHz, for computing the Singing Power Ratio.

between the periods of adjacent cycles divided by the mean period. It is thus an F_0 (fundamental frequency)-related measurement. For shimmer, a similar computation is made on peak-to-peak amplitudes. Voice breaks must always be excluded. For pathologic voices, the coefficients of variation of jitter and shimmer measurements on a sustained /a/ are in the order of 20 to 30%

for successive single trials as well as trials on different days.[37] A general limitation is that the system employed for acoustic analysis cannot (or not in a reliable way) analyze strongly aperiodic acoustic signals: this is related to the criteria for identifying individual periods. Perturbation measures less than about 5% have been found to be reliable.[38] Only "quasiperiodic" voices are suited for perturbation analysis. Therefore, a visual control of the period definition on the microphone signal is always necessary. Even in regular voices, a strong harmonic or subharmonic may account for erratic values. Alternatives from the field of nonlinear dynamics, as the coefficient of Lyapunov, have been proposed for analyzing "chaotic" or "bifurcated" signals.[39]

For signal-to-noise ratio computations (NNE: normalized noise energy, HNR: harmonics to noise ratio, cepstrum peak, etc), there is currently insufficient standardization of the optimal algorithm(s), as well as insufficient knowledge about normative values, for widely spread clinical use. Harmonics-to-noise ratio was also found to be a less suited parameter for demonstrating the effects of voice therapy.[40]

Examples of Specific Application in Singers

Aperiodicity is significantly lower on a sustained /a:/, at all SPL-levels, in children with trained singing voices than in normal controls (Figure 9–6).[41]

Vocal warm-up was found to significantly reduce frequency perturbation and amplitude perturbation values and to significantly improve the noise-to-harmonics ratio. It also increases the singer's formant amplitude.[42]

Phonetography/Voice Range Profile

The phonetogram plots the dynamic range (dBA) as a function of fundamental frequency range (Hz), documenting the extreme possibilities of voice, which is relevant for voice classification. These extremes of the dynamic range are important for professional voice users, especially singers,[43] but they must be interpreted with care[44] because the acoustic energy is related to spectral distribution. Normative values for children and teachers have been defined by Heylen.[45] From a methodologic point of view, as the boundaries of the phonetogram represent "extreme" performances, they are, as well as MPT and CV, very sensitive to learning and fatigue effects. Computerized systems make possible real-time measurement and display of fundamental frequency versus SPL and also of quality parameters such as jitter. Jitter results in various color gradations within the voice area, showing specific altered zones, or register boundaries (Figure 9–7). Such computerized systems can also provide range profiles of current speech, possibly coupled with provocation tests, such as the task of reading at a controlled, louder intensity. These profiles are expected to be relevant for occupational voice users.

The highest and lowest frequencies and the softest intensity (dBA at 30 cm) seem most sensitive for changes in voice quality[46–49]: the latter being related to phonation threshold pressure.[25,44]

Example of Specific Application in Singers

The voice range profile has been used to demonstrate significant positive effects of vocal training on the singing voice in students.[50]

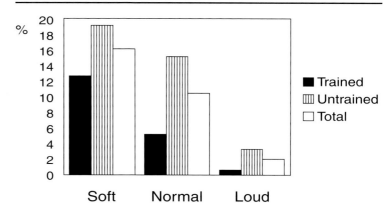

Figure 9–6. Irregularity of F_0, as measured on a sustained /a:/, as a function of intensity of voicing. Average values of 38 children trained in singing (high level choir) and 43 normal, untrained children. Irregularity means the percentage of frequency pairs (adjacent cycles) with a cycle-to-cycle F_0-variation which is larger than 10.96% of the mean F_0 value. Aperiodicity clearly decreases when intensity increases.

Figure 9–7. Computerized phonetogram (voice range profile), with a gray scale indicating the amount of jitter (normal female voice). The more jitter, the darker the area. Horizontal axis: fundamental frequency in Hz (or musical tones on a keyboard). Vertical axis: Sound pressure level, measured at 30 cm (dBA). This plot combines information about extreme possibilities of voice as well as an aspect of voice quality.

Rhinophonia Measurement

Rhinophonia is an abnormality of voice resonance in the nasal cavity. It can appear as an isolated problem or in combination with an articulatory disorder (rhinolalia). Hyperrhinophonia means that vowels and voiced consonants are excessively resonated in the nasal cavity. This excessive resonance occurs when the velopharyngeal port remains open during production of phonemes other than the nasal consonants. The increase in nasal resonance may or may not be accompanied by excessive nasal air emission. Hyporhinopho-nia is the lack of nasal resonance when it is normally present, as in nasal consonants /m/, /n/, and /ng/. Hyporhinophonia is caused by an overclosure of the velopharyngeal port or an obstruction of the nasal cavity. The easiest way to identify rhinophonia is the nasal mirror test (showing air escape) with selected nasal and denasal phonemes and sentences. Some commercially available systems (Nasal Oral Ratiometry System, Laryngograph Limited, Laryngograph, London, UK) display nasal airflow waveforms and oral airflow waveforms in "real time," using a dual-chamber mask assembly. Acoustic devices (Nasometer by Kay Elemetrics,

Lincoln Park, NJ; Nasal View by Tiger Electronics) can compute in quasi-real time a ratio of the acoustic energy emanating from the nose to the total acoustic energy emanating from the nose and mouth together. This ratio is averaged and expressed as a percentage.[51] It is very useful for objectivizing treatment effects.[52]

Example of Specific Application in Singers

It is known that the velopharyngeal port is closed significantly longer in singing than in speaking samples. The amount of time the velopharyngeal port is opened diminishes as the singer ascends in pitch.[53]

REFERENCES

1. Nair G. *Voice Tradition and Technology: A State-of-the-Art Studio.* San Diego, Calif: Singular Publishing Group;1999.
2. Howes P, Callaghan J, Davis P, Kenny D, Thorpe W. The relationship between measured vibrato characteristics and perception in Western operatic singing. *J Voice.* 2004;8:216-230.
3. Hirano M. Objective evaluation of the human voice: clinical aspects. *Folia Phoniatr.* 1989;41:89-144.
4. Neiman GS, Edeson B. Procedural aspects of eliciting maximum phonation time. *Folia Phoniatr.* 1981;33:285-293.
5. Kent RD, Kent JF, Rosenbek JC. Maximum performance tests of speech production. *J Speech Hear Res.* 1987;52:367-387.
6. Rau D, Beckett RL. Aerodynamic assessment of vocal function using hand-held spirometers. *J Speech Hear Dis.* 1984;49:183-188.
7. Morris S, Jawad MSM, Eccles R. Relationships between vital capacity, height and nasal airway resistance in asymptomatic volunteers. *Rhinology.* 1992;30:259-264.
8. Hirano M. *Clinical Examination of Voice.* New York, NY: Springer; 1981.
9. Verdolini K. Voice disorders. In: Tomblin JB, Morris HL, Spriesterbach OC, eds. *Diagnosis in Speech-Language Pathology.* San Diego, Calif: Singular Publishing Group; 1994:247-306.
10. Colton RH, Casper JK. *Understanding Voice Problems.* Baltimore, Md: Williams & Wilkins; 1996.
11. Woo P, Colton RH, Shangold L. Phonatory airflow analysis in patients with laryngeal disease. *Ann Otol Rhinol Laryngol.* 1987;96:549-555.
12. Woo P, Casper J, Colton R, Brewer D. Aerodynamic and stroboscopic findings before and after microlaryngeal phonosurgery. *J Voice.* 1994;8:186-194.
13. Schutte HK. *The Efficiency of Voice Production.* [thesis]. Kemper: University of Groningen; 1980.
14. Schutte HK. Integrated aerodynamic measurements. *J Voice.* 1992;6:127-134.
15. Hirano M, Koike Y, von Leden H. Maximum phonation time and air usage during phonation. *Folia Phoniatr.* 1968;20:185-201.
16. Fritzell B, Hallen O, Sundberg J. Evaluation of Teflon injection procedures for paralytic dysphonia. *Folia Phoniatr.* 1974;26:414-421.
17. Murry T, Bone RC. Aerodynamic relationships associated with normal phonation and paralytic dysphonia. *Laryngoscope.* 1978;88:100-109.
18. Sabol JW, Lee L, Stemple JC. The value of vocal function exercises in the practice regimen of singers. *J Voice.* 1995;9:27-36.
19. Rothenberg M. A new inverse filtering technique for deriving the glottal airflow during voicing. *J Acoust Soc Am.* 1973;53:1632-1645.
20. Sapienza CM, Stathopoulos ET, Dromey C. Approximations of open quotient and speed quotient from glottal and EGG waveforms: effects of measurement criteria and sound pressure level. *J Voice.* 1998;12:31-43.
21. Sulter AM, Wit HP. Glottal volume velocity waveform characteristics in subjects with and without vocal training, related to gender, sound intensity, fundamental frequency and age. *J Acoust Soc Am.* 1996;100:3360-3373.
22. Sundberg J, Thalen M, Alku P, Vilkman E. Estimating perceived phonatory pressedness in singing from flow glottograms. *J Voice.* 2004;18:56-62.
23. Rothenberg M. Interpolating subglottal pressure from oral pressure. *J Speech Hear Dis.* 1982;47:218-224.
24. Baken RJ, Orlikoff R. *Clinical Measurement of Speech and Voice.* San Diego, Calif: Singular Thomson Learning; 2000.
25. Titze IR. Phonation threshold pressure—a missing link in glottal aerodynamics. *J Acoust Soc Am.* 1992;91:2926-2935.
26. Jiang J, O'Mara T, Conley D, Hanson D. Phonation threshold pressure measurements during phonation by airflow interruption. *Laryngoscope.* 1999;109:425-432.
27. Colton RH, Woo P. Measuring vocal fold function. In: Rubin JS, Sataloff RT, Korovin GS, et al, eds. *Diagnosis and Treatment of Voice Disorders.* New York, NY: Igaku-Shoin;1995:290-315.

28. Brown WS Jr, Rothman HB, Sapienza CM. Perceptual and acoustic study of professionally trained versus untrained voices. *J Voice.* 2000;14:301–309.

29. Diaz JA, Rothman HB. Acoustical comparison between samples of good and poor vibrato in singers. *J Voice.* 2003;17:179–184.

30. Bartholomew WT. A physical definition of "good voice quality" in the male voice. *J Acoust Soc Am.* 1934;6:25–33.

31. Sundberg J. *The Science of the Singing Voice.* DeKalb: Northern Illinois University Press; 1987.

32. Cleveland TF, Sundberg J, Stone RE. Long-term-average spectrum characteristics of country singers during speaking and singing. *J Voice.* 2001;15:54–60.

33. Omori K, Kacker A, Carrol LM, Riley WD, Blaugrund SM. Singing power ratio: quantitative evaluation of singing voice quality. *J Voice.* 1996;10:228–235.

34. Dejonckere PH, Remacle M, Fresnel-Elbaz E, Woisard V, Crevier Buchman L, Millet B. Differentiated perceptual evaluation of pathological voice quality: reliability and correlations with acoustic measurements. *Rev Laryngol Otol Rhinol.* 1996;117:219–224.

35. Dejonckere PH, Lebacq J. Acoustic, perceptual, aerodynamic and anatomical correlations in voice pathology. *ORL J Otorhinolaryngol Relat Spec.* 1996;58:326–332.

36. Wolfe V, Fitch J, Martin D. Acoustic measures of dysphonic severity across and within voice types. *Folia Phoniatr Logop.* 1997;49:292–299.

37. Speyer R, Wieneke GH, Dejonckere PH. Documentation of progress in voice therapy: perceptual, acoustic and laryngostroboscopic findings pretherapy and posttherapy. *J Voice.* 2004;18:325–339.

38. Titze I, Liang H. Comparison of Fo extraction models for high precision voice perturbation measurements. *J Speech Hear Res.* 1993;36:1120–1133.

39. Yu P, Ouaknine M, Giovanni A. Clinical significance of calculating the coefficients of Lyapunov in the objective assessment of dysphonia. *Rev Laryngol Otol Rhinol (Bord).* 2000;5:301–305.

40. Speyer R, Wieneke GH, Dejonckere PH. The use of acoustic parameters for the evaluation of voice therapy for dysphonic patients. *Acta Acustica united with Acustica.* 2004;90:520–527.

41. Dejonckere PH, Wieneke GH, Bloemenkamp D, Lebacq J. F_0-perturbations and F_0/loudness dynamics in voices of normal children, with and without education in singing. *Int J Pediatr Otorhinolaryngol.* 1996;35:107–115.

42. Amir O, Amir N, Michaeli O. Evaluating the influence of warm-up on singing voice quality using acoustic measures. *J Voice.* 2005;19:252–260.

43. Schultz-Couion HJ. *Stimmfeldmessung.* Berlin, Germany: Springer-Verlag; 1990.

44. Titze IR. Acoustic interpretation of the voice profile (phonetogram). *J Speech Hear Res.* 1992;35:21–34.

45. Heylen L , Wuyts FL, Mertens F, De Bodt M, Dan de Heyning PH. Normative voice range profiles of male and female professional voice users. *J Voice.* 2002;16:1–7.

46. Heylen L, Wuyts F, et al. Evaluation of the vocal performance of children using a voice range profile index. *J Speech Lang Hear Res.* 1998;41:232–238.

47. Van de Heyning PH, et al. Research work of the Belgian study group on voice disorders. *Acta Oto-Rhino-Laryngologica Belg.* 1996;50:321–386.

48. Wuyts F, De Bodt M, Molenberghs G, et al. The Dysphonia Severity Index: an objective measure of quality based on a multiparameter approach. *J Speech Lang Hear Res.* 2000;43:796–809.

49. Speyer R, Wieneke GH, van Wijck-Warnaar I, Dejonckere PH. Effects of voice therapy on the voice range profiles of dysphonic patients. *J Voice.* 2003;17:544–556.

50. Mendes AP, Rothman HB, Sapienza C, Brown WS Jr. Effects of vocal training on the acoustic parameters of the singing voice. *J Voice.* 2003;17:529–543.

51. Haapanen ML. A simple clinical method of evaluating hypernasality. *Folia Phoniatr.* 1992;43:122–132.

52. Dejonckere PH, van Wijngaarden, HA. Retropharyngeal autologous fat transplantation for congenital short palate: a nasometric assessment of functional results. *Ann Otol Rhinol Laryngol.* 2001;110:168–172.

53. Austin SF. Movement of the velum during speech and singing in classically trained singers. *J Voice.* 1997;11:212–221.

Chapter 10

PERCEPTUAL ATTRIBUTES AND ASSESSMENT OF THE SINGER'S VOICE

Rahul Shrivastav
Judith Wingate

Vocal performance is unique in that the performer *is* the instrument. Further, each singer's instrument is distinct from all others due to differences such as body size and vocal tract configuration. The singer's voice is a product of his or her individual experiences, emotions, training, and perceptions. The singer learns, in large part, by means of the teacher's perceptions and his or her own perception of the teacher's instructions and feedback. Therefore, understanding of the singing voice, perception of the singing voice and its role in both performance and clinical assessment is important in the care of the singer's voice.

The development of singing pedagogy in the Western European tradition had its origins in the seventeenth century Italian "bel canto" method. The method was largely dependent on perceptual assessment, relying on the "ear" of the teacher and the ability of the student to understand and respond to the teacher's instructions. The method was enhanced by the use of imagery by the teacher to elicit vocal changes from the student. In order to replicate the desired sound consistently, the student had to rely on memory as well as kinesthetic and auditory feedback when a "target" voice was achieved. This feedback based on perception continued throughout the performer's training. The significance of perceptual feedback and memory on the singing performance cannot be underestimated and its relevance in singing has been summarized well by Vennard[1(p80)]:

Learning to sing is a slow and patient undertaking, in which a good ear is the prerequisite, the imagery is an aid supplied by the teacher, and the experience is gradually accumulated until it is so powerful that merely calling up the memory will reproduce it.

In spite of technological advances in speech and voice science and instrumentation, much singing instruction continues to follow the methods used by the early teachers of bel canto singing. Teachers typically teach in the same manner as that used by their own teacher. These traditions are passed on orally over the years in a master-to-apprentice fashion. As many of the structures involved in singing cannot be visualized without invasive means, the tradition has largely persisted, requiring singing teachers to rely heavily on perceptual methods.

Perceptual assessment continues to play a key role in the clinical assessment of singing voice as well. Each of us assesses the voices around us without conscious awareness of how we perform this task. Listeners have a referent for normal voice quality and are easily aware of a voice when it deviates from this referent. However, perceptual assessment of voice may be further refined by following a systematic approach based upon our knowledge of the auditory perceptual process. Such a method can help identify the consistencies and inconsistencies in perceptual judgments and assists in comparing these observations to the information gathered in the instrumental assessment of voice. Additionally, a thorough knowledge of how vocal fold physiology, voice acoustics, and perception relate to each other can benefit clinicians in understanding the voice problems faced by a singer in its entirety and in developing an appropriate rehabilitation program. Perceptual assessment also serves as an important measure of treatment outcome as it gives the clinician a picture of the patients' functional capabilities. Because many problems for the singer will be those of function, observation in a variety of contexts is important[2] and should include assessment of the speaking voice concurrent with the singing assessment.

This chapter is divided into two sections. The first section provides an overview of the research related to the auditory perceptual process, with an emphasis on the singing voice. This is followed by more specific guidelines that may be useful in the perceptual assessment of the singing voice.

THE AUDITORY PERCEPTUAL PROCESS

Understanding the relationship between a physical stimulus and its perception has been the focus of much research over the last century and has resulted in a distinct branch of cognitive psychology called *psychophysics*. The origin of psychophysical research dates back to the work of Weber and Fechner in the mid-19th century. Psychophysical experiments typically deal with two distinct but related questions: (1) what is our "sensory capability?" and (2) what is our "response proclivity?"[3] Sensory capability refers to the resolving power of a sensory system. For example, we may be interested in knowing the lowest sound pressure level that can be detected by the human ear. In contrast, response proclivity refers to the tendency of an observer to respond in a specific manner. For

example, when a listener is asked to assign a score to reflect the loudness of a signal, he may choose a specific ratio based on factors such as his pervious experiences, training, characteristics of the sensory system, and so forth.

Psychophysical experiments use a variety of methods to investigate perceptual phenomena. The experimental paradigms include tasks such as determination of thresholds (the smallest perceivable magnitude), difference limens (the smallest perceivable difference), identification (assigning stimuli to unique categories), judgments of equality (the magnitude at which two stimuli appear equal in some aspect), ranking (ordering a set of stimuli based on specific perceptual attribute), and others. The findings from such experiments have helped us understand how the characteristics of a physical stimulus are related to its perceptual attributes.

In the context of voice assessment our primary interest is in the vocal acoustic signal produced by the singer. There are three major components related to the perception of an acoustic signal. These include its pitch, loudness, and quality (or timbre).

Pitch

Pitch is one of the most fundamental perceptual attributes of sound. It is defined as "that attribute of auditory sensation in terms of which sounds may be ordered on a musical scale."[4] When listeners are asked to judge pitch, they can represent sounds on a single scale varying from low to high. In this aspect, pitch is often regarded as a one-dimensional perceptual attribute. Considerable research has been done to understand the processes underlying the perception of pitch and how it is influenced by changes in the physical properties of the acoustic signal.

The pitch of pure tones is related primarily to its frequency (F). Similarly, the pitch of complex periodic signals, such as those observed in speech and music, is related primarily to its fundamental frequency (F_0). As the F or the F_0 of a signal increases, it is perceived to have a higher pitch. However, this relationship is not linear. In other words, if the frequency of a tone were to change by a certain proportion, the corresponding change in pitch is not of the same proportion. For example, doubling the frequency of a tone may not result in a doubling of pitch. Although pitch is a perceptual correlate of frequency, the two terms cannot always be used synonymously.

Certain other characteristics of the sound also influence its pitch. For example, experiments have shown that the pitch of a pure tone may be affected by its loudness.[5] Although individuals differ in their responses, most experimental findings show that with increasing level the pitch of low frequency pure tones (below 2 kHz) decreases whereas that of high frequency tones (above 2 kHz) increases slightly. However, tones between 1 and 2 kHz do not show a significant change with level.

Theories to explain the perception of pitch take one of two forms. The "place theory" views the cochlea (within the inner ear) as a frequency analyzer. It suggests that each frequency stimulates a different part of the basilar membrane in the cochlea, thereby stimulating different neurons. The activity of different neurons translates into differences in pitch. In contrast, the "temporal theory" suggests that pitch information is obtained from the timing by which nerve fibers in the auditory system are excited by a particular sound. However, neither of these theories is capable of explaining all aspects of pitch perception. Instead, most experts believe both of these mechanisms contribute to the perception of pitch. The perception of low frequencies (below 5 kHz) can be explained by timing theories, but frequencies above 5 kHz can only be explained by place theory.

Understanding how listeners perceive pitch is important in music and song. This is because the perception of musical scales is related to their pitch. Sounds that differ in frequency by one octave sound similar and are given the same name on the musical scale. Other notes in Western classical music generally hold some simple relationship to the octave, such as 3/2 or 5/4 (although others, such as Indian classical music, may utilize ratios that deviate from the conventional musical scale). Similarly, experiments have shown that when listeners are asked to adjust the frequency of a test tone (F_t) so that it is perceived to be an octave higher in pitch than a standard (F_s), they generally adjust F_t to be *twice* the frequency of F_s. These findings have led some researchers to theorize that musical pitch has two components—"tone height" (which is related to the frequency of the tone) and "tone chroma" (which is related to the musical note assigned to the tone).[6] Interestingly, however, the ability to judge octave relationship between tones has been found to hold true only when both sounds (F_s and F_t) are below 5 kHz in frequency. Above this frequency listeners are unable to make such judgments consistently.[7] Fortunately, this does not pose serious concerns in singing because the pitch of most songs and musical instruments is well below this range.

A systematic variation of pitch during singing is necessary for the perception of appropriate intonation and vibrato. Intonation is cued by relatively slow changes in pitch that occur over long phrase or sentence boundaries. These changes in pitch generally co-occur with changes in loudness and duration of specific syllables. Appropriate intonation is necessary not only for melody, but also for cueing linguistic information such as syllable stress. On the other hand, vibrato results from relatively faster modulation of pitch. If the rate and extent of the vibrato remain relatively low and if the sung vowel is relatively long in duration, then the modulation of F_0 does not affect the overall pitch of the vowel. This is because the overall pitch of a frequency modulated tone appears to be related to a weighted average of short samples.[8,9] If the rate of vibrato is too slow (below ~4 Hz), listeners tend to hear a modulation in pitch.

Loudness

Loudness is the perceptual attribute of auditory sensation in terms of which sounds may be ordered on a scale extending from quiet to loud.[10(p127)] Loudness, like pitch, is generally viewed as a one-dimensional percept. The loudness of a sound is related primarily to the sound pressure level (SPL) of that sound. In general, sounds with greater SPL are perceived to be louder while those with a lower SPL are perceived to be softer. However, loudness is a subjective phenomenon and may be affected by factors other than its SPL alone. Further, the relationship between SPL and loudness is not linear. Therefore, the terms loudness and SPL (or intensity) cannot always be used synonymously.

As loudness is a subjective entity, it cannot be measured directly. Instead, the perception of loudness has been studied using a variety of techniques. The most commonly used methods to study loudness include loudness "scaling" and "matching." In scaling techniques such as magnitude estimation, listeners hear sounds with known acoustic characteristics and assign each a rating on a specific scale. The assigned rating represents the perceived loudness of that signal. In matching techniques, listeners are asked to match the loudness of a sound to that of another sound (called the "standard"). These experiments allow listeners to manipulate the level of the standard until they achieve a match in terms of the loudness of the two sounds. The effects of various acoustic parameters, such as frequency or spectral shape, on perceived loudness can be inferred by systematically varying the sound characteristics during such experiments.

Loudness of pure tones varies as a function of their frequency. In other words, pure tones of different frequency result in different loudness even when these are presented at the same SPL. Although the exact results vary significantly across different experiments, they show the same general tendencies. At low SPL, pure tones in the mid-frequency range (approximately 500–4000 Hz) elicit the greatest loudness. Tones of frequencies below and above this range need significantly greater SPL to elicit the same loudness (for example, see Fletcher and Munson, 1933[11]). However, at higher SPL these differences tend to disappear and tones of all frequencies result in approximately equal loudness at the same SPL. This means that the growth of loudness with increasing SPL varies with the frequency of the tone. The effects of such differences in loudness growth become evident in many practical applications. For example, if a sung vowel is amplified and reproduced at high SLP, the amplified sound often appears to have a "bassy" sound quality. This effect arises from the fact that loudness growth of low-frequency sounds differs from than that of higher frequency sounds, thereby affecting the overall quality of the sound. However, most modern amplifiers minimize this effect by amplifying the low and high frequencies in a manner that preserves the sound quality.

Loudness of pure tones also depends on its duration. If listeners are presented two tones of the same frequency but different durations, then the tone with a longer duration is perceived to be louder than the one with a smaller duration. However, this effect is only seen for tones that are very brief in duration (less than 100–200 milliseconds). For tones greater than about 200 ms, duration appears to have no effect on loudness.[12]

The loudness of complex sounds such as speech and music is related not only to its overall SPL, but also to the spectral shape of the complex signal. Several experiments have studied the change in loudness that occurs when the bandwidth of a signal is increased but its total energy is kept constant. These experiments show that an initial increase in the bandwidth of a broadband noise does not affect the loudness of the sound. However, once the bandwidth of the noise exceeds a certain threshold (called the critical bandwidth), an increase in loudness is perceived. The critical bandwidth has been found to be narrow when the low center-frequency of the noise is low, and it increases with an increase in the center-frequency of the noise.[13] These effects are believed to result from the way sounds are processed by the auditory system. Models to explain such effects have recently been utilized to develop "loudness meters." Such calculations provide significantly better correlates of perceived loudness than older methods that used specific weighing functions with the measured sound pressure level (eg, the A- or C-weighting scale on a sound level meter).

The overall loudness of speech or song is related primarily to the SPL of a few dominant harmonics of the signal.[14,15] Most often, the SPL of the fundamental frequency and/or the harmonics corresponding to the first formant frequency are most closely related to the overall loudness of the vowel. However, as explained above, the best method to quantify loudness is through the use of the critical band concept, which is often implemented in "loudness meters."

Quality or Timbre

Sound quality or timbre is defined as that attribute of auditory sensation in terms of which a listener can judge two sounds having the same pitch and loudness as being dissimilar.[16] Like pitch and loudness, the quality of a sound is a subjective experience. However, unlike pitch and loudness, the quality of a sound cannot be described using a single scale. In other words, when asked to sort a group of sounds or voices based on their quality, listeners cannot organize them using a single scale. Rather, listeners use a larger set of perceptual attributes or descriptors to organize voices in terms of their quality. Therefore, the quality of a sound is considered to be a multidimensional percept.

The quality of a sound is hypothesized to be related to two general properties of the sound. First, quality depends on how energy changes as a function of frequency. This refers to the spectral envelope or the spectral shape of the sound. Second, the quality of a sound also depends upon how energy changes over time. This refers to the temporal envelope of the sound. Most sounds, including speech and music, are characterized by simultaneous variations in their spectral and temporal envelopes. Thus, quantification of vocal quality requires attention to multiple changes that occur in the signal.

In the context of speech and song, the term "quality" is used to describe two different concepts.[14] One aspect, called "vowel quality," refers to the vowel being produced by the speaker. The other, called "voice quality," refers to the personal characteristics of a particular speaker's voice. Vowel quality is a phonemic property and affects the intelligibility of speech. For example, the words "beat" and "boot" differ in terms of their vowel quality and signal a change in the meaning of the word. Voice quality, on the other hand, is relatively unique to individual speakers and allows listeners to obtain paralinguistic information such as the speaker's identity, age, gender, emotional status, and so forth. Although classification of the singing voice appears to be based primarily upon its pitch, voice quality also plays a role in this regard.[14,17]

The quality of steady-state sounds is primarily related to its spectral envelope. Vowel quality, for instance, is cued primarily by the frequency of the first two or three formants. However, in certain instances the vowel spectrum fails to provide information about the vowel formants. For example, vowels sung with a high fundamental frequency are characterized by widely separated harmonics. The vowel formant frequency may not be easily noticeable in the spectrum of such vowels.[14] In such instances, listeners appear to judge the vowel identity based on changes in the formant frequency at the consonant-vowel boundary (this is called the "formant transition").

A speaker's voice quality may be affected by a number of factors that affect its spectral and temporal envelope. The vocal fold vibration affects the spectral envelope of the sound generated at the glottis. For example, voices may differ in terms of their spectral slope and in terms of the level of "aspiration noise" present in the voice. The vocal fold vibration generally has some degree of aperiodicity, which results in changes in the temporal envelope of the voice. The

sound generated at the glottis is further modified by the characteristics of the vocal tract. For instance, differences in vocal tract length and the configuration of the tongue, jaw, lips, pharyngeal cavity, and the velopharyngeal port can affect the formant frequencies considerably, further modifying the spectral envelope of the voice. Although speakers can modify the frequency of the lower formants by manipulating the lips, tongue, and jaw position, it is difficult to manipulate the higher formants as easily. These higher formants are partly responsible for each singer's unique vocal characteristics. The presence of a "singer's formant" in many singers further affects the spectral envelope, thus affecting voice quality.

Figure 10-1 shows the spectrogram of an /ɑ/ vowel produced by a male singing at 233 Hz. The singer's formant is illustrated by the increased energy around 3000 Hz. Figure 10-2 shows the same vowel sung by a female at the same fundamental frequency.

Although we have discussed pitch, loudness, and quality as independent perceptual constructs, these are often interrelated. Changes in one parameter may result in a corresponding change in another. Some of these relationships result from how speech is produced. For example, a change in the F_0 affects how closely a specific harmonic aligns with the formant frequency of the vowel. The resulting "formant tuning," may affect the overall spectral shape, and thereby affect vocal quality. Similarly, attempts to increase the loudness of the voice also affect the spectral shape of the sound generated by the vocal folds. As a speaker increases the loudness of a sung or a spoken vowel, the higher harmonics gain greater energy than the lower harmonics. This results in a decrease in the spectral slope at higher SPL.

Singers rely heavily on auditory feedback during singing. However, the quality of one's own voice when it is heard live (ie, when a speaker hears his or her own voice during singing/speaking) is perceived to be very different from the quality of the same voice when it is recorded and played back to the speaker. There are at least two reasons for this phenomenon. First, when a speaker hears his or her voice live, the sound is being transmitted to the ear primarily through "bone conduction." In effect, the sound travels through the bones of the skull and stimulates the ear directly. In contrast, when listening to a recorded sample of the same voice, the sound reaches the ear primarily through "air

Figure 10-1. Spectrogram of an /a/ vowel sung by a male singer at 233 Hz.

Figure 10-2. Spectrogram of an /a/ vowel sung by a female singer at 233 Hz.

conduction," or by traveling through space in air. As these two mechanisms affect the spectrum of the voice differently, they affect the perceived vocal quality. A second reason for this phenomenon is related to the nature of the sound propagation in air. For a speaker to hear his or her voice live, the sound needs to travel around the head back toward the ears. How-

ever, low- and high-frequency sounds do not propagate in all directions equally, thereby affecting the overall-spectrum of the sound reaching the ear. These spectral differences may further result in differences in quality between live and recorded voice.[18] Additionally, it is likely that the characteristics of the recording instrument itself distort the speech signal to some degree.

PERCEPTUAL ASSESSMENT OF THE SINGING VOICE

The following section identifies and defines parameters that should be considered for perceptual assessment of the singing voice. It should be noted that there are no defined standards for perceptual assessment of the singing voice. This creates difficulty as an anchor point of normalcy must be agreed on to compare any voice to the expected normal quality. Therefore, it is not surprising that perceptual assessment is often limited by poor agreement and reliability across different raters. For example, it has been observed that ratings of voice quality made by different listeners show very poor agreement across listeners.[19] However, this variability largely reflects differences in how individual raters interpret and use the rating scale.[20] Although reliability and agreement between raters can be improved significantly in an experimental setup, perceptual evaluation using rating scales in a clinical setting is often limited in terms of the sensitivity and consistency of perceptual judgments. Nevertheless, adequate training and experience can help the clinician in developing the auditory skills necessary to adequately perform a perceptual voice assessment.

In order to assess the voice of a singer, it is necessary to have the singer perform several songs and vocalises. The selections will vary according to the level of the singer and the type of music typically performed. Information should also be gathered on the singer's previous training, their personal goals regarding singing, how often they rehearse, and general vocal hygiene habits. Finally, it is also important to pay attention to any vocal problems noted in the speaking voice.

Intonation

The singer must accurately reproduce a sequence of pitches indicated by the composer during performance. Accurate production of pitch requires excellent auditory skills and constant laryngeal adjustment in response to the auditory feedback. The singer must be aware of the intonation necessary for the sung piece and adjust the pitch accordingly. While instrumentalists must also do this to some degree, singers are required to respond with constant physical adjustments to aural and kinesthetic feedback regarding intonation. Singers must match the pitch produced by any accompanying instruments as well as tune to other singers when in an ensemble or choral settings. Intonation is an important factor to consider when assessing the singer, especially in an untrained singer. It is also an important consideration for aging singers that may have loss of hearing acuity, because it may affect their ability to hear their own voices or the accompanying music.

Vibrato

Vibrato is an important component of overall vocal quality and is described as a regular variation around a fundamental frequency of less than a semitone.[21] The current standard for vibrato in classical singing is between 4 to 7 cycles per second.[15,21] Rates slower than this will often be described as a wobble (less than 5.5 Hz) with faster rates (7.5 Hz or higher) being classified as a tremolo. Tremolo and wobble result from emotional state, vocal fatigue, and/or technical problems, especially excessive tension and poor breath support.[21,22] In assessing vibrato, the examiner should look for jaw or chin shaking that occurs simultaneously with the vibrato as these may be indicators of poor technique.

Overall Quality

Voice quality, or timbre, refers to the overall sound of the voice. As described previously, quality is largely related to the spectral and temporal envelope of the signal. It is generally described subjectively, often using contrastive terms such as dark/bright, heavy/light, breathy/pressed, and clear/fuzzy. From a clinical perspective, a prime concern is the consistency of the timbre throughout the range of fundamental frequency. Large inconsistencies in vocal quality may be indicators of: (1) poor technique, particularly if heard in the passagio, (2) tension, if heard in the upper range, or (3) changes in subglottal pressure related to poor breath management. Assessment of voice quality during speaking should also be included during assessment. The overall voice quality observed in singing and speaking should be similar. If not, any incongruities observed may be indicators of potential vocal problems.

Voice Onset

The manner in which the voice is initiated should be considered as part of the evaluation. In general, onsets may be hard or gentle. The hard onset is initiated with increased subglottal pressure and is characterized by a fast intensity rise-time. Such onset is not considered to be healthy as it increases the force of vocal fold impact and is believed to be a contributor to edema and, over time, to vocal fold pathologies. In contrast, an excessively easy onset may result in an extremely breathy sound. The preferred onset pattern is a balanced onset, between these two extremes. Vennard[1] advocates the use of an imaginary aspirate to achieve the preferred onset. This may allow the singer to "sing on the breath" without increasing laryngeal tension. Voice onset in the speaking voice should be examined concurrently. For example, a singer may use a balanced onset in singing but frequent hard voice onsets when speaking. Over time, these hard glottal onsets may lead to vocal fold edema. This, in turn, may lead to difficulties with both singing and speaking.

Classification

Voice classification is discussed at length in the singing literature. The terms used in voice classification have their origins in Italian opera and are termed "Fachs" in German. The Fach designation allowed opera house agents to specify the type of singer needed for a particular role. The Fach terminology is still used and includes terms such as coloratura, lyric, dramatic, and spinto.

These terms are usually combined with the more familiar labels of soprano, mezzo-soprano, contralto, tenor, baritone, and bass.

Classification of the singing voice is generally done by the singing teacher using perceptual means. This classification may not be completed until the voice has completely matured. Classification of the singing voice is based on a number of perceptual factors. These include judgments of voice quality, pitch (based on fundamental frequency), pitch range that can be achieved by the singer (based on the phonation frequency range), passagio demarcation (which is related to the fundamental frequency at which the singer's voice changes from one vocal register to another), and tessitura (or the average pitch of a given song). The range of frequency expected for various voice types is well documented[2,15,21] and generally follow those listed in Table 10-1.

The pitch where the passagio, or the transition from one register to another, occurs is another factor used to determine voice classification. Although the reported frequency of the transition areas differs slightly from one author to another, these tend to follow the general trend shown in Table 10-2.[15] Voice breaks and subtle difficulties in the passagio are frequent indicators of vocal difficulty and should be examined carefully in a perceptual assessment.

The last component to be considered in voice classification is tessitura. This is the area in which the voice performs with special ease.[23] It may also be defined as the average pitch level of a song or part of a song in relation to the overall phonation range.[15] So, the voice classification depends in part

Table 10-1. Range Expectations for Voice Types

Voice Type	Low Note	Frequency	High Note	Frequency
Soprano	G_3	196 Hz	D_6	1175 Hz
Mezzo-Soprano	E_3	165 Hz	A_5	880 Hz
Contralto	D_3	147 Hz	E_5	659 Hz
Tenor	C_3	131 Hz	C_5	523 Hz
Baritone	G_2	98 Hz	G_4	392 Hz
Bass	E_2	82 Hz	E_4	330 Hz

Table 10–2. Passagio Points for Voice Types

Voice Type	First Passagio	Frequency	Second Passagio	Frequency
Soprano	$D\#_4$	311 Hz	$F\#_5$	740 Hz
Mezzo-Soprano	$F\#_4$	370 Hz	F_5	698 Hz
Contralto	G_4	392 Hz	E_5	659 Hz
Tenor	$C\#_4$	277 Hz	$F\#_4$	370 Hz
Baritone	$A\#_3$	233 Hz	$D\#_4$	311 Hz
Bass	$G\#_3$	208 Hz	D_4	294 Hz

on the singer's ability to sustain certain pitch ranges over the course of an aria or an entire opera. For example, the dramatic soprano would be expected to deal with the tessitura of the role of Brunhilde in Wagner's *Die Walkure*.

When assessing the student singer or the elite professional, it is important to determine if the literature being performed is appropriate for the singer's voice classification. If there is a serious mismatch, particularly if the voice is classified in one of the higher categories, the singer may be more prone to strain, and ultimately, to vocal pathologies.[22]

Resonance

Resonance is best described as a reinforcement of specific frequencies in the acoustic spectrum. As described previously, the frequencies that resonate in the vocal tract depend on the size and shape of the vocal tract and affect the overall spectral shape. This varies with vowel positions and typically requires some vowel modification to maintain a consistent vocal quality. The desired quality is a brilliance, or ring to the voice, which correlates with the singer's formant. The singer's formant refers to an emphasis or frequencies around 3000 Hz, which allows the voice to be heard over an orchestra or background noise.[14,18]

The ring of the voice is not to be confused with excessive nasality which may be a problem for some amateur singers. The degree of nasality is typically judged in the singing and speaking voice. Denasality,

the sound that is produced by nasal congestion or stuffiness, if heard in the absence of congestion, should also be considered abnormal.

Dynamics

A healthy singer uses a variety of loudness, or dynamic levels, when singing. These loudness levels are indicated by the composer in most types of music. The loudness levels are relative to each other and will vary depending on the type of performance and the singer's skill. Most trained singers should also be able to perform the messa di voce task throughout their entire singing range.[21] The messa di voce is performed on a sustained pitch with a crescendo followed by a decrescendo. The trained singer can change the loudness level smoothly without changing the pitch level. The messa di voce requires excellent physical control over the voice and may be used as a method of assessing a singer's dynamic control and, to some degree, his or her control of pitch. A singer's inability to vary loudness may indicate poor vocal technique, vocal fold pathologies, difficulty regulating subglottal or breath pressure, or problems with neural control.

Rhythmic Accuracy

Healthy singers can replicate rhythmic patterns indicated by the composer with accuracy. This requires rapid adjustment of the entire mechanism, especially at the laryngeal level and with the articulators. There may be occasional singers who exhibit difficulty with rapid articulation. When they do this consistently, it may be the first sign of a neurologic disease.

Phrasing

Musical phrasing is similar to phrasing for speech in that breaks for breath or for emphasis should occur in linguistically appropriate places. Difficulty with this may indicate poor breath control or vocal fatigue.

Diction

Because singing involves conveying meaning with both text and music, the singer must demonstrate clear, understandable pronunciation across languages. Vowels are often changed in the upper registers, especially by sopranos, to allow for ease of singing and this may sacrifice some intelligibility. As described earlier, the vowel quality in these singers may be cued by formant transitions. Therefore, identification of the vowels may be easier in a sung piece than during production of sustained vowels.

Posture

Because the singer's body is the instrument, it is important to assess posture while singing. Performance usually occurs in a standing position. Therefore, the singer's stance should be assessed for proper spinal alignment with no evidence of excessive tension. Tension in the body, particularly resulting from misalignment of the neck, shoulders, or pelvis will have direct impact on the vocal quality.

Gesture

The singer typically makes use of hand and arm gestures when singing most types of vocal literature. This should be included in the perceptual assessment and is purely subjective. Facial expression is also related and should be congruent with the emotion conveyed in the text.

There is a need for a more formalized scheme for perceptual assessment of the singer, especially in clin-

ical settings. However, few examples of such assessment protocols exist. Some authors have developed checklists that may provide clinicians a systematic method for doing a perceptual evaluation of the singer's voice.[24] Another recent study found that listeners could reliably judge specific perceptual attributes of the operatic voice using both, rating-scales and visual-analog scales.[25] Such research shows that a systematic approach to perceptual evaluation can provide reliable and useful information about a singer's voice. A possible outline for the perceptual evaluation of voice is shown in Figure 10–3.

Self-Perception and the Singer

During all singing, but especially in performance settings, the singer must rely on his or her own perceptions from multiple sources to monitor the vocal production and to make adjustments as needed to maintain the desired quality. Figure 10–4 shows the many different factors that may affect a listener's self-perception of his or her voice. In addition to the auditory feedback of one's own voice, the singer receives some feedback from the audience, which is typically visual. As the singer is communicating via music, the visual feedback from the audience informs the singer that the message is being heard and that the appropriate emotions are being conveyed. Another auditory feedback, typically in the form of applause, allows the singer to know if the product is appreciated. The singer also receives auditory feedback of his or her own voice in the form of reflected sound from the room or perhaps from monitor speakers. This feedback gives the singer information regarding intonation, dynamics, and voice quality. Although singers do not hear themselves as others hear them, the auditory feedback is helpful for many aspects of the performance.

The most important feedback comes from internal sensations such as proprioceptive and kinesthetic feedback. The singer must constantly monitor posture to make sure that it is maintained appropriately. The singer should monitor for sites of tension and make a conscious effort to keep all parts of the vocal mechanism in a state of "active" relaxation. Additionally, vibratory sensations that accompany the "target" voice quality must be monitored and compared to those sensations that have been learned over time as being desirable.

Name: _____ **Date:** _____

Voice Classification: _____ **Evaluator:** _____

Songs performed: _____

Vocalises performed: _____

Messa di voce: _____

Instructions: Rate each parameter based on performance of songs, vocalises, and messa di voce.

Intonation
Under pitch ♭	On-pitch	above pitch #

Vibrato
Wobble	Normal	Tremolo

Voice Quality
Dark	Unremarkable	Bright

Voice Onset
Hard	Normal	Gentle

Passagio
Rough	Some good transitions	Smooth

Resonance
Denasal	Normal	Nasal

Dynamics
None	Expressive	Excessive

Rhythmic Accuracy
Inaccurate	Semi-accurate	Accurate

Phrasing
Poor	Adequate	Appropriate

Diction
Sloppy	Moderately pronounced	Articulate

Posture
Too relaxed	Balanced	Stiff

Gesture
Too little	Adequate	Excessive

Facial Expression
Too little	Appropriate	Excessive

Figure 10–3. Perceptual Assessment of Singing Voice. This form may be used to assess the singer's voice after hearing the singer perform songs from her or his repertoire.

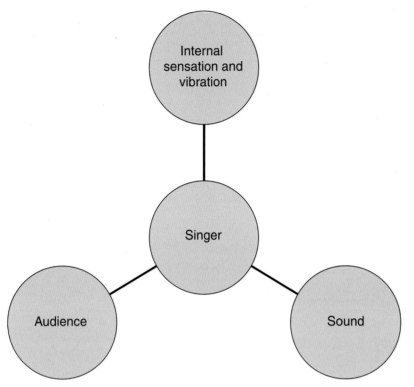

Figure 10-4. Factors that affect a singer's perception of his or her voice.

Another component that a singer must attend to during performance is breath management. While the singer will have practiced appropriate phrasing and breath control in rehearsal, factors such as anxiety, room size, and distraction during performance may all affect breath control. As a result, the singer may run out of breath before the end of an important phrase. Therefore, breath management necessitates conscious attention to placement of an appropriate pause for breath without destroying phrasing and disrupting the musicality of the performance.

As can be seen from the above, the singer must be successful at performing multiple perceptual tasks in a performance setting. So, the singer must be adept at assessing his or her own perceptions and responding accordingly. The ultimate result is a beautiful song, one that both the singer and the audience enjoy.

REFERENCES

1. Vennard W. Singing: *The Mechanism and the Technique.* New York, NY: Carl Fischer, Inc., 1967.

2. Benninger MS, Jacobson BH, Johnson AF. *Vocal Arts Medicine: The Care and Prevention of Professional Voice Disorders.* New York, NY: Thieme Medical Publishing; 1994.

3. Watson CS. Psychophysics. In: Wolman BB, ed. *Handbook of General Psychology.* Englewood Cliffs, NJ: Prentice Hall, Inc; 1973.

4. American Standards Association. *American Standard Acoustical Terminology.* New York, NY: Author; 1960.

5. Stevens SS. The relation of pitch to intensity. *J Acoust Soc Am.* 1935;6:150-154.

6. Bachem A. Tone height and tone chroma as two different pitch qualities. *Acta Psych.* 1950;7: 80-88.

7. Ward WD. Subjective musical pitch. *J Acoust Soc Am.* 1954;26:369-380.

8. Feth LL, O'Malley H, Ramsey JJ. Pitch of unresolved, two-component complex tones. *J Acoust Soc Am.* 1982;72:1403-1412.

9. Shonle JI, Horan KE. The pitch of vibrato tones. *J Acoust Soc Am.* 1980;67:246-252.

10. Moore CJ. *An Introduction to the Psychology of Hearing.* 5th ed. San Diego, Calif: Academic Press; 2003.

11. Fletcher H, Musnon WA. Loudness, its definition, measurement, and calculation. *J Acoust Soc Am.* 1933;5:82-108.
12. Buus S, Florentine M, Poulsen T. Temporal integration of loudness, loudness discrimination, and the form of the loudness function. *J Acoust Soc Am.* 1997;101:669-680.
13. Moore BCJ, Glasberg BR, Baer T. A model for the prediction of thresholds, loudness and partial loudness. *J Audio Eng. Soc.* 1997;45:224-240.
14. Sundberg J. Perceptual aspects of singing. *J Voice.* 1994;8(2):106-122.
15. Titze IR. *Principles of Voice Production.* Englewood Cliffs, NJ: Prentice Hall, Inc; 1994.
16. American National Standards Institute. *American Standard Acoustical Terminology.* New York, NY: Author; 1960.
17. Bloothooft G, Plomp R. The timbre of sung vowels. *J Acoust Soc Am.* 1988;84:847-860.
18. Sundberg J. *The Science of the Singing Voice.* Dekalb, Ill: Northern Illinois University Press; 1987.
19. Kreiman J, Gerratt BR, Kempster GB, Erman A, Berke GS. Perceptual evaluation of voice quality: review, tutorial, and a framework for future research. *J Speech Hear Res.* 1993;36(1):21-40.
20. Shrivastav R, Sapienza C, Nandur V. Application of psychometric theory to the measurement of voice quality using rating scales. *J Speech Lang Hear Res.* 2005;48(2):323-335.
21. Ware C. *Basics of Vocal Pedagogy: The Foundations and Process of Singing.* Boston, Mass: McGraw Hill; 1998.
22. McKinney J. *The Diagnosis and Correction of Vocal Faults.* Nashville, Tenn: Broadman Press; 1982.
23. Doscher B. *The Functional Unity of the Singing Voice.* Lanham, Md: The Scarecrow Press, Inc; 1994.
24. Carroll LM, Sataloff RT. The singing voice. In: Sataloff RT, ed. *Professional Voice: The Science and Art of Clinical Care.* New York, NY: Raven Press; 1991.
25. Oates JM, Bain B, Davis P, Chapman J, Kenny D. Development of an auditory-perceptual rating instrument for the operatic singing voice. *J Voice.* 2006;20(1):71-81.

Chapter 11

REFLUX AND THE PERFORMER'S VOICE

Albert L. Merati

Of all the known and suspected villains responsible for laryngeal dysfunction, gastroesophageal reflux maintains a conspicuous position; the spectrum of ailments and abnormalities ascribed to this disorder results in the performer undergoing evaluation and treatment by a variety of physicians, often with conflicting views about its management. Although science has provided a remarkable understanding of both disease pathophysiology and medical/surgical treatment, controversy persists particularly as it relates to laryngeal manifestations of reflux.[1,2] In this chapter, the problem is defined and the predilection of performers who suffer from this problem discussed. Additionally, contemporary knowledge regarding the manifestations of reflux is reviewed, with particular attention to laryngopharyngeal reflux (LPR), a useful term for the constellation of symptoms and signs related to the upper aerodigestive tract. The role of diagnostic testing in LPR, including laryngoscopy, esophagoscopy, pH probe testing, and impedance testing is examined.

Medical and surgical treatments are available for the management of reflux disease. Although the most important steps that performers can take include significant behavioral changes, the majority of patients presenting to a medical laryngology practice are prescribed medication.[3]

Several key points should be recognized at the outset as they provide structure to the discussion. First, regardless of the challenges and controversies,

reflux is clearly a significant contributor to laryngeal dysfunction. As an extreme example of this relationship, a recent case-control study demonstrated that LPR symptoms such as cough and hoarseness better predict the presence of esophageal adenocarcinoma[4] than patients with "typical" GER symptoms such as heartburn. Second, the impact of reflux on the upper aerodigestive tract may not be solely dependent on refluxate reaching the pharynx or larynx. The neural interrelatedness of the foregut and its derivatives[5,6] may play an important part in the function and dysfunction as it relates to reflux and the performer.

WHAT IS REFLUX?

The original derangement at the "heart" of heartburn and related symptoms depends on the reverse flow of gastric contents into the esophagus (Figure 11–1). These contents may include food at various stages of digestion and acidification, liquid and gas. It is believed that gastroesophageal reflux (GER) results in daily symptoms for 7% of adults, weekly in 20%, and up to 36% having symptoms at least once a month.[7,8] The incidence of "asymptomatic" reflux is not known but would understandably be higher. The local pathophysiology resulting from reflux has primarily been ascribed to acidic injury to the lower esophagus. Disordered

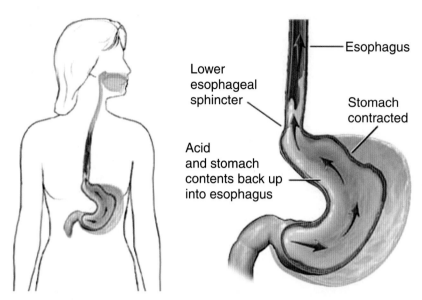

Figure 11-1. Basic concept of gastroesophageal reflux (GER).

states resulting from this injury to the esophagus are properly referred to as gastroesophageal reflux disease, or GERD. This should be distinguished from the impact of reflux on the *upper* aerodigestive tract (Table 11-1). These conditions are collectively referred to as laryngopharyngeal reflux, or LPR.

The basis for injury is believed to be related to stomach acid and digestive enzymes, namely *pepsin*, causing tissue damage to the epithelium of the esophagus, larynx, and other structures. Whether or not other agents such as bile salts can cause laryngeal injury has been debated. Until recently, the bulk of experimental evidence has not supported the concept

Table 11-1. Manifestations of Laryngopharyngeal Reflux

Chronic laryngitis
Vocal nodules
Reinke's edema
Dysphagia
Cricopharyngeal dysfunction
Globus pharyngeus
Laryngotracheal stenosis
Asthma
Laryngeal ulcer/granuloma

of biliary injury to the larynx and pharynx[9]; this is important for several reasons. It has been suggested that the persistence of symptoms despite aggressive antacid therapy may be ascribed to the presence of injurious nonacidic chemicals, such as bile salts. A recent breakthrough, however, was presented by Sasaki et al; in their report, laryngeal tissue injury at neutral or near-neutral pH was demonstrated in an animal model[10] following exposure to bile salts. (pH relates to the degree of acid in the stomach, esophagus, or larynx. Pure water has a pH of 7; lemon juice and vinegar have a pH of approximately 2.) The significance of the controversy regarding nonacidic reflux has not been well defined, although it is commonly discussed when reviewing sources of treatment failure for acid suppression.

WHAT ARE THE BODY'S NATURAL DEFENSE MECHANISMS AGAINST REFLUX?

There are several mechanical and chemical safeguards in place to prevent the inflammation and tissue injury from refluxed gastric contents. The mechanical protections include the lower and upper esophageal sphincters, the angle of the esophageal hiatus at the diaphragm, and gravity. Great precision and discretion is demanded of the sphincters in particular—they are asked to allow food to pass appropriately, in one direction only—yet the sphincters must permit the forceful emptying of the stomach and esophagus during belching and emesis. In addition, the innate motility of the esophageal body and its peristalsis work against reflux.

Derangement of the lower esophageal sphincter (LES) function interrupts its tonic contraction working to keep stomach contents from backflow. This sphincter may be affected by medications such as calcium channel blockers (prescribed for hypertension and cardiac disease) and progesterone, as well as by tobacco, alcohol, and caffeine. All of these contribute to acid reflux.

Chemical protection from refluxed material begins with salivary bicarbonate, which serves as a buffer to neutralize acidic material. When salivary flow is compromised and less bicarbonate is available in the alimentary tract, whatever acid is present has a greater opportunity to effect damage. The prototypical example would be in Sjögren's syndrome, in which the salivary glands are not able to produce adequate volumes of saliva.[11] A similar effect may also be seen as a by-product of aging or medical therapy; dry mouth from reduced salivation is a common side effect of many various medications, including antihistamines, antidepressants, and some diuretics. This is why singers are cautioned about the use of antihistamines whether prescribed or bought over the counter.

The esophagus' innate ability to clear itself of ingested and refluxed materials depends on its motility, including peristalsis and secondary swallows. It has been hypothesized that one of the key differences between patients with laryngeal and pharyngeal symptoms and "typical" reflux patients reflects differences in esophageal motility.[12-14] There is some controversy, however, regarding the nature of the differences; one common theme is that patients with LPR tend to be daytime or "upright refluxers," in contrast to the GERD patients, who have more classic nighttime supine reflux.

Finally, intracellular defenses may play a key part in understanding the clinical presentation and variability of symptoms in patients. Pepsin, the principal digestive enzyme, has been found intracellularly in LPR patients[15,16] but not in the normal subjects studied. This was accompanied by finding a relative depletion of carbonic anhydrase, a natural buffer against injury. It is unknown exactly what the contribution of intracellular defenses are in the differing clinical manifestation of LPR and GERD, but these promising studies may explain much in the future. Impairment of any of these physical or chemical safeguards makes the larynx more susceptible to injury from reflux.

WHO GETS REFLUX?

While the prototypical patient with GERD may be the overweight male, perhaps acutely or chronically stressed, the majority of patients do not fit into this category. Tobacco use and alcohol consumption, through their reduction of lower esophageal sphincter pressure, are well-established behavioral risk factors for reflux.[17] On the other hand, several widely held beliefs regarding LPR may be more controversial. One example of this is body habitus. Within the general reflux literature, several papers have shown the association[18,19] between obesity and GERD. For patients with laryngeal and pharyngeal symptoms, a recent retrospective review of 500 patients undergoing 24-hour pH probe testing (see below under Diagnostic Testing), those with abnormal *pharyngeal* reflux events did not have a higher mean body-mass index (BMI) than those with normal studies.[20] A significantly higher percentage of *esophageal* reflux events was, however, seen in obese versus nonobese participants. The authors concluded that pharyngeal reflux is not associated with increasing BMI or obesity in LPR patients; abnormal esophageal reflux (GERD), in contrast, is associated with increasing BMI and obesity, as noted in the above references.

Pregnancy, a well-appreciated risk factor for reflux, presents an interesting study of the potential interplay of physical and chemical issues related to reflux. It is quite easy to imagine the impact of a near-term pregnancy on abdominal physiology; the increased pressure affects the bladder, bowels, and the gastroesophageal junction. This is not a complete picture, however. Hormonal alterations in pregnancy likely play the dominant role in relaxation of the protective action of the LES.[21] Progesterone, reaching high levels in pregnancy's second term, has a potent relaxing effect on the LES, thus promoting reflux. In normally menstruating women, however, the association with reflux has been suspected but not proven.[22]

WHY ARE PEFORMERS PARTICULARLY AT RISK FOR REFLUX?

Sataloff has written several excellent reviews of this topic; in the third edition of his compendium on voice care,[17] the connection between performers and reflux is thought to be related to several physical and behavioral factors. First, singing requires significant abdominal contraction for "breath support," superimposed on the known impact of exertion on reflux.[23] A recent report regarding a series of Italian singers demonstrated an increase in reflux issues during the act of singing[24]; this was ascribed to a "rapid decrease in subglottal pressure, with an abrupt and prolonged increase in intra-abdominal pressure."

Behaviorally, performers may exacerbate their problems by eating large meals late in the evening after performances. Finally, although vocal professionals have no monopoly on psychosocial stress, the lifestyle of the performer is certainly one prone to pressure and challenge. It is well known that psychological stress may result in hyperacidity and motility issues.[25] Recently, an interesting study was published which noted the effect of stress on the perception of reflux symptoms in volunteers with heartburn.[26]

CLINICAL MANIFESTATIONS OF REFLUX

Symptoms

Although the cardinal symptom of GERD is heartburn, it is not present in the majority of patients with laryngeal and pharyngeal complaints related to reflux. In Koufman's landmark treatise in 1991, only 43% of the studied patients had complaints of heartburn or acidic regurgitation.[27] Furthermore, when analyzed by otolaryngologic-presenting symptom, the rates of positive pH-probe testing were quite high; 58% of patients with a globus sensation, 45% of dysphagia patients, and 52% of those with chronic cough demonstrated abnormal pH testing. It is in fact unlikely that the patient with the clinical diagnosis of reflux complains of heartburn.[27,28]

The spectrum of laryngeal complaints secondary to reflux also includes hoarseness, throat clearing, dysphagia, globus pharyngeus, and laryngospasm. A recent publication reviewed one very common otolaryngology complaint, *postnasal drip*. In a large group of subjects with a presenting complaint of postnasal drip and no evidence of rhinologic disease on nasal endoscopy or computed tomography of the sinuses, there were a higher than expected number of acid-exposure events than in controls without postnasal drip.[29] This study introduces the probability that a portion of postnasal drip complaints may be related to reflux.

In an attempt to standardize reporting and allow for further study, Belafsky and colleagues at Wake Forest designed and tested the Reflux Symptom Index (RSI). This was subsequently validated as a tool in the clinical management of LPR.[30] The symptom questions asked are presented in Table 11–2. The RSI distinguishes between patients with laryngeal and pharyngeal complaints (mean RSI 22) and normals (mean RSI 11) as well as demonstrating sensitivity to reflux treatment. In the patients with the clinical diagnosis of LPR, RSI fell to the levels of asymptomatic normals following a course of medical therapy.

Signs: Laryngoscopy

Although nonlaryngeal, nonpharyngeal physical findings, such as dental erosion, have been described in reflux patients, the dominant clinical information comes from laryngoscopy. Despite the presence of consistent evidence supporting the association between laryngeal findings on endoscopy and the clinical diagnosis of reflux, few areas have been as controversial or contentious. In an important early paper, Hanson et al demonstrated that the examination findings of patients with chronic laryngitis can be recorded and shown to change in response to medical and behavioral treatment.[31] The key findings in Hanson's paper were posterior laryngeal erythema, of both the arytenoid mucosa and the vocal folds. This was also found to be significant in a group of patients whose laryngeal findings were prospectively video-documented and followed after therapy.[32] "Blinded" observation demonstrated changes in laryngeal inflammation following a 6-week course of pantoprazole, a proton-pump inhibitor (see below under Treatment of Reflux, Medical).

The importance of laryngeal findings in the clinical evaluation of reflux was advanced significantly in

Table 11-2. Reflux Symptom Index.

Within the last MONTH, how did the following problems affect you:	0 = No Problem 5 = Severe Problem
1. Hoarseness or a problem with your voice	0 1 2 3 4 5
2. Clearing your throat	0 1 2 3 4 5
3. Excess throat mucus or postnasal drip	0 1 2 3 4 5
4. Difficulty swallowing food, liquid, or pills	0 1 2 3 4 5
5. Coughing after you ate or after lying down	0 1 2 3 4 5
6. Breathing difficulties or choking episodes	0 1 2 3 4 5
7. Troublesome or annoying cough	0 1 2 3 4 5
8. Sensations of something sticking in your throat or a lump in your throat	0 1 2 3 4 5
9. Heartburn, chest pain, indigestion, or stomach acid coming up	0 1 2 3 4 5

From Belafsky et al, 2002[30]

2001 with the publication of Belafsky's Reflux Finding Score (RFS).[33] In that report, a scoring paradigm for reflux-attributable findings (Table 11-3) was designed and validated. The interobserver reproducibility was quite good, with high correlation coefficients. One of the strengths of this study is that it reviewed only patients with positive pH studies. Indeed, later work by Oelschlager et al described laryngoscopy as "complementary" to pH-probe testing.[34] Patients with positive RFS (in combination with positive probe tests) were much more likely to be responders to medical treatment than those with a low RFS.

Concerns have been raised regarding the significance of laryngoscopy and laryngeal findings in the support of the clinical diagnosis of reflux. Branski et al,[35] published a compelling report in 2002 in which reflux findings were noted by 5 observers reviewing videotaped examinations. The conclusions were important; there was significant intra-and interobserver variability in describing reflux-attributable findings. This study has been widely cited in criticizing the assertion that physical examination of the larynx is an unpredictable or even fruitless exercise in the clinical evaluation of LPR. Some features of this study deserve comment, however. First, the subjects were predominantly dysphonia patients; fully 50% had vocal lesions. Thus, it is

Table 11-3. Reflux Finding Score.

Subglottic edema	0 = absent 2 = present
Ventricular	2 = partial 4 = complete
Erythema/hyperemia	2 = arytenoids only 4 = diffuse
Vocal fold edema	1 = mild 2 = moderate 3 = severe 4 = polypoid
Diffuse laryngeal edema	1 = mild 2 = moderate 3 = severe 4 = obstructing
Posterior commissure hypertrophy	1 = mild 2 = moderate 3 = severe 4 = obstructing
Granuloma/granulation tissue	0 = absent 2 = present
Thick endolaryngeal mucus	0 = absent 2 = present

From Belafsky et al, 2001[33]

not surprising that there was a great deal of variability in the examiner's findings related to reflux as these patients were not likely to have reflux injury as a source of their dysfunction.

Perhaps the best-known paper in this area was published in 2002 by Hicks et al from the Cleveland Clinic.[1] In this important paper, 100 "normal" volunteers underwent laryngoscopy. These video examinations were then reviewed by speech pathologists and otolaryngologists to estimate the incidence of "reflux-attributable" lesions in the general public. A major point was revealed here—that a vast majority of subjects (nearly 80%) were felt to have a significant interarytenoid "bar" or hypertrophy. This appropriately calls into question the significance of this one finding. Unfortunately, this notable revelation has been taken as an indication that laryngoscopy in general is not useful in the clinical evaluation of reflux disease.

On balance, findings on laryngoscopy are predictive in patients with the clinical diagnosis of LPR. A recent paper regarding the outcomes of medical treatment reinforced the findings of Hanson et al years earlier; Park et al reported that, two laryngeal findings—interarytenoid mucosal erythema and vocal fold abnormalities—were found to be predictive of symptomatic improvement following medical therapy.[36]

DIAGNOSTIC TESTING

Probably the most common "diagnostic test" for reflux is an empiric course of medical therapy; this is discussed below in the treatment section. Specific diagnostic tests associated with the management of reflux are pH probe testing, impedance testing, and esophagoscopy.

pH Probe Testing

For years, the "gold-standard" for the diagnostic evaluation of GERD and LPR has been the 24-hour pH probe, in which a catheter is placed transnasally into the esophagus, with one detector, or "probe" just above the LES and another at or above the upper esophageal sphincter (UES).[27,37] The probe is left in place for 24 hours to provide an adequate time sample

to detect acidic events. Of course, the test is limited by patient tolerance of a catheter being placed (and left to remain) from the nose down to the stomach for 24 hours.[27] This had led to the advent of the Bravo device, a small pH detector implanted endoscopically on the esophageal mucosa.[38] Telemetry from this device provides 24 or even 48-hour[39] information about esophageal acid exposure without a transnasal catheter. Its role in pharyngeal disease is being evaluated.

Double pH probe testing has also been the subject of much debate with regard to the evaluation of LPR. Several studies have questioned the utility and reliability of the upper probe.[40,41] One of the typical shortcomings of individual studies of pH probe findings in otolaryngologic disorders is study size; it is difficult for any one investigation to achieve statistical significance when reporting the incidence of abnormal pH probe testing in controls versus patients with laryngeal disorders. A recent meta-analysis was published to better describe findings in the literature as they relate to the upper probe methodology and findings.[37] Indeed, in a statistical review of 16 publications, the upper probe methodology was found to be quite consistent and a significant difference was found between controls and patients with the clinical diagnosis of LPR.

The exact role and timing of pH testing is not agreed on; most practitioners use it to confirm the diagnosis of patients who are symptomatic nonresponders after medical therapy. It is at this point that the discussion of nonacid reflux often arises; the larynx, being more sensitive to acid than the esophagus, may be injured at pH 5. Currently, most pH probe events are scored as abnormal when the pH reaches 4. The significance of "low-acidity" injury in laryngeal reflux is being explored.[42] Despite these controversies, it should be re-emphasized that the probe's capacity for detection of acid at the upper probe are generally reliable; with recalibration of the suspected injurious pH level from 4 to 5, this may reveal a high rate of "low-acid" exposure and potential for damage as pepsin is still active at pH 5.[16]

Impedance Testing

Impedance testing detects changes in the ionic conduction of the space being investigated. In this case, it would be the pharyngeal or esophageal lumen. Solid, liquid, and gas reflux may be detected by the impedance process. In a nonacidic belch, for example, a reflux "event" may occur without the pH probe noting it. When applied to the study of LPR, impedance testing may be an important tool in measuring *nonacidic* reflux or events with minor changes in pH. A recent study by Kawamura et al examined 3 groups of patients: controls, patients with known GERD, and those with reflux-attributed laryngeal disorders.[43] Interestingly, gaseous reflux events were quite common, particularly in patients with the laryngeal findings. The events were weakly or nonacidic. This modality shows some promise in this clinical arena.

Esophagoscopy

There are several reasons to perform esophagoscopy in patients with suspected reflux. The dominant one is to evaluate for the presence or absence of cancer. The association between esophageal malignancy and reflux is well established. It bears repeating that the symptoms related to the larynx and pharynx may be more predictive of the presence of esophageal cancer than the classic GERD complaints.[4] Esophagoscopy is indicated to examine the digestive tract whenever malignancy is suspected, such as in patients with significant dysphagia, weight loss, or constitutional symptoms related to the presence of cancer. Of course, the presence of risk factors for the development of esophageal carcinoma, such as tobacco use, alcohol, and/or caustic ingestion, should further press the issue. Beyond that, its role in LPR patients has been debated. Some reports have concluded that esophagitis or other abnormal esophageal findings are not predictive of the presence or absence of laryngeal reflux[13,28]; in contrast, a series of papers has shown a high level of mucosal disease noted during esophagoscopy on LPR patients. These include a recent paper in which 52% of the "ear, nose and throat" patients had erosive esophagitis on endoscopy compared to 38% of the "typical" GERD patients.[44] The rate of Barrett's metaplasia, a transforming step as the esophageal mucosa is replaced by gastric lining, was noted in about 5% of both groups. This is alarming as Barrett's metaplasia is the main risk factor for adenocarcinoma of the esophagus.

One technical development that will likely affect clinical practice is the advent of transnasal esophagoscopy (TNE).[45] With this technology, an unsedated examination of the esophagus and stomach is performed through a smaller scope. This may indeed lower the threshold for examination and biopsies being performed. TNE has been shown to be equivalent to standard sedated esophagoscopy for the detection of premalignant lesions of the esophagus,[46] so the patient may have the same diagnostic benefit with relative comfort and safety.[47]

TREATMENT OF REFLUX

Behavioral

In reviewing some of the key risk factors for reflux—tobacco use, alcohol, and diet—it is easy to see that the impact of behavior on GERD and LPR is immense. It is also easy to see why this disease may have a significant effect on the performer's voice. Mechanical measures, such as avoiding large or late meals and placing blocks under the bed frame to raise the head of the bed may be useful in many patients. Indeed, Hanson et al showed that behavioral treatment alone leads to clinical improvement but not necessarily resolution in over 50% of patients with chronic laryngitis.[48] In the same study, however, the response rates rose to over 70% and 95%, respectively, when histamine blockers (eg, ranitidine, cimetidine) or proton-pump inhibitors (eg, omeprazole) were used.

The damage to the vocal folds and larynx caused by irritant exposure may be multifactorial. Cigarette smoke promotes reflux by its effect on the LES; it may also alter regulatory protection of the UES and the glottis itself and subsequently make the smoker's larynx and upper airway more susceptible to reflux injury.[49,50] Despite the clear benefit from behavioral adjustment, these important measures are not usually sufficient in most patients, either due to the severity of the clinical issue or patient compliance.

Medical

Drugs are the mainstay of treatment for reflux.[3,51] The dominant class of therapeutics is the proton-pump inhibitors (PPI). The PPIs include omeprazole, lansoprazole, pantoprazole, rabeprazole, and esomeprazole. Although PPI treatment of laryngeal and pharyngeal dysfunction related to reflux is effective, several important points should be made. First, in many of the controlled studies investigating the treatment of LPR with PPIs, there may be significant resolution with observation or even a placebo effect.[52,53] In addition, as in many areas related to LPR, the treatment benefit has been controversial. Despite this, an empiric trial of twice-daily PPIs is not only considered reasonable *treatment* for suspected laryngeal and pharyngeal dysfunction related to reflux, it has been recommended as a reasonable *diagnostic* measure in the management of reflux.[36,44,54] A positive response to treatment confirms the clinical suspicion that the symptoms being treated are related to reflux.

As noted above, Hanson first demonstrated the clinical improvement in the treatment of chronic laryngitis in over 90% of patients treated with both behavior modification and PPIs.[48] Few authors have matched this success rate in controlled studies, although the results have been promising in many studies. There have been some notable limitations to the studies that have been executed; each adds a piece to the puzzle but few have comprehensive conclusions. One example may be illustrative; Steward et al published a prospective trial in 2004 in which a significant placebo response (as reported above) was detected after 2 months of blinded treatment[53]; interestingly, no difference was seen between the placebo and the twice-daily PPI treatment group in terms of laryngeal findings or symptomatology. Behavioral modification was found to be a strong predictor of improvement, however. Park and colleagues, on the other hand, reported significant improvements in another study when comparing twice-daily to once-daily treatment.[36] In the Park study, the treatment period was 4 months, with improvement occurring in the second 2-month period. Although this was not a blinded or placebo-controlled study, it does offer some insight into the impact of medical treatment and its effectiveness in suspected laryngeal manifestations of reflux.

Although there is no clear benefit of one PPI over the others, some comparative studies have demonstrated certain advantages such as speed of onset; in the management of a long-term issue such as LPR, it is likely that patient compliance with medication and

behavior are much more important than which pill is selected. One common error made is the timing of PPI therapy in relation to a meal. The ideal time is about 15 to 30 minutes prior to eating[55]; despite this, there remains a great deal of confusion among patients and practitioners which may in turn affect treatment.[56]

As a class, the PPIs have a tremendous track record for safety.[57] This fact is important for the performer who might shy away from pharmaceutical intervention in general. When negative effects occur, they are typically self-limiting, such as abdominal cramping and headache. The initial fear that long-term PPI use would lead to carcinoid tumors, as seen in early animal studies, have not been borne out.[58] Finally, another recent concern has been raised about the long-term effect of eliminating gastric acid and the subsequent effect on GI flora. It has been suggested that the nature and even the frequency of aspiration pneumonia may be affected in patients on acid suppression. In a recent investigation of the critically ill, the presence or absence of PPI treatment was not found to be an independent risk factor for the development of hospital-acquired pneumonia.[59]

The H2-blockers, such as ranitidine and cimetidine, provided important relief to patients prior to the advent of the PPIs in the late 1980s. They have largely been supplanted by the PPIs but may have a role in patients who do not tolerate the PPIs due to side effects or even cost. A resurgence of use of H2-blockers followed studies that demonstrated that they may be better for nocturnal acid breakthrough.[60,61] These studies resulted in many patients being on an additional dose of an H2-blocker at night in addition to twice-daily PPIs. Although this has not been well studied in patients with LPR, Park[36] showed that H2-blockers in patients with laryngeal and pharyngeal complaints did not add any benefit to a regime of twice-daily PPIs.

It is not known what the ideal duration of medical treatment is in the management of LPR. It is reasonable to treat patients for a minimum of 3 to 6 months if their clinical picture (history and laryngeal findings) is compelling. Certain predictors of treatment response, such as posterior laryngitis and vocal fold abnormalities,[36,48] may compel the treating physician to stay the course even if early results are not promising. It should be noted that improvement in physical findings may lag behind symptomatic improvement.[62] Once a patient has improved, a common course of action is to maintain the current regime and begin to taper therapy downward, from twice-daily to once-a-day. From that point, there is no established method for stopping therapy. Some practitioners discontinue medications completely, although patients should be warned to expect some transient rebound acidity.

Other important treatments include alginate preparations, such as found in Gaviscon (GlaxoSmithKline). Alginate serves as a mechanical antireflux barrier; this may reduce both acid and nonacid reflux events and impede the proximal migration of esophageal refluxate.[63] If taken in conjunction with PPIs, the low acid environment does not appear to impede alginate's ability to form a protective barrier against mucosal injury.[64]

Surgical

Surgical management of reflux is an evolving field. After initial enthusiasm, the role of operative intervention for reflux disease has waned somewhat. Many studies have shown benefit for patients with GERD; in patients with LPR, the outcomes have been generally positive, although not to the degree as for "typical" reflux symptoms. For the performing artist or professional vocalist, the additional considerations related to surgery, such as the need for translaryngeal and nasogastric intubation, must factor in the decision for referral to a surgeon.

Nissen fundoplication is the principal operation performed for the surgical management of reflux disease.[65] In this procedure, the fundus, or upper part of the stomach, is wrapped around the LES in the upper abdomen in order to achieve a snug lower esophageal valve mechanism (Figure 11–2A and 2B). It is performed laparoscopically in the vast majority of cases. So et al showed in 1998 that the outcomes of fundoplication for laryngeal and pharyngeal disease were not as great as in "typical" cases of GERD.[66] Nonetheless, a significant portion of these patients did benefit. Toohill and colleagues reported a higher success rate for symptom relief, with 26 of 29 LPR patients benefitting from fundoplication after one year.[67] Despite these promising results, it is not know what the long-term benefit of the procedures will be on patients with laryngeal and pharyngeal symptoms.

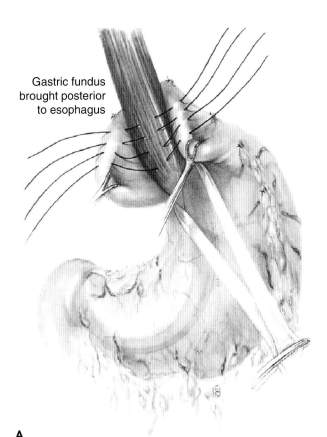

Gastric fundus brought posterior to esophagus

A.

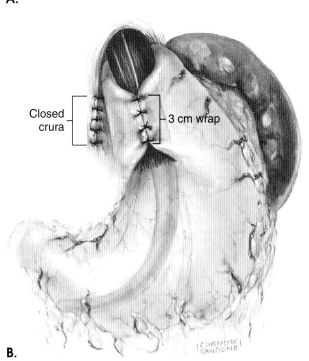

Closed crura

3 cm wrap

B.

Figure 11–2. Nissen fundoplication just before **A.** and after wrap **B.**

REFLUX OR REFLEX?

One theme that may serve to unite future discussions of reflux and its effect on the larynx is the neural inter-relatedness of the foregut and its derivatives (larynx, pharynx, esophagus, stomach).[5] It was noted earlier that smoking results in a two-fold impact on laryngeal injury; not only does it directly lower LES pressure, but smoking alters the natural neural protection by blunting the UES closure reflex. From a functional standpoint, the association of muscle tension dysphonia with reflux has been noted[68]; when significant vocal fold changes are noted, such as edema, it is easy to imagine the impact on phonation. When structural changes are minimal, it is possible that there are neural connections which contribute to this dysfunction. The esophagoglottal closure reflex[6] may be one example of such a connection. In this reflex, esophageal distension or acidification results in glottic closure. It is easy to see the protective nature of this function; taken to the extreme, this may be responsible for laryngospasm and even aberrant inspiratory closure, such as in paradoxical vocal fold dysfunction.[69,70] In a chronic or less severe form, glottic tension may be a direct result of esophageal afferent stimulus from reflux; this would be a mechanism by which reflux could contribute to laryngeal dysfunction without clinically apparent structural alteration to the organ itself. This is an area of active investigation.

SUMMARY

The reflux of gastric and duodenal contents into the esophagus, larynx, and pharynx occurs in many performers due to lifestyle, diet, and performance itself. Reflux is a significant and treatable source of laryngeal dysfunction causing performers to complain of hoarseness. Most patients with LPR present with dysphonia, throat clearing, and even a globus sensation. Laryngeal findings on examination, particularly as related to the vocal folds, are quite reliable and even predictive of treatment outcome.

Much controversy exists over the diagnosis and management of laryngeal dysfunction secondary to reflux. An important consideration is the variability of cell defenses against injury; perhaps identical acid exposures in larynges with differing resistance to injury results in varying levels of damage.

Diagnostic testing may include a 24-hour double pH probe and esophagoscopy; their exact role in the initial care of these patients is not clear. Endoscopy of the digestive tract is important for the evaluation of precancerous conditions. Patients with alarming indicators, such as dysphagia, weight loss, significant tobacco/alcohol use, or a strong family history, should be evaluated at the outset of symptoms.

On a practical level, empiric therapy with twice-daily proton-pump inhibitors is typically the appropriate first step in the management of suspected laryngopharyngeal reflux. Even long-term PPI treatment appears to be safe for the vast majority of patients. This approach should be maintained for at least 3 to 4 months in conjunction with an aggressive vocal hygiene regime. In patients with milder symptoms, once-daily therapy may be initiated. In time, it should be the goal of each physician to get the patient off the medications once they are no longer necessary. Antireflux surgery has little role in the initial or even early treatment of the performer. In patients with a good response to medication, Nissen fundoplication may be an option as an alternative to long-term medical therapy.

REFERENCES

1. Hicks DM, Ours TM, Abelson TI, Vaezi MF, Richter JE. The prevalence of hypopharynx findings associated with gastroesophageal reflux in normal volunteers. *J Voice.* 2002;16(4):564-579.
2. Vaezi MF. Laryngitis and gastroesophageal reflux disease: increasing prevalence or poor diagnostic tests? *Am J Gastroenterol.* 2004;99(5):786-788.
3. Altman KW, Stephens RM, Lyttle CS, Weiss KB. Changing impact of gastroesophageal reflux in medical and otolaryngology practice. *Laryngoscope.* 2005;115(7):1145-1153.
4. Reavis KM, Morris CD, Gopal DV, Hunter JG, Jobe BA. Laryngopharyngeal reflux symptoms better predict the presence of esophageal adenocarcinoma than typical gastroesophageal reflux symptoms. *Ann Surg.* 2004;239(6):849-856; discussion 856-858.

5. Shaker R, Hogan WJ. Normal physiology of the aerodigestive tract and its effect on the upper gut. *Am J Med.* 2003;115(Suppl 3A):2S-9S.

6. Shaker R, Dodds WJ, Ren J, Hogan WJ, Arndorfer RC. Esophagoglottal closure reflex: a mechanism of airway protection. *Gastroenterology.* 1992; 102(3):857-861.

7. Nebel OT, Fornes MF, Castell DO. Symptomatic gastroesophageal reflux: incidence and precipitating factors. *Am J Dig Dis.* 1976;21(11):953-956.

8. Locke GR, 3rd, Talley NJ, Fett SL, Zinsmeister AR, Melton LJ 3rd. Prevalence and clinical spectrum of gastroesophageal reflux: a population-based study in Olmsted County, Minnesota. *Gastroenterology.* 1997;112(5):1448-1156.

9. Vaezi MF, Richter JE. Duodenogastroesophageal reflux and methods to monitor nonacidic reflux. *Am J Med.* 2001;111(Suppl 8A):160S-168S.

10. Sasaki CT, Marotta J, Hundal J, Chow J, Eisen RN. Bile-induced laryngitis: is there a basis in evidence? *Ann Otol Rhinol Laryngol.* 2005;114(3):192-197.

11. Belafsky PC, Postma GN, The laryngeal and esophageal manifestations of Sjögren's syndrome. *Curr Rheumatol Rep.* 2003;5(4):297-303.

12. Knight RE, Wells JR, Parrish RS. Esophageal dysmotility as an important co-factor in extraesophageal manifestations of gastroesophageal reflux. *Laryngoscope.* 2000;110(9):1462-1466.

13. Koufman JA. Laryngopharyngeal reflux is different from classic gastroesophageal reflux disease. *Ear Nose Throat J.* 2002;81(9 Suppl 2):7-9.

14. Postma GN, Tomek MS, Belafsky PC, Koufman JA. Esophageal motor function in laryngopharyngeal reflux is superior to that in classic gastroesophageal reflux disease. *Ann Otol Rhinol Laryngol.* 2001;110(12):1114-1116.

15. Johnston N, Bulmer D, Gill GA, et al. Cell biology of laryngeal epithelial defenses in health and disease: further studies. *Ann Otol Rhinol Laryngol.* 2003;112(6):481-491.

16. Johnston N, Knight J, Dettmar PW, Lively MO, Koufman J. Pepsin and carbonic anhydrase isoenzyme III as diagnostic markers for laryngopharyngeal reflux disease. *Laryngoscope.* 2004;114(12): 2129-2134.

17. Sataloff R. *Professional Voice: The Science and Art of Clinical Care.* Vol 2. 3rd ed. San Diego, Calif: Plural Publishing; 2005:591-652.

18. Smith KJ, O'Brien SM, Smithers BM, et al. Interactions among smoking, obesity, and symptoms of acid reflux in Barrett's esophagus. *Cancer Epidemiol Biomarkers Prev.* 2005;14(11 pt 1): 2481-2486.

19. Stein DJ, El-Serag HB, Kuczynski J, Kramer JR, Sampliner RE. The association of body mass index with Barrett's oesophagus. *Aliment Pharmacol Ther.* 2005;22(10):1005-1010.

20. Halum SL, Postma GN, Johnston C, Belafsky PC, Koufman JA. Patients with isolated laryngopharyngeal reflux are not obese. *Laryngoscope.* 2005; 115(6):1042-1045.

21. Richter JE. Gastroesophageal reflux disease during pregnancy. *Gastroenterol Clin North Am.* 2003; 32(1):235-261.

22. Alvarez-Sanchez A, Rey E, Achem SR, Diaz-Rubio M. Does progesterone fluctuation across the menstrual cycle predispose to gastroesophageal reflux? *Am J Gastroenterol.* 1999;94(6):1468-1471.

23. Clark CS, Kraus BB, Sinclair J, Castell DO. Gastroesophageal reflux induced by exercise in healthy volunteers. *JAMA.* 1989;261(24):3599-3601.

24. Cammarota G, Elia F, Cianci R, Galli J, Paolillo N, Montalto M, Gasbarrini G. Worsening of gastroesophageal reflux symptoms in professional singers during performances. *J Clin Gastroenterol.* 2003; 36(5):403-404.

25. Bhatia V, Tandon RK. Stress and the gastrointestinal tract. *J Gastroenterol Hepatol.* 2005;20(3):332-339.

26. Naliboff BD, Mayer M, Fass R, et al. The effect of life stress on symptoms of heartburn. *Psychosom Med.* 2004;66(3):426-434.

27. Koufman JA. The otolaryngologic manifestations of gastroesophageal reflux disease (GERD): a clinical investigation of 225 patients using ambulatory 24-hour pH monitoring and an experimental investigation of the role of acid and pepsin in the development of laryngeal injury. *Laryngoscope.* 1991;101(4 pt 2 Suppl 53):1-78.

28. Koufman JA, Belafsky PC, Bach KK, Daniel E, Postma GN. Prevalence of esophagitis in patients with pH-documented laryngopharyngeal reflux. *Laryngoscope.* 2002;112(9):1606-1609.

29. Loehrl TA, Smith TL, Merati A, Torrico-Brusky L, Hoffman RG, Toohill RJ. Pharyngeal pH probe findings in patients with postnasal drainage. *Am J Rhinol.* 2005;19(4):340-343.

30. Belafsky PC, Postma GN, Koufman JA. Validity and reliability of the reflux symptom index (RSI). *J Voice.* 2002;16(2):274-277.

31. Hanson DG, Jiang J, Chi W. Quantitative color analysis of laryngeal erythema in chronic posterior laryngitis. *J Voice.* 1998;12(1):78-83.

32. Habermann W, Eherer A, Lindbichler F, Raith G, Friedrich G. Ex juvantibus approach for chronic posterior laryngitis: results of short-term pantoprazole therapy. *J Laryngol Otol.* 1999;113(8):734-739.

33. Belafsky PC, Postma GN, Koufman JA. The validity and reliability of the reflux finding score (RFS). *Laryngoscope.* 2001;111(8):1313-1317.

34. Oelschlager BK, Eubanks TR, Maronian N, et al. Laryngoscopy and pharyngeal pH are complementary in the diagnosis of gastroesophageal-laryngeal reflux. *J Gastrointest Surg.* 2002;6(2):189-194.

35. Branski RC, Bhattacharyya N, Shapiro J. The reliability of the assessment of endoscopic laryngeal findings associated with laryngopharyngeal reflux disease. *Laryngoscope.* 2002;112(6):1019-1024.

36. Park W, Hicks DM, Khandwala F, et al. Laryngopharyngeal reflux: prospective cohort study evaluating optimal dose of proton-pump inhibitor therapy and pretherapy predictors of response. *Laryngoscope.* 2005;115(7):1230-1238.

37. Merati AL, Lim HJ, Ulualp SO, Toohill RJ. Meta-analysis of upper probe measurements in normal subjects and patients with laryngopharyngeal reflux. *Ann Otol Rhinol Laryngol.* 2005;114(3):177-182.

38. Wong WM, Bautista J, Dekel R, et al. Feasibility and tolerability of transnasal/per-oral placement of the wireless pH capsule vs. traditional 24-h oesophageal pH monitoring—a randomized trial. *Aliment Pharmacol Ther.* 2005;21(2):155-163.

39. Tseng D, Rizvi AZ, Fennerty MB, et al. Forty-eight-hour pH monitoring increases sensitivity in detecting abnormal esophageal acid exposure. *J Gastrointest Surg.* 2005;9(8):1043-1052.

40. Bauman NM, Bishop WP, Sandler AD, Smith RJ. Value of pH probe testing in pediatric patients with extraesophageal manifestations of gastroesophageal reflux disease: a retrospective review. *Ann Otol Rhinol Laryngol Suppl.* 2000;184:18-24.

41. Vaezi MF. Therapy Insight: gastroesophageal reflux disease and laryngopharyngeal reflux. *Nat Clin Pract Gastroenterol Hepatol.* 2005;2(12):595-603.

42. Postma GN, Belafsky PC, Aviv JE, Koufman JA. Laryngopharyngeal reflux testing. *Ear Nose Throat J.* 2002;81(9 Suppl 2):14-18.

43. Kawamura O, Aslam M, Rittmann T, Hofmann C, Shaker R. Physical and pH properties of gastroesophagopharyngeal refluxate: a 24-hour simultaneous ambulatory impedance and pH monitoring study. *Am J Gastroenterol.* 2004;99(6):1000-1010.

44. Poelmans J, Feenstra L, Demedts I, Rutgeerts P, Tack J. The yield of upper gastrointestinal endoscopy in patients with suspected reflux-related chronic ear, nose, and throat symptoms. *Am J Gastroenterol.* 2004;99(8):1419-1426.

45. Postma GN, Cohen JT, Belafsky PC, et al. Transnasal esophagoscopy: revisited (over 700 consecutive cases). *Laryngoscope.* 2005;115(2):321-323.

46. Saeian K, Staff DM, Vasilopoulos S, et al. Unsedated transnasal endoscopy accurately detects Barrett's metaplasia and dysplasia. *Gastrointest Endosc.* 2002;56(4):472-478.

47. Sharma A, Price T, MierzwaK, Montgomery P, Qayyum A, Bradnam T. Transnasal flexible laryngo-oesophagoscopy: an evaluation of the patient's experience. *J Laryngol Otol.* 2006;120(1):24-31.

48. Hanson DG, Kamel PL, Kahrilas PJ. Outcomes of antireflux therapy for the treatment of chronic laryngitis. *Ann Otol Rhinol Laryngol.* 1995;104(7):550-555.

49. Dua K, Bardan E, Ren J, Sui Z, Shaker R. Effect of chronic and acute cigarette smoking on the pharyngo-upper oesophageal sphincter contractile reflex and reflexive pharyngeal swallow. *Gut.* 1998;43(4):537-541.

50. Dua K, Bardan E, Ren J, Sui Z, Shaker R. Effect of chronic and acute cigarette smoking on the pharyngoglottal closure reflex. *Gut.* 2002;51(6):771-775.

51. Book DT, Rhee JS, Toohill RJ, Smith TL. Perspectives in laryngopharyngeal reflux: an international survey. *Laryngoscope.* 2002;112(8 pt 1):1399-1406.

52. Eherer AJ, Habermann W, Hammer HF, Kiesler K, Friedrich G, Krejs GJ. Effect of pantoprazole on the course of reflux-associated laryngitis: a placebo-controlled double-blind crossover study. *Scand J Gastroenterol.* 2003;38(5):462-467.

53. Steward DL, Wilson KM, Kelly DH, et al. Proton pump inhibitor therapy for chronic laryngo-pharyngitis: a randomized placebo-control trial. *Otolaryngol Head Neck Surg.* 2004;131(4):342-350.

54. Gaynor EB. Laryngeal complications of GERD. *J Clin Gastroenterol.* 2000;30(3 Suppl):S31-S34.

55. Richter JE. Medical management of patients with esophageal or supraesophageal gastroesophageal reflux disease. *Am J Med.* 2003;115(Suppl 3A):179S-187S.

56. Barrison AF, Jarboe LA, Weinberg BM, Nimmagadda K, Sullivan LM, Wolfe MM. Patterns of proton

pump inhibitor use in clinical practice. *Am J Med.* 2001;111(6):469–473.

57. Reilly JP. Safety profile of the proton-pump inhibitors. *Am J Health Syst Pharm.* 1999;56(23 Suppl 4):S11–S17.

58. Robinson M. Review article: current perspectives on hypergastrinaemia and enterochromaffin-like-cell hyperplasia. *Aliment Pharmacol Ther.* 1999; 13(Suppl 5):5–10.

59. Mallow S, Rebuck JA, Osler T, Ahern J, Healey MA, Rogers FB. Do proton pump inhibitors increase the incidence of nosocomial pneumonia and related infectious complications when compared with histamine-2 receptor antagonists in critically ill trauma patients? *Curr Surg.* 2004;61(5): 452–458.

60. Peghini PL, Katz PO, Castell DO. Ranitidine controls nocturnal gastric acid breakthrough on omeprazole: a controlled study in normal subjects. *Gastroenterology.* 1998;115(6):1335–1339.

61. Xue S, Katz PO, Banerjee P, Tutuian R, Castell DO. Bedtime H2 blockers improve nocturnal gastric acid control in GERD patients on proton pump inhibitors. *Aliment Pharmacol Ther.* 2001;15(9): 1351–1356.

62. Belafsky PC, Postma GN, Koufman JA. Laryngopharyngeal reflux symptoms improve before changes in physical findings. *Laryngoscope.* 2001;111(6): 979–981.

63. Zentilin P, Dulbecco P, Savarino E, et al. An evaluation of the antireflux properties of sodium alginate by means of combined multichannel intraluminal impedance and pH-metry. *Aliment Pharmacol Ther.* 2005;21(1):29–34.

64. Dettmar PW, Little SL, Baxter T. The effect of omeprazole pre-treatment on rafts formed by reflux suppressant tablets containing alginate. *J Int Med Res.* 2005;33(3):301–308.

65. Westcott CJ, Hopkins MB, Bach K, Postma GN, Belafsky PC, Koufman JA. Fundoplication for laryngopharyngeal reflux disease. *J Am Coll Surg.* 2004;199(1):23–30.

66. So JB, Zeitels SM, Rattner DW. Outcomes of atypical symptoms attributed to gastroesophageal reflux treated by laparoscopic fundoplication. *Surgery.* 1998;124(1):28–32.

67. Lindstrom DR, Wallace J, Loehrl TA, Merati AL, Toohill RJ. Nissen fundoplication surgery for extraesophageal manifestations of gastroesophageal reflux (EER). Nissen fundoplication surgery for extraesophageal manifestations of gastroesophageal reflux (EER). *Laryngoscope.* 2002;112(10): 1762–1765.

68. Altman KW, Atkinson C, Lazarus C. Current and emerging concepts in muscle tension dysphonia: a 30-month review. *J Voice.* 2005;19(2):261–267.

69. Patel NJ, Jorgensen C, Kuhn J, Merati AL. Concurrent laryngeal abnormalities in patients with paradoxical vocal fold dysfunction. *Otolaryngol Head Neck Surg.* 2004;130(6):686–689.

70. Maschka DA, Bauman NM, McCray PB, Jr, Hoffman HT, Karnell MP, Smith RJ. A classification scheme for paradoxical vocal cord motion. *Laryngoscope.* 1997;107(11 pt 1):1429–1435.

Chapter 12

ELECTROMYOGRAPHY FOR THE SINGER'S VOICE

Glendon M. Gardner

Electromyography (EMG) is the measurement of electrical activity within muscles achieved by inserting a needle into the muscle fibers. Contraction of a muscle fiber is associated with changes in the electrical potential across the cell membrane wall. The needle is connected to an oscilloscope, which provides a graphic display of the electrical activity at the needle tip as well as audio output. Both are important in interpreting the test.

Abnormalities of the central nervous system, the peripheral nerves, and the muscles themselves will yield characteristic findings on EMG.

Laryngeal electromyography (LEMG) is applied in otolaryngology for a few select reasons:

1. Diagnosis of a paralyzed vocal fold versus a fixed vocal fold.
2. Diagnosis of neurologic disease (upper motor neuron versus lower motor neuron).
3. Site of lesion determination: vagus nerve versus superior and/or recurrent laryngeal nerves.
4. Prognosis in the case of a paralyzed vocal fold:
   a. Will the vocal fold function recover?
   b. Will it recover completely?
   c. When will it recover?
5. Biofeedback.
6. Intraoperative monitoring during cervical surgery.
7. Confirming placement of the needle in a muscle for Botox injection.

In the context of a singer, the application of LEMG is very similar to its use in the general population. Singers are just as likely to suffer from neurologic diseases, idiopathic vocal fold paralysis, and trauma to the neck as nonsingers. For nonsingers, the prognosis for vocal fold function recovery may not be as critical as for singers, as nonsingers can often function in their vocation without an optimal voice. For the singer, then, LEMG may often be used whereas the nonsinger may choose to simply wait for recovery rather than employ LEMG to prognosticate.

The use of LEMG during cervical surgery (thyroidectomy, anterior cervical approach to the cervical vertebrae, carotid endarterectomy) is not standard. Endotracheal tubes with integrated LEMG electrodes help monitor stimulation of the vagus and recurrent laryngeal nerves.[1] A singer may request such monitoring to help lessen the likelihood of injury to the nerves during such surgery. The stakes are certainly higher in the professional singer in these cases than in the nonprofessional.

One of the most useful applications of LEMG is localization of muscles for Botox injections, which are typically performed for spasmodic dysphonia (SD), an uncommon neurologic disease of the larynx characterized by episodes of spasm of the vocal folds. As SD is uncommon in the population at large, it would also be expected to be uncommon in professional singers. There are other professional voice users with SD. One well-known radio talk show host regularly undergoes Botox injections to control her adductor spasmodic dysphonia and her career continues successfully.[2] LEMG allows for confirmation of the placement of the tip of the needle in the vocalis muscle to ensure proper injection of the Botox.

BASIC ELECTROMYOGRAPHY

The basic unit of neuromuscular function is the single motor unit. One neuron innervates a specific number or array of muscle fibers. When the neuron fires, a group of muscle fibers contract simultaneously. The result is a single motor unit action potential which has specific characteristics. The motor unit constitutes the smallest functional element of contraction.[3]

When interpreting LEMG, we generally look at several characteristics: presence of normal motor units, recruitment patterns, insertional activity, presence of fibrillation potentials, positive sharp waves, and polyphasic waveforms.

When the normal patient exerts more effort, more units will be recruited to contribute to the contraction, which results in the recruitment or interference pattern. Absence of any recruitment indicates that there is no communication between the cerebral cortex and the muscle. This is a bad sign and may mean that the nerve to the vocal fold has been cut. If recruitment is reduced, then the nerve is definitely still intact, but not functioning at 100% activity.

When a nerve is severely injured and no longer sending impulses to the muscle fiber, that muscle is denervated. Denervated muscle is unstable, which leads to several characteristic findings on EMG. When the needle is inserted into the muscle, it destabilizes the fiber and, being inherently unstable, it takes longer than usual for the fiber to re-establish its normal electrical potential across the membrane, resulting in prolonged insertional activity. This unstable muscle fiber may fire spontaneously and sporadically yielding fibrillation potentials (fibs) or positive sharp waves (PSW). These findings are indicative of denervation and do not bode well for recovery of normal function. Although lack of recruitment will be seen immediately after an injury, fibs and PSW do not appear until 10 to 14 days after injury.

If a nerve has been injured, the axons have been disrupted in some way. As the nerve recovers, the axons may reconnect with muscle fibers in a disorganized pattern rather than the very precise organization before injury. The resultant waveform is broader or longer on the time scale with more deflections and is known as a polyphasic waveform.[4] This is a sign of reinnervation (see Table 12–1).

LARYNGEAL ELECTROMYOGRAPHY PROCEDURE

Diagnostic LEMG is often performed in the Neurology EMG suite with a neurologist certified in EMG. LEMG can be performed via the transoral or percutaneous route. The transoral route is done with curved needles and a laryngeal mirror or telescope. It requires more cooperation from the patient, but one can be more certain of the location of the needle. The more common route is percutaneously. The needle is inserted

Table 12–1. Electromyography Waveforms and Their Significance

Insertional Activity	Spontaneous Activity	Volitional Activity	Significance
Fibrillation potential Prolonged activity	Fibrillation potential PSW	No recruitment	Denervation
Brief activity	None	Decreased recruitment Polyphasic MUPs	Reinnervation
Brief activity	None	Normal recruitment	Normal

PSW, positive sharp wave; MUP, motor unit potential.

through the skin overlying the cricothyroid membrane where it can access both the cricothyroid and thyroarytenoid (vocalis) muscles (see Figure 12–1). This is a more consistently successful technique and requires little patient cooperation, but is a blind technique with less assurance that the needle is properly located.

The muscles usually tested are the thyroarytenoid (TA), innervated by the recurrent laryngeal nerve (RLN), and the cricothyroid (CT), innervated by the superior laryngeal nerve (SLN).[5] The TA is active with phonation and cough and silent during quiet respiration. The CT demonstrates low activity during low-pitch phonation and increased activity during high-pitch phonation. The posterior cricoarytenoid, which is responsible for opening or abducting the vocal folds, is also innervated by the RLN, but is not often tested. It is accessible by rotating the larynx and approaching laterally. It is relatively silent during phonation and active with sniffing and respiration.

In many clinics, an otolaryngologist inserts the EMG needles while a neurologist interprets the waveforms. There are experienced members of both specialties who are competent to do the entire procedure themselves.[5] Working together, however, provides an excellent environment for education for both groups and takes advantage of the strengths of both specialties.

Potential complications of LEMG include hematoma of the skin and/or vocal fold, mucosal laceration, or infection. These are considered "potential" complications because the author has never seen any of these

nor are they reported in the literature. In fact, Parnes, who published one of the first reports on LEMG for prognosis, had a 0% complication rate, and complications are rarely mentioned in subsequent articles on the subject.[6] But, they must be considered, especially in the professional performer. By withdrawing the needle before repositioning the tip, the serious potential complications of lacerations and bleeding can be avoided.

INDICATIONS FOR LARYNGEAL ELECTROMYOGRAPHY

As stated at the beginning of this chapter, there are various reasons to perform LEMG. The most common is when a vocal fold is immobile or severely hypomobile. This topic is covered in detail in another chapter. The contribution of LEMG to the workup can be critical.

Occasionally, the cause and severity of the vocal fold immobility (VFI) is known, such as the sacrifice of the RLN during surgery for thyroid or lung cancer. In this case, recovery of normal RLN function will not occur and LEMG is unnecessary. Most cases, however, are not so clear. After surgery of the neck or chest, the vocal fold may be immobile, but the surgeon is confident that the RLN is intact. In other cases, a patient may awaken with a breathy voice, feeling otherwise completely healthy, or perhaps with upper respiratory

Figure 12–1. Laryngeal procedure. The bipolar concentric needle is inserted through the skin at the cricothyroid membrane where it can be directed toward the cricothyroid muscle or inserted through the membrane to access the thyroarytenoid muscles.

tract infection symptoms. The patient is noted to have an immobile vocal fold. The workup in these latter patients is first aimed at determining the cause of the VFI.[7] The cause of a vocal fold paralysis is often a much more important health issue for a patient than the paralysis itself.[8]

The vagus nerve (cranial nerve X) exits the skull base via the jugular foramen and descends in the neck. It sends a branch to the pharyngeal plexus, which innervates the soft palate and the pharyngeal constrictors. Still high in the neck, it gives off the superior laryngeal nerve which splits into an extrinsic branch, which supplies motor innervation to the cricothyroid muscle, and the intrinsic branch, which supplies sensory innervation to the supraglottis. The vagus nerve continues down into the chest where the recurrent laryngeal nerve arises at the level of the subclavian artery on the right and the aortic arch on the left. While the course of the vagus nerve terminates at the stomach, the RLN returns (or recurs) to the neck along the tracheoesophageal groove en route to the larynx

where it supplies motor innervation to the intrinsic muscles of the larynx and sensory innervation to the glottis and subglottis (see Figure 12–2).

The physical examination can sometimes tell us if there is a high vagal lesion by noting activity of the palate. Assessing the status of the superior laryngeal nerve purely with the physical examination is not consistent. LEMG can determine the site of the lesion and guide the remainder of the workup by differentiating between an isolated TA paralysis (indicating a RLN lesion) or a combined TA and CT paralysis (indicating a problem within the neck, but not the chest). When the problem is in the neck, evaluation of the skull base and neck with imaging will reveal any serious causes, such as tumors. With an isolated RLN problem, the focus should be on the neck and chest. In most practices, however, LEMG is not used early in the workup. Most clinicians will proceed with a thorough radiologic workup first.

Unless a dislocated arytenoid is strongly suspected, LEMG should not be done before 2 weeks after onset.

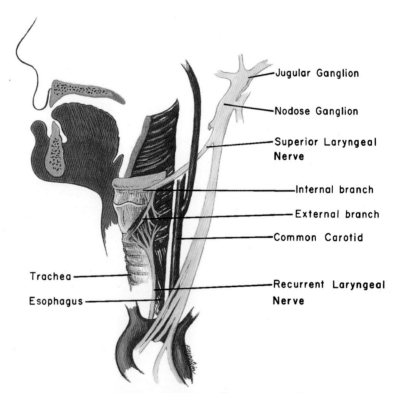

Figure 12–2. Course of the vagus and laryngeal nerves. (Reprinted with permission from Benninger M, Gardner GM, Schwimmer C, Divi M. Laryngeal neurophysiology. In: Rubin J, Sataloff RT, Korovin G. eds. *Diagnosis and Treatment of Voice Disorders.* 3rd ed. San Diego, Calif: Plural Publishing; 2006:109.)

This allows the development of fibrillation potentials which indicate denervation. If done earlier, it is sometimes difficult to know whether there is electrical silence due to denervation or the needle may have simply missed the thyroarytenoid muscle.

A traumatic intubation is considered the most likely cause of an acute arytenoid dislocation.[9,10] Scarring of the cricoarytenoid joint (due to long-term intubation or inflammatory disease such as rheumatoid arthritis) will also cause VFI. In these cases the vocal fold is immobile and the LEMG is normal.

After determining whether the vocal fold is, in fact, immobile due to a neural injury, LEMG may provide a prognosis of neural function recovery. Important factors to consider when performing LEMG for prognosis are the timing of the exam relative to the onset of the injury and the findings, especially the waveforms discussed earlier.[4,6,11,12]

Seeing recruitment and normal or polyphasic motor unit potentials is a good prognostic sign and indicates the nerve is intact, although not functioning normally. The earlier this is seen after onset, say at 2 months, the more likely the vocal fold is to recover motion. With the same positive LEMG findings at 6 months, but still an immobile vocal fold, there is less likelihood of recovery of motion. Fibs, PSW, and lack of recruitment are all bad prognostic signs. These findings at 6 months are more predictive of lack of recovery than at 2 months. In general, negative results are more accurately predictive of functional outcome than positive results.

It is important to know that recovery of electrical activity does not necessarily lead to recovery of normal vocal fold motion. Abnormal reinnervation may occur with neurons that should stimulate muscles that abduct the vocal folds connecting with muscles that adduct or tense the vocal folds and vice versa. This results in synkinesis of the laryngeal muscles, which would cause the vocal fold to have good tone, but remain immobile.[13,14] This abnormal reinnervation and resultant synkinesis is probably the main reason that LEMG is not as accurate in predicting prognosis as we would like it to be.

The literature on LEMG has mostly focused on the prognostic aspect of the technique. Unfortunately, the various studies lack much standardization and the results of these studies reflect that inconsistency. There are studies that demonstrate 100% predictive

value with certain findings and others that show little correlation.[15] The basic guidelines just discussed are the most important to remember.

VOCAL FOLD PARESIS AND SUPERIOR LARYNGEAL NERVE PALSY

For most patients undergoing LEMG, the symptoms and physical findings are obvious. The voice is very rough or breathy and the vocal fold is immobile. Singers, however, can have very subtle abnormalities that cause them significant problems. Two conditions that can do this while being difficult to diagnose are vocal fold paresis and superior laryngeal nerve injury.

Paresis means that a muscle is working at less than 100% activity. This can occur after a formerly paralyzed vocal fold has partially recovered or it can occur without the vocal fold having been completely paralyzed. The causes of the latter situation are not clear. A patient with vocal fold paresis may note a slight breathiness always or perhaps just after much use. Loss of range or early vocal fatigue may be the presenting symptoms as well as diplophonia and odynophonia. Initial physical examination often seems normal. Sometimes a slight asymmetry of vocal fold motion, vocal fold bowing, or a small glottal gap are apparent. Some patients will develop compensatory hyperkinetic disorders with excessive compression of the false vocal folds. These hyperkinetic conditions can mask the fact that the underlying problem is one of hypokinesis.[16] Videostroboscopy is extremely helpful in this situation.[17]

Signs of paresis on LEMG include decreased recruitment or decreased amplitude of MUPs. Occasionally signs of reinnervation (polyphasic motor unit potentials) will be seen. The results of electromyography are not easily quantified and this point is particularly true with paresis. Often the only sign of an abnormality is the difference in recruitment between the two thyroarytenoid muscles. When the differences are minimal, this can be a difficult and somewhat subjective judgement. Additionally, the technique, specifically needle placement within the muscle, can influence the results and cloud the diagnosis. An experienced laryngeal electromyographer can make this diagnosis, however. Once paresis has been diagnosed, the patient should undergo voice therapy and, if indicated, surgery. This is discussed in another chapter.

Superior laryngeal nerve palsy is another condition that is difficult to diagnose. This can occur from an injury during thyroid or parathyroid surgery, from external trauma, or after an upper respiratory infection. It can also be a sign of other neurologic disease.[18] The cricothyroid muscle is responsible for bringing the anterior aspects of the thyroid and cricoid cartilages together, thereby stretching and tightening the vocal folds. Loss of this ability leads to the complaint of loss of the upper range, something much more problematic for singers than for nonsingers. A variety of other less specific voice complaints may be present as well. There is disagreement as to whether the physical examination can reliably diagnose SLN palsy.[19-21] Asymmetric tilting of the epiglottis during high-pitch phonation and bowing of an otherwise mobile true vocal fold are some of the signs considered indicative of SLN palsy. Vocal fold lag (sluggish motion) was the most consistent finding in a series of 126 LEMG confirmed cases of superior laryngeal paresis or paralysis.[18] Decreased sensation of the supraglottis, due to dysfunction of the internal branch of the SLN, supports the diagnosis of SLN paresis or paralysis.

LEMG can show obvious evidence of denervation or, as in the case of true vocal fold paresis discussed above, less obvious signs of paresis of the cricothyroid muscle. Once the diagnosis is confirmed and the etiology determined, the singer should undergo voice therapy. Some patients will develop compensatory muscle tension dysphonia that can be even more detrimental, in the long run, than the SLN problem. Treatment of this problem is discussed in chapter 17.

Patients who present with dysphonia and any signs of vocal fold motion abnormalities should be evaluated with LEMG. Although LEMG alone will not answer all the questions, it can be a powerful tool used in conjuction with others in managing these patients.[22-24]

REFERENCES

1. Hermann M, Hellebart C, Freissmuth M. Neuromonitoring in thyroid surgery: prospective evaluation of intraoperative electrophysiological responses for the prediction of recurrent laryngeal nerve injury.[see comment]. *Ann Surg.* 2004;240:9–17.
2. Rehm D. *Finding My Voice.* Herndon, Va: Capital Books, Inc; 1999.
3. Kimura, J. *Electrodiagnosis in Diseases of Nerve and Muscle.* 2nd ed. Philadelphia, Pa: FA Davis; 1989.
4. Koufman JA, Postma GN, Whang CS, et al. Diagnostic laryngeal electromyography: The Wake Forest experience 1995-1999. *Otolaryngol Head Neck Surg.* 2001;124:603–606.
5. Halum SL, Patel N, Smith TL, Jaradeh S, Toohill RJ, Merati AL. Laryngeal electromyography for adult unilateral vocal fold immobility: a survey of the American Broncho-Esophagological Association. *Ann Otol Rhinol Laryngol.* 2005;114:425–428.
6. Parnes SM, Satya-Murti S. Predictive value of laryngeal electromyography in patients with vocal fold paralysis of neurogenic origin. *Laryngoscope.* 1985; 95:1323–1326.
7. Benninger MS, Crumley RL, Ford CN, et al. Evaluation and treatment of the unilateral paralyzed vocal fold. *Otolaryngol Head Neck Surg.* 1994; 111:497–508.
8. Gardner GM, Shaari C, Parnes S. Long-term morbidity and mortality in patients undergoing surgery for unilateral vocal cord paralysis. *Laryngoscope.* 1992;102:501–508.
9. Sataloff RT. Arytenoid dislocation: techniques of surgical reduction. *Op Tech Otolaryngol Head Neck Surg.* 1998;9:196–202.
10. Rubin AD, Hawkshaw MJ, Moyer CA, Dean C, Sataloff RT. Arytenoid cartilage dislocation: a 20 year experience. *J Voice.* 2005;19:687–701.
11. Munin MC, Murray T, Rosen CA. Laryngeal electromyography: diagnostic and prognostic applications. *Otolaryngol Clin North Am.* 2000;33:759–770.
12. Sittel C, Stennert E, Thumfart WF, Dapunt U, Eckel HE. Prognostic value of laryngeal electromyography in vocal fold paralysis. *Arch Otolaryngol Head Neck Surg.* 2001;127:155–160.
13. Crumley RL. Laryngeal synkinesis revisited. *Ann Otol Rhinol Laryngol.* 2000;109:365–371.
14. Benjamin B. Vocal cord paralysis. *ANZ J Surg.* 2003;73:784–786.
15. Sataloff RT, Mandel S, Mann EA, Ludlow CL. Practice parameter: laryngeal electromyography (an evidence-based review). *Otolaryngol Head Neck Surg.* 2004;130:770–779.
16. Koufman JA, Postma GN, Cummins MM, Blalock PD. Vocal fold paresis. *Otolaryngol Head Neck Surg.* 2000;122:537–541.

17. Rubin AD, Praneetvatakul V, Heman-Ackah Y, et al. Repetitive phonatory tasks for identifying vocal fold paresis. *J Voice.* 2005;19:679-686.

18. Dursun G, Sataloff RT, Spiegel JR, Mandel S, Heuer RJ, Rosen DC. Superior laryngeal nerve paresis and paralysis. *J Voice.* 1996;10:206-211.

19. Koufman JA, Walker FO, Joharji GM. The cricothyroid muscle does not influence vocal fold position in laryngeal paralysis. *Laryngoscope.* 1995;105:368-372.

20. Woodson GE. Configuration of the glottis in laryngeal paralysis. I. Clinical study. *Laryngoscope.* 1994;103:1227-1234.

21. Woodson GE, Murry MP, Schweizer V, Hengesteg, Chen N, Yeung D. Unilateral cricothyroid contraction and glottic configuration. *J Voice.* 1998;12:335-339.

22. Altman KW. Laryngeal asymmetry on indirect laryngoscopy in a symptomatic patient should be evaluated with electromyography. *Arch Otolaryngol Head Neck Surg.* 2005;131:356-359.

23. Postma GN. The promise of LEMG. *Arch Otolaryngol Head Neck Surg.* 2005;131:359.

24. Sulica L. LEMG and laryngeal asymmetry. *Arch Otolaryngol Head Neck Surg.* 2005;131:359-360.

Chapter 13

ACUTE ASSESSMENT OF PROFESSIONAL SINGERS

Josef Schlömicher-Thier
Matthias Weikert

Professional singing must be regarded as a high-performance sport; it requires special training conditions and top physical performance. Singing is an athletic activity and as such requires good physical fitness and coordinated interaction. The vocal mechanism is a finely tuned, complex instrument. Maladies of any part of the body may be reflected in the voice and undermine the power source of the voice. Inappropriate compensation maneuvers result in vocal dysfunction. Stricken by sudden illness, the professional singer is under enormous time pressure, as the première sets him a precise deadline. In case of illness, a variety of individual factors arise. The decision to recast is made more difficult by responsibility toward the other members of the cast, anxiety on the part of the management, exertion of influence by the conductor and the director; recording contracts are tempting, and—last but not least—the audience wishes to see a radiant hero or heroine. In such cases the physician in attendance assumes a high degree of responsibility. It is his or her duty to protect the singer affected by a disorder from further damage which might have a fatal effect on the singer's future career. The physician must also devise an effective treatment algorithm that will enable the patient to make full use of his or her voice again within the shortest possible time. Any unduly prolonged "voice rest for safety" entails unnecessary cancellations. The singer risks losing income and even

further contracts. On the other hand, a rest time that is too short will also constitute a danger. Finding the adequate treatment variables requires knowledge of the performer's world. This chapter presents the findings from a major laryngology practice in Austria where singers come from around the world to perform under demanding conditions. The examinations are often done in the theater or acutely in the office.

Professional singers are expected to meet very special demands. As freelance artists, they may have a full diary of engagements in opera houses and at music festivals all over the world, and only air travel enables them to attend rehearsals in one place and concerts in another. This demands a stable physical and psycho-emotional constitution, a first-class vocal and musical training in a **clearly defined vocal category**, and great flexibility in adapting to new situations in stage-direction and casting.

Demanding roles with text and music to learn require timely (if sometimes brief) preparation before the start of rehearsals. But professional singers are subject to illness from the same causes as other people, such as acute viral and bacterial infection, allergies, faulty diet, environmental influences at work (on stage), side effects of medication, hormonal factors (especially for female singers), psychological strain due to family or social circumstances, personal crises, overwork, and overexertion in the course of working life.

WHAT IS EXPECTED OF A VOICE DOCTOR WHO LOOKS AFTER SINGERS?

The voice doctor has to be aware of the possible causes that can put the singer's voice at risk and damage a singing career. He or she has to know the heavy demands made on the singer in respect of physical and psychological strain, artistic sensibility, individuality, and empathy for the greatest possible expressive capability and interpretation. He or she will know from experience that the ever increasing strain on "jet-setting" singers includes frequent change of location in air-conditioned airplanes, living in dry and often noisy hotel rooms with a variety of allergens, and adverse atmospheric conditions on stage (dust, heat, sensitizing substances). All these factors make the vocal organs particularly susceptible to the harmful influences mentioned above.

THE SITUATION OF THE VOICE DOCTOR—HOW TO PROCEED IN A VOCAL EMERGENCY

The primary concern is the singer's medical history, which must be ascertained even under extreme circumstances and pressure of time. The overall condition of the singer is of prime importance to determine voice capacity. The vocal and physical demands of the performance in question—that is, the theatre, concert hall, or festival must always be taken into account.

Specific Questions

Time of indisposition—gradual or possibly chronic preceding symptoms

Nature and severity of the reaction to the disorder and its effect on the voice

Medication taken

Personal disposition and estimate of current stress

Point in menstrual cycle for female singers under vocal stress

Environmental influences (also on stage) which might lead to acute vocal and physical reactions or decompensation and thus indisposition.

Cancellation Policy

The voice doctor is the mediator between the singer and the manager of the opera house or festival. He must show circumspect empathy for the well-being of the singer, while retaining the confidence of both sides—singer and manager. Overprotective "safety advice" at every incipient infection ("Better stay at home for a week, and then we'll see how you're doing") only causes both sides to lose out: the singer loses his or her fee and the manager has to pay for a replacement.

Only if the physician, the singer, and the manager collaborate in the best interests of the singer's situation, is it possible to find a suitable solution in an emergency. Reorganizing rehearsal schedules, or possibly hiring a "standby" replacement to sing in the orchestra pit while the indisposed singer acts out the complicated movements on stage should be considered. It is also important for the physician to inform the manager as soon as possible that a replacement or a standby may be required. This way, the singer is relieved of the burden of responsibility and the manager is placed under less pressure. On account of the economic pressure of today's concert and festival business, the motto here can be quite realistic: **Save the singer's fee, but avoid health risks.**

THE VOICE DOCTOR'S ROLE IN THE TREATMENT OF SINGERS

Medical care at the workplace (theater stage/concert platform) may be required from time to time. ENT medical examination for the purpose of establishing the vocal constitution and suitability for the part played in the performance may be necessary.

Professional and competent application of vocal physiology for the patient at the workplace, although difficult, must be considered as part of the voice doctor's role. In general, the physician does not make artistic judgments nor influence the singer, but should guide and lead with the greatest possible empathy in emergency situations when decisions have to be made regarding disposition or indisposition. Singers are usually extremely able-bodied and efficient—a "class apart" in health.

PSYCHOPHYSICAL AND PSYCHOSOMATIC BACKGROUND OF THE ENDANGERED ARTIST

If this robust quality of the singer is endangered by acute infection, psychological disturbance, or overtaxing of the vocal capacity, as for instance through a heavy rehearsal schedule or difficult repertoire, then the singer no longer feels able to operate at maximum efficiency, which is necessarily the basic approach to artistic performance. This means that even the slightest disturbance will automatically put the singer in a stress situation in which he or she may show physical and psychological reactions that create additional strain. At this point the professional will immediately ask whether he or she "can sing at all," and is thus in a borderline situation where realistic self-assessment is no longer possible.

Factors Triggering the Stress Situation

These include chronic, initially slight disorders which may decompensate, acute infections, vocal difficulties either occurring acutely during performance or of longer duration. Worrying about domestic circumstances due to frequent changes of venue, and often strenuous travel entailing separation from family also contribute to the singer's stress. Workplace problems on stage or concert platform through conflicts with directors, stage partners, or ensemble colleagues may contribute or increase an already stressed individual.

Factors such as the psychophysical reserves of the patient are important to assess. The patient may activate his or her own physical and psychological reserves sufficiently to feel capable of singing the performance, or may lapse into uncertainty that may affect the voice adversely so that an indisposition threatens, in which case a phoniatrician, or voice specialist, will be required for emergency treatment. The physician must be aware that the singer has doubts about being able to sing the performance, as even a slight cold coupled with the fear of indisposition can lead to considerable feelings of stress. If we look at the increase in these feelings of stress as the performance draws near, we can imagine how nervous the singer becomes, and the consequent increase in physical symptoms, such as muscular tension. The voice—always a highly sensitive indicator of emotion—threatens to fail. Pressure and tension heighten and the singer decides in sudden panic that he cannot sing. The pressure is considerable—the audience is arriving, the curtain will soon rise.

In this crisis, the singer shows signs of regression. He or she feels weakened, exposed, overwhelmed and threatened by the situation. Feeling helpless, he or she relinquishes part of his independence and lapses into regression. This regressive phase projects the patient back into childhood, so that he is prepared to accept help from a parent-figure, in this case the voice specialist.

The **singer in regression** looks for help, security, and guidance; indeed, he or she demands it, though not in so many words. This is now the important task and the opportunity for the voice doctor. The more the singer abdicates his or her independence in this situation, and the more he lapses into crippling regression, the more the physician can assume guidance, which in turn demands great empathy.

The voice doctor has to put him- or herself psychologically in the situation of the singer, whose inner monologue goes something like this: Does the doctor recognize my weakness, does he understand my fear? I'm ashamed and frightened of disgracing myself in my eyes and those of the others and the audience. The physician has to approach the singer at this psychological low point with complete openness and self-effacement, but with a clear mandate for guidance. The doctor shows the singer that he or she understands his helplessness and takes him seriously, that the singer need not feel ashamed, that no one finds him ridiculous. In this extreme situation of having to accept basically undesired medical help, the singer is encouraged to retain his dignity. Thus, in this phase, the singer must feel that the doctor is competent to help, and absolute discretion is necessary.

Once this psychological block is overcome, one can proceed to the actual medical examination, in order to reach a clear evaluation and decision as to whether in this situation sufficient fortification and therapy can be provided in time for the patient to sing the role on stage.

Medical Examination

The voice doctor has to carry out a series of tasks to make the diagnosis and develop a treatment plan that is appropriate for the time. This includes the following tasks:

Ascertaining the patient's medical history;

Obtaining information on symptoms that might point to a general disorder;

Evaluating the singer's psychological and physical situation;

Making a specific ENT-oriented diagnosis with a rapid assessment of vocal problems;

Reaching a clear decision on moderate therapeutic measures appropriate to the situation;

Maintaining contact with those responsible for the impending performance such as manager, conductor, technical team, and possibly other singers and ensemble members.

The medical history often has to be established quickly. An important question here is whether the singer has had similar experiences of singing with this kind of indisposition. How did he or she master the situation? Has he or she ever suffered vocal breakdown on stage in the past? There is often too little time for further diagnosis. The main task is to evaluate the singer's vocal function and the capacity of the voice in relation to the role to be sung. This is done by summing up the symptoms against the possibility of a general acute illness, such as hypertonia, an acute allergic reaction. In this case, a specific ENT examination is necessary, carried out in private so that during questioning and examination the doctor is alone with the singer (who may of course wish to have close friends present) and absolute discretion can be assured. The more quickly and specifically the doctor is able to diagnose the disorder, the more effective the therapy will be. If the vocal function is essentially normal, well-directed and effective treatment of bronchial catarrh or acute nasal obstruction may be sufficient. This is not infrequent in jet-set singers. Both of these disorders can have a disastrous effect on voice production. The larynx is healthy, but the resonance cavities are considerably impaired. These can, however, very often be restored fairly quickly.

In addition to a brief psychotherapeutic intervention, exercises from the field of vocal and respiratory therapy can be helpful. The voice doctor should not adopt a demanding or patronizing attitude, but should remain sympathetic, providing **courteous but authoritative support**, as the singer's unassuming coach. It is important to provide psychological guidance. Skillfully directing and increasing concentration on the approaching performance can mobilize forces in the singer to counteract the indisposition. The doctor must, of course, make a realistic estimate of the role and the singer's vocal potential.

If the singer can be convinced that he is capable of giving an adequate performance, then his biological processes will alter accordingly. Muscular tension will ease, vegetative processes will be influenced for the better. The singer's state of mind and thus his efficiency will be enhanced. Here the singer has abdicated some of his independence to the physician, who should remind him of times when he was singing well, thus creating a positive attitude toward his voice. These are all verbal interventions incorporated in the routine medical rituals of examination and designed to absorb and remedy the singer's regression. The physician provides the singer with a feeling of security.

EQUIPMENT THE VOICE DOCTOR HAS AT THE WORKPLACE (THEATER/CONCERT HALL)

Emergency phoniatric treatment often takes place in the green-room; friends, ensemble members, and theater personnel should generally leave the room. The doctor should develop an instinct for deciding whether close friends or family may stay. The doctor will have his or her ENT emergency equipment case on hand. Nowadays this will contain small LEDs, nasal specula, otoscope, and disposable instruments such as spatulas. Besides the physician's trained eye, the most useful diagnostic instrument is his or her trained ear, for listening to medical history and assessing the voice. He or she also requires manual skills, as specific sensitive manipulation of neck, throat, and larynx can be useful. In addition, the physician should have an assured bearing and a steady voice, in order to inspire confidence and a feeling of security.

THE PROBLEM OF ACUTE MEDICATION AT THE WORKPLACE (THEATER/CONCERT HALL) ONE DAY OR ONLY HOURS BEFORE A PERFORMANCE

The voice doctor must be familiar with the effect of medication on the singing voice. Not only medication, but also environmental factors can influence the extremely complex and highly sensitive equilibrium of the singer. Physical strain, emotional sensibility, and maximum expressive ability must be taken into account. In prescribing medication, the general principles of pharmacodynamics and pharmacokinetics have to be observed. This means that dosage must be individually assessed, according to age, weight, organic functions, lifestyle, and means of application. The physician should ascertain any so-called "initiation rites" of singers—individual habits such as the use of milk, herbal teas, honey, raw eggs, chewing-gum, gargles, grated apple, or even medication before a performance. It is best to avoid expressing contempt or ridiculing these tried and tested "harmless" aids. On the contrary, a moment of reflection on such activities can be important for inducing a stable emotional situation to settle the voice. This is regarded as a vocal rite of initiation. However, the voice doctor must be aware that some of these so called "harmless aids" may actually be harmful if they counteract other prescribed medications or if they unduly change the singer's internal sensations.

CASE REPORTS

Case Report 1: Sensitizing Materials on Stage

During rehearsals, a molding material was used for a stage figure which released aromatic diisocyanate as it dried. The soloists and chorus singers were mostly placed around this figure, and rapidly developed symptoms such as hoarseness, coughing, and breathing difficulties, which abated only after the stage figure was removed.

Case Report 2: Sensitizing Substances on Stage

At an opera rehearsal, cork bark was used to form a stage landscape over which the singers were required to crawl as they sang. To prevent dust forming, the bark was regularly sprayed with water. After a time, the singers complained of coughs and a burning sensation in eyes and mouth. An allergy test showed evidence of mold. The cork bark contained molds, which were activated by humidification, and the symptoms disappeared only after the bark had been removed.

Case Report 3: Reflux Attacks with Case Presentation

A young soprano, singing the role of Pamina in *The Magic Flute*, attended the party following the successful première at 11 PM. As she did not wish to risk harming her voice by eating late in the evening, she drank only two glasses of sparkling wine. During the night she woke with a sore throat and a need to cough. She said that she prefers to sleep prone. The following morning she had a husky speaking voice and a feeling of excessive mucus, and her throat was still sore. When she started her vocal warm-up exercises, her voice responded only to increased pressure, and she had problems with her top register. A videostroboscopic examination showed an inflammation of the arytenoid cartilages, a diffuse glassy texture of the mucous membrane, and streaky vascularization in the vocal folds on both sides, with a mucilaginous coating and slight interarytenoid hyperplasia. The singer was breast-feeding, so initially only inhalations and therapy for protection of the mucous membrane were prescribed. Her sore throat worsened during the night, and a checkup showed edematous vocal folds on both sides. A 4-day PPI therapy with cortisone and Wobenzym brought considerable improvement. She also changed her sleeping position. The next performance, 5 days later, went perfectly.

Case Report 4: Cancellation Policy in a Case of a Vocal Fold Hematoma with Polyps

During a rehearsal, a 47-year-old mezzo-soprano suddenly lost her voice, and came for a consultation. She was cast for two roles during the summer festival: one in a Mozart opera, the other in a modern opera (*Le Grand Macabre*) by Ligeti. Rehearsals were just starting for the premières 3 weeks later. For 4 days she had been taking about 1,000 mg of aspirin daily for repeated migraine attacks. A videostroboscopic examination showed a vocal fold hematoma with a polypoid swelling on the left side. The singer agreed that the manager should be informed. The therapy consisted of prednisolone in decreasing doses, Reparil lozenges, and inhalations. After a voice rest of 10 days, the

hematoma disappeared, but the polyp was still visible on the left side. The question was then whether the singer would have to cancel her appearances in both operas or whether she could still sing the Ligeti. It was recommended that the patient should try some cautious warm-up exercises over a few hours, then an aria from the Ligeti opera. That afternoon, I listened to her singing the Ligeti aria, which required nothing above the middle register, and she managed it beautifully. We decided that she should sing the Ligeti role, but not the Mozart, which had a much higher tessitura. Thus, half the fee was saved, at least.

EVALUATION OF 74 PROFESSIONAL SINGERS AT THE SALZBURG FESTIVAL OVER 5 FESTIVAL SEASONS (2001–2005)

The following figures are derived from an extensive history of caring for singers. They include the main causes necessitating emergency intervention and the treatments given. Although this may not reflect the typical otolaryngologic or voice center practice, it does provide a basis for expectation.

Figure 13–1 shows the distribution of singers according to voice type, with a striking predominance

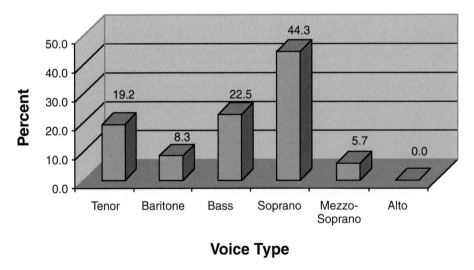

Figure 13-1. The distribution by voice type of 74 singers treated for voice complaints over 5 seasons at the Salzburg Festival.

of soprano voices. Half the singers selected for comparison were male and half were female (Figure 13-2). This leads to the conclusion that, of the female voices, the soprano, is more vulnerable.

A retrospective statistical evaluation of 74 singers was carried out on vocal problems arising during rehearsals and performances over five festival seasons. Figure 13-3 lists the symptoms mentioned by the singers during consultation; there may be several concurrent symptoms. The majority (47.3%) complained of acute cold symptoms; in 40% of cases, the vocal problems were in the upper register. 23% showed distinct hoarseness in the speaking voice. Singers could give more than one answer; hence, the total percentage is more than 100%.

As shown in Figure 13-4, the onset of a disorder is classified as acute (within 1-2 days), intermediate (within 2-5 days), or as a chronic problem (more than 1 week); 64.9% of symptoms occurred as acute The laryngostroboscopic examination showed 70% acute

Figure 13-2. Gender distribution of 74 singers treated over 5 festival seasons.

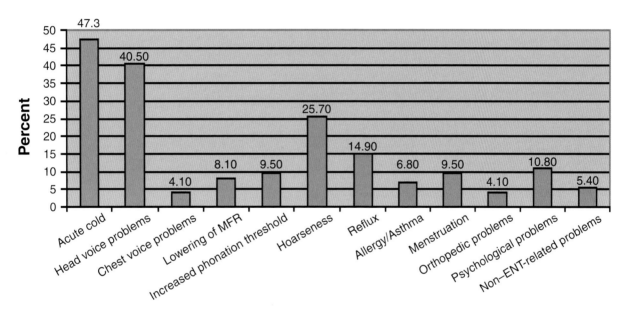

Figure 13-3. Symptoms displayed by the 74 singers who were treated over 5 festival seasons.

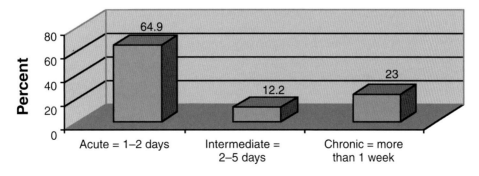

Figure 13-4. Onset of voice problems displayed by the 74 singers who were treated.

change in the mucosa, such as superficial edema or redness, and 32.4% chronic laryngeal changes, such as chronic reflux symptoms, polyps, or nodes (Figure 13-5).

Figure 13-6 displays principal causes of the singers' disorders, with the possibility of several factors occurring together, such as an acute infection exacerbated by rehearsal stress (external factor) or acute infection

with previous reflux symptoms and premenstrual tension. It is evident that approximately 48.6% of the disorders reported are caused by rehearsal stress and vocal pressure despite an incipient cold infection. In conjunction with environmental influences on stage (6.8%), rehearsal and performance stress constitute 55.4% of causes; this balances approximately the acute

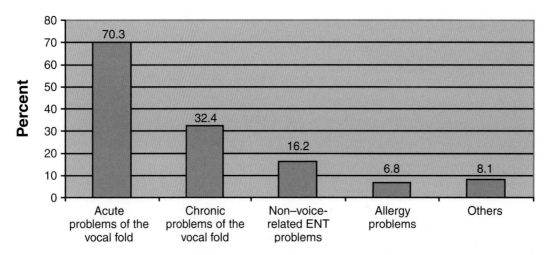

Figure 13-5. Distribution of diagnoses across the 74 singers treated over 5 festival seasons. Because some singers had more than one problem, the total percentage is more than 100%.

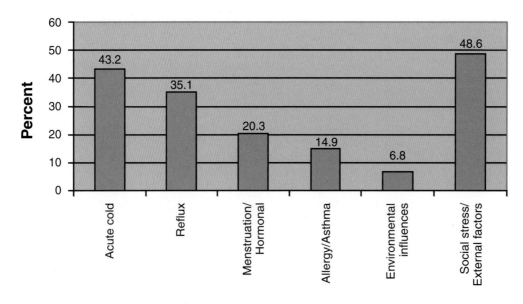

Figure 13-6. Causes of singing-voice disorders for 74 singers seen during the 5 festival seasons (2001-2005). Because some singers had more than one disorder, the total percentage is more than 100%.

causes (infection, allergy, 58%). Reflux (35.1%) is also a prominent cause; this is a lifestyle disorder, and indicates the importance of consistent measures to maintain good vocal health. The question of vocal technique and casting is not significant as a cause of illness, as the singers at the Festival are selected and experienced performers with mature technique and clearly defined vocal category. Figure 13-7 shows that 32.43% of the disorders in the female singers occurred during the premenstrual period or during menstruation. This demonstrates hormonal influence as a significant cofactor in female disorders.

Figure 13-8 underlines the necessity of applying several therapeutic modalities at the same time, such as inhalation together with reflux medication and nonsteroid antirheumatic drugs (NSAIDs) or antitussive medication. Sixty percent of therapies consist of 3 or 4 concurrent therapies (multimodal), as opposed to 9.46% monomodal. This indicates the necessity of a synergetic therapy concept.

The frequency of therapies applied is shown in Figure 13-9. Inhalation therapy (78.4%) is of outstanding importance for vocal disorders, followed by NSAIDs (64%) and reflux medication (40.5%). Antibiotics (9.5%) and corticosteroids (16.2%) are prescribed only when their use is clearly indicated.

An evaluation of 74 professional male and female singers (Figure 13-10) showed that, with appropriate therapy for an illness with an acute onset of 1 to 2 days, the average voice rest time needed before the next performance was up to 3 days for more than 55% of the singers. 22% of the singers needed a Voice Rest Time (VRT) of 4 to 7 days; 6.7% of the singers had a VRT of more than 7 days. In the majority of these cases, the symptoms had been sudden and acute. It may be concluded that immediate medicinal intervention in the acute phase of illness achieved a good response relative to a chronic process, which required a longer voice rest time.

32.43

67.57

■ no
■ yes

Figure 13-7. Occurrence of singing-voice disorders in female singers in relation to menstruation.

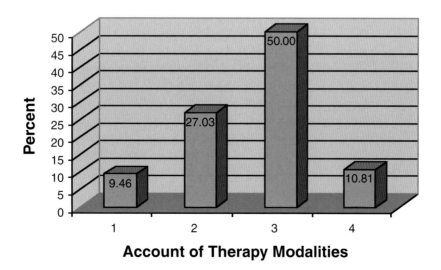

Account of Therapy Modalities

Figure 13-8. Monomodal versus multimodal therapies prescribed for 74 singers over 5 festival seasons.

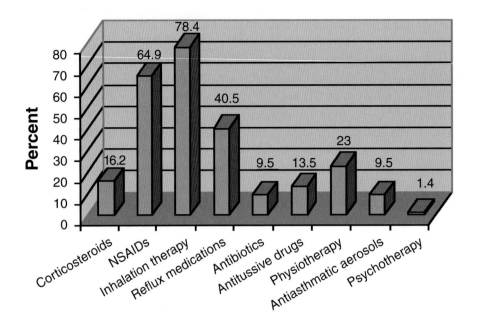

Figure 13-9. Medications prescribed in treating 74 singers over 5 festival seasons. Because some singers had more than one medication, the total percentage is more than 100%.

Figure 13-10. Distribution of voice rest prescribed for 74 singers over 5 festival seasons.

SUMMARY

When clarification of a singer's indisposition at the workplace (theater/concert hall) is required, the circumstances are of a special nature. The time available is short. The voice doctor must make a rapid diagnosis and often important decision. The conditions for examination will be emergency ones, in all senses, and the voice doctor must feel comfortable in these situations to put the singer at ease. The singer's reaction to the physician's therapeutic intervention is often unpredictable because the singer is in an exceptionally stressful situation. The voice doctor must be ready to deal with unexpected questions and behaviors. The doctor's task is to emanate calmness and security, and to offer the singer guidance. This can be done only if the physician:

A. Is familiar with the singer's area of work;
B. Is well-informed about opera and concert performances in the relevant venue, or can gather this information quickly;
C. Can assess the difficulties entailed in specific roles (vocal range, passaggio, dynamics, particular movements on stage);
D. Knows the effect of medication on the singing voice; and
E. Communicates well with both singer and management.

SUGGESTED READING

1. Seidner W, Wendler J. *Die Sängerstimme*. Berlin, Germany: Henschel; 2004.
2. Seidner W. Phoniatrische Notbehandlung bei Sängern und Schauspielern. *HNO aktuell*. 2004; 12(4)
3. Richter B. Harmful substances on the opera stage. *J Voice*. 2002;16(1):72-80.
4. Fussi F. *La Voce del Cantante*. Torino, Italy: Omega Edizioni; 2000.
5. Sataloff RT. *Professional Voice: The Science and Art of Clinical Care*. 3rd ed. San Diego, Calif: Plural Publishing, Inc; 2005.
6. Wendler J, Seidner W, Kittel G, Eysholdt U. *Lehrbuch der Phoniatrie und Pädaudiologie*. Stuttgart, Germany: Thieme;1996.
7. Rubin JS, Sataloff RT, Korovin GS. *Diagnosis and Treatment of Voice Disorders*. New York, NY: Igaku-Shoin; 1995.
8. Flach M. Indisposition und akute Dysphonie beim Berufssänger. *Laryngo-Rhino-Otol*. 1992;71:233-235.
9. Joussen K. Wirkung von Medikamenten auf die Sängerstimme. Sprache-Stimme-Gehör. 1999;23: 98-104.

Part III

Pharmacologic Treatment

Chapter 14

MEDICATIONS: THE POSITIVE AND NEGATIVE IMPACT ON VOICE

David M. Alessi
Audrey Crummey

Drugs can have an effect on laryngeal physiology in a number of ways. These effects are on the mucosa of the vocal folds, the lamina propria, the musculature of the larynx, and its innervation (Tables 14–1 and 14–2).

ANTIHISTAMINES

Antihistamines are commonly prescribed to treat allergies. They include a broad variety of pharmacologic agents, from first-generation H_1-receptor antagonists (eg, diphenhydramine) to the newer, nonsedating H_1 blockers (eg, loratadine). Histamines are compounds that serve as mediators of the allergic response. They are released when allergens interact with surface IgE antibodies on mast cells. Histamines act on H_1-receptors, inducing vasodilation, edema, pain, and other symptoms in affected tissues.

Most H1-receptor antagonists, such as diphenhydramine have significant anticholinergic effects. These agents cause increased viscosity of secretions in the respiratory tract.[1-3] This drying effect leads to decreased vocal fold lubrication, increased throat clearing, and frequent coughing.[4] Furthermore, they also have a sedative effect, which may also decrease the ability for singers to perform successfully. Newer antihistamines such as loratadine, fexofenadine, and desloratadine are highly selective for H1-receptors, and have less of an effect on the central nervous system. They have been reported to have no anticholinergic effect,[2] and cause less drowsiness as well.[5] The drying effect for the newer H_1-blockers appears to be less than older antihistamines, but can still be bothersome. The sedation seen with diphenhydramine is sometimes felt to be beneficial for the insomniac performer. However, it prevents stages 3 and 4 of sleep, and can thus leave the patient more sleep deprived.

Another alternative for singers is a leukotriene-inhibitor such as montelukast. Leukotrienes, like histamines, are released by mast cells and regulate the immune response. Leukotriene inhibitors, like antihistamines, may be effective in treating both asthma and allergic rhinitis.[6-8] However, they do not appear to have the side effects of respiratory dryness and drowsiness.

Singers should be aware that antihistamines have been deregulated by the Food and Drug Administration (FDA), and thus can be found in many common medications. Some over-the-counter sleep aids and treatments for motion sickness such as meclizine contain antihistamines, and should be avoided.[1,3]

Table 14–1. Quick Reference Guide to Recommended Drug Therapy for Singers

Common Complaint	Recommended Drug Therapy
Acid Reflux	Twice-a-day esomeprazole, lansoprazole, omeprazole, pantoprazole, rabeprazole; if no response in 6 weeks, add ranitidine twice, three, or four times per day, or metoclopramide twice or four times per day
Acute Bacterial Laryngitis	cefuroxime, cefdinir, moxifloxacin, gatifloxacin, levofloxacin, telithromycin, high-dose amoxicillin/clavulanate
Asthma	montelukast—AVOID INHALED CORTICOSTEROIDS
Laryngeal Inflammation	For same day performances, oral or intramuscular dexamethasone; for next day performances, prednisone or intramuscular triamcinolone; for more severe problems, methylprednisolone or 5 days of prednisone; AVOID DIURETICS
Dry Mouth (Xerostomia)	Cevimeline and water consumption
Allergies	loratadine, fexofenadine, desloratadine, montelukast; AVOID DIPHENHYDRAMINE
Mucus and Congestion	Expectorants (guaifenesin); AVOID DECONGESTANTS
General Aches and Pains	Acetaminophen; AVOID NSAIDS
Smoking Cessation	Buproprion; AVOID NICOTINE SUPPLEMENTS

DECONGESTANTS

Decongestants act as vasoconstrictors, helping to reduce secretion production by shrinking mucous membranes.[2] Misuse of decongestants like phenylpropanolamine (found in over-the-counter cough medications), as with antihistamines, can cause excessive respiratory dryness.[9] However, some decongestants also contain expectorants, such as guaifenesin.[10] Expectorants act as mucolytics, thinning and increasing secretions. Such agents like high-dose guaifenesin do not have a drying effect on the voice, and may actually help to counteract the drying effects of decongestants. They are often sold as antitussives and may be helpful to singers suffering from overly viscous mucus or postnasal drip.[1] Singers should be mindful that many antitussives may contain antihistamines and other drying ingredients.[3] As with all respiratory dryness, there is no substitute for adequate water consumption, which is the best way to maintain adequate lubrication.

Singers may want to consider using a saliva-stimulating agent to help counteract the effects of respiratory dryness. There has been some success with cevimeline for this purpose. This cholinergic agent with muscarinic agonist activity is often prescribed for severe xerostomia as seen with Sjögren's syndrome. However, it is often useful in performers with dryness issues when simple hydration and mucolytics are not enough.

INHALED CORTICOSTEROIDS

Inhaled corticosteroids (ICSs) are anti-inflammatory drugs often prescribed to treat asthma. They act as vasoconstrictors, reducing respiratory mucosal edema and thickening that follow allergen exposure.[11,12] Long-term use of ICSs may reduce the number of mast cells in the mucosa, and decrease immediate response to allergens.[13] However, inhaled steroids have been known to cause vocal symptoms such as dysphonia, hoarseness, cough, and increased throat clearing.[14] The estimated rate of these symptoms varies widely, and has been reported as between 5 and 50% of

Table 14–2. Drugs That May Induce Dryness

Drug Type	Examples That Induce Dryness	Safe Alternatives
Antihistamines	diphenhydramine	loratadine, fexofenadine, desloratadine, leukotriene inhibitors like montelukast
Decongestants	phenylpropanolamine	Expectorants such as guaifenesin, Antitussives
Inhaled Corticosteroids	Inhalers to treat asthma (eg, fluticasone, budesonide)	Leukotriene inhibitors (eg, montelukast)
Diuretics	Treatments for menstrual fluid retention	Corticosteroids (either oral or intramuscular) can help reduce laryngeal edema
Tricyclic antidepressants	doxepin, clomipramine, amitriptyline	No viable substitutes
Selective Serotonin Reuptake Inhibitors (SSRIs)	fluoxetine, sertraline, paroxetine	No viable substitutes
Antipsychotics	Phenothiazines	No viable substitutes
Major tranquilizers and anxiolytics	alprazolam, diazepam, lorazepam, benzodiazepines, chlorpromazine, thioridazine, haloperidol	No viable substitutes
Antihypertensives	reserpines, agents of the methyldopa group, thiazides, loop diuretics like furosemide, alpha-adrenergic agonists such as clonidine	Ganglionic blocking agents, alpha-adrenergic antagonists
Vitamin C	n/a	No viable substitutes
Anti-influenza drugs	amantadine	oseltamivir, zanamivir, rimantadine
Certain antacids and antispasmodic drugs	phenobarbital, prochlorperazine, isopropamide, propantheline bromide, members of the belladonna alkaloid group	Proton pump inhibitors (esomeprazole, lansoprazole, omeprazole, pantoprazole, rabeprazole)
Lifestyle drugs	caffeine, cocaine, amphetamine	No viable substitutes
Nicotine supplementation	nicotine patches, nicotine gum	bupropion

patients, especially in those susceptible to vocal strain like singers.[11,15,16] This wide reported range of symptom prevalence is probably due to varied methods of data collection, and the higher rates of 50% or more were probably reached through questionnaire rather than through clinical measurement.[13]

ICSs seem to cause dysphonia via local inflammation, but the mechanism of this inflammation is not entirely understood. It is possible that some property of ICSs irritates the airway, leading to the inflammatory response. Such symptoms are probably dose-dependent; in fact, twice-daily regimens show fewer side effects than when ICSs are administered four times daily.[16,17] Furthermore, there is some evidence that the steroid, and not the propellant, is the cause of these symptoms.[17] Generally, once use of the inhaler is withdrawn, dysphonia and other vocal symptoms cease. In certain cases, use of ICSs can induce a vocal fold deformity leading to bowing upon phonation.[18] When bowing occurs, a gap is left between the folds during phonation, leaving room for air to escape. We have seen mucosal thinning on the vocal folds with long-term ICS use that can be severe and may take up to a year to resolve.

In short, ICSs are not a good choice for the professional singer. Alternatives for the treatment of asthma are leukotriene inhibitors.

SYSTEMIC CORTICOSTEROIDS

Systemic corticosteroids are potent anti-inflammatory agents, and can be used to treat laryngeal edema.[2] Thus, they are quite effective in alleviating inflammation caused by acute laryngitis and other laryngeal disorders.[19] Prednisone is a corticosteroid that is administered orally. Methylprednisolone has about the same potency, and can be given either orally or intramuscularly. Dexamethasone is the most potent corticosteroid, having approximately 5 times the strength of prednisone and methylprednisolone. It is the most effective of the corticosteroids in reducing this type of inflammation.[2] However, steroids must be prescribed with great care. If the injection is not given intramuscularly or allowed to seep into surrounding fatty tissue, a deep steroid dimple may occur from the fatty wasting at the site of the injection. This is especially true with triamcinolone injection. The dosage of steroid should be significant, such as prednisone 60 mg daily for the treatment of acute laryngeal edema. The timing of the administration is important also. A shorter-acting but rapid-onset steroid would be used on a performer singing the same evening as opposed to one with a slower onset. The physician should be sure to rule out the presence of vocal fold hemorrhage, acute laryngitis, and ulceration of vocal fold mucosa before steroid treatment. Also, steroids can cause gastric irritation, which could have further negative effects on the voice. Furthermore, as corticosteroids are so effective in treating laryngeal inflammation, singers may have a tendency to overuse them.[1] Thus, use of steroids should be closely monitored by the singer's physician.

DIURETICS

Diuretics are agents that decrease systemic levels of water and can help relieve edema. They are commonly used by women to help counteract the fluid retention that occurs during the premenstrual period. During this time, circulating levels of estrogen and progesterone are decreased, which leads in turn to increased circulating antidiuretic hormone. This is what causes fluid retention in Reinke's space and other tissues.[1] Female singers often request diuretics from their gynecologists in an effort to counteract these effects in laryngeal tissues.[4] However, water in vocal fold tissues is protein bound, and diuretics cannot effectively remobilize this fluid. Rather, diuretics only serve to cause dehydration and increased viscosity of secretions, and in turn make singing an increasingly difficult task.[9,20] Thus, they should not be prescribed to alleviate symptoms of menses, and their use for any other purposes should be closely monitored. An alternative is to use corticosteroids, which affect protein-bound water directly.[3]

PSYCHOACTIVE DRUGS

Psychoactive drugs are commonly prescribed, and many have potentially deleterious side effects for the vocalist. One particularly relevant category is the tricyclic antidepressants. These agents are strongly anticholinergic, and block the reuptake of both norepinephrine and serotonin. They often cause drying of the upper respiratory tract mucosa, and can lead to hoarseness.[2,3,21,22] Another type of antidepressants is selective serotonin reuptake inhibitors (SSRIs). These are some of the most commonly prescribed drugs to treat depression, and include fluoxetine, sertraline, and paroxetine. These are weakly anticholinergic, but are well known to cause xerostomia and can have a dehydrating effect on laryngeal tissues.[2] Monoamine oxidase inhibitors (MAOIs), also prescribed to treat depression, inhibit the breakdown of serotonin and norepinephrine by monoamine oxidase. MAOIs may not have as substantial a drying effect on the vocal folds. However, they can have strong adverse interactions with many medications, including decongestants and nasal sprays.[1] Therefore, use of MAOIs should always be monitored closely by a physician.

In addition to antidepressants, there are also some antipsychotic drugs that can have adverse effects on the voice. The phenothiazines, which are prescribed to treat conditions such as schizophrenia and mania, almost always lead to dryness of the vocal tract mucosa.[2,3] Furthermore, patients taking phenothiazines and other antipsychotics, are occasionally known to exhibit tremor, which can affect the vocal fold muscles. Approximately 14% of patients who take antipsychotic agents for longer than 7 years will develop tardive dyskinesia, especially of the head, neck, and tongue.[1] Of course, such conditions would be quite detrimental to a vocalist's career.

Major tranquilizers are another type of medication that can lead to vocal fold dryness. These agents are often prescribed for pain management and for sedative purposes. One type of the major tranquilizers is the benzodiazepines, which include aprazolam, diazepam, lorazepam, and others. Other common tranquilizers are chlorpromazine, thioridazine, and haloperidol.[3]

Many vocalists may try to use anxiolytic drugs to help alleviate performance anxiety, commonly known as "stage fright." Use of these drugs should be considered very carefully by both the singer and his or her physician. For one, some anxiolytics, particularly major tranquilizers like benzodiazepines, should be avoided because they induce vocal fold dryness. In addition, anxiety can serve a crucial role for vocalists. Extreme anxiety can be debilitating, but mild anxiety can actually enhance performance. There is some evidence that small doses of beta-adrenergic stimulators (commonly known as beta-blockers) can effectively treat performance anxiety, but in high doses detract from performance.[23] It seems that some degree of nervousness is what gives singers a competitive edge, and can be necessary for a successful performance. Generally, preperformance anti-anxiety medicines should be avoided. It is preferred that both the laryngologist and the vocal coach instill confidence in the performer that everything is fine.

ANTIHYPERTENSIVE AGENTS

Antihypertensives are commonly prescribed, and most types have the potential to negatively affect the voice.

Antihypertensives vary considerably in their mechanism of action, so it is usually possible to find a type that minimizes adverse side effects for the singer. Almost all the current agents have some parasympathomimetic action, and thus result in dryness of mucous membranes in the upper respiratory tract.[3] This effect is seen in particular for reserpines and agents of the methyldopa group.[23]

Diuretics are also commonly used to treat high blood pressure. As previously discussed, diuretics can cause increased viscosity of secretions secondary to systemic decrease in water. Thiazides cause a decrease in sodium, potassium, and water.[2] Loop diuretics, such as furosemide, have a similar effect.

Alpha-adrenergic agonists, such as clonidine, act centrally to reduce blood pressure.[2] They act on presynaptic neurons to inhibit norepinephrine activity. As a result, they can have drying effects on the respiratory tract secretions similar to those of other anticholinergic agents.

There are some antihypertensive agents that have minimal side effects for the voice. For example, angiotensin-converting enzyme inhibitors do not cause drying of mucosal secretions.[2] However, they can induce coughing, which may be caused by the release of prostaglandins. Coughing can lead to vocal fold trauma, and in turn may cause Reinke's edema. Beta-blocking agents are also used to treat high blood pressure. They are sympatholytic agents; consequently, they do not affect the vocal tract. However, as previously discussed, anxiolytics can have adverse effects on a singer's ability to sing at his or her best during a performance. Finally, ganglionic blocking agents and alpha-adrenergic antagonists are options to treat hypertension without drying effects on the vocal fold.

HORMONES

Hormones can have significant impact on a singer's voice. These changes in voice can be brought on by either endogenous or exogenous causes.[24] Endogenously, tumors of the ovary or adrenal gland can produce androgenic hormones that lead to masculinization of the voice. However, these are quite rare. More commonly, virilization is caused exogenously by the administration of androgens for medical purposes.[2,3] The effects of androgens can cause lowering of fundamental frequencies, huskiness, hoarseness, and coarsening of the voice.[24,25] Furthermore, these effects are often permanent, depending on the subject's age, the treatment duration, and the amount of drug given.[26,27] It seems that the female voice is most sensitive to virilization during puberty and menopause, when hormonal levels are already in flux.[28] Voice changes are found to accompany hormonal treatment in 5 to 10% of patients.[25] In particular, this effect has been found with danazol, but is also applicable to other agents similar in structure to testosterone. Anabolic steroids, which are often abused for the sake of enhancing athletic performance, have been shown to cause an often irreversible deepening of the voice in women.[28-30]

Hormonal agents are prescribed to treat a variety of conditions. Nandrolone decanoate (Decadurabolin) is an anabolic steroid often prescribed as a treatment for osteoporosis, and it too has been shown to irreversibly lower vocal pitch of female patients.[28,31] Androgen therapy is often prescribed by gynecologists as a treatment for endometriosis and dysmenorrhea.[2,3,25] Chemotherapy for women with breast cancer can also include androgenic hormone therapy as part of the treatment.[3]

In the past, oral contraceptives were seen as a threat to a singer's voice.[32] Earlier formulations of birth control pills contained relatively high amounts of progesterone, and were thus more likely to lead to masculinization of the voice.[3,33] In fact, some types of birth control from Europe may still have significant dosages of anabolic steroids. However, most modern oral contraceptives in the United States have tended toward lower hormone levels, and voice side effects are seen in only about 5% of patients.[1] These changes tend to be temporary, and normal voice is usually restored when use of birth control pills is discontinued. The "morning-after pill" is becoming more commonly used in the United States and abroad, and mifepristone (RU-486) is an antiprogestin that may also have an androgenic effect on the voice; however, the effects of these substances have not been clearly studied.

When a female singer reaches menopause and hormone levels begin to change, she may notice adverse changes in her voice. Such changes are quite typical. Estrogen replacement therapy is often helpful in counteracting these changes, and should be offered by the physician at the time of menopause.[1]

Men may also experience voice changes as a result of exogenous hormones, although these scenarios are less common. Estrogens in men can lead to feminization of the voice. In particular, this situation can arise in men who are being treated palliatively with diethylstilbestrol for prostatic carcinoma.[2]

Dysfunction in endocrine function can cause vocal changes, and hormone therapy is often successful as a remedy for these effects. Hypothyroidism causes mucopolysaccharides to accumulate in tissues, including the vocal folds.[2] This leads to a decrease in vocal efficiency and "ring."[1] Thyroid hormone replacement therapy helps counteract this process, thereby restoring normal vocal function. Men with impaired pituitary secretion of gonadotropins tend to have higher than normal fundamental vocal frequency because gonadotropins regulate the production of sex steroids. There is some evidence that this can be ameliorated by testosterone treatment.[34]

Thyroid hyper- or hypofunction can have a deleterious effect on laryngeal function. Mucosal thinning or thickening can occur as well as increased dryness, to name a few of the known effects. Thus, testing for thyroid function is a key part of any dysphonia workup. This is especially important when a patient is already on thyroid supplementation. The appropriate amount of exogenous thyroid hormone needs to be adjusted carefully with the use of serial thyroid function tests.

VITAMIN C

It is quite common for physicians to encounter singers who are taking large quantities of ascorbic acid (vitamin C) in an effort to prevent colds or shorten their duration.[3] There is evidence that vitamin C (at 4000 milligrams per day) can be useful in limiting the duration of the common cold.[35,36] There is evidence that the rhinovirus receptor in the nasal mucosa (ICAM receptor) is inhibited by ascorbic acid. However, in some of these patients there has been found a drying effect of too high dosages of vitamin C.[1,3] These effects are diuretic in nature, and are comparable to the effects of a mild antihistamine. Therefore, the use of high-dose vitamin C should be limited to exposure to or the onset of a cold.

TREATMENTS FOR ACUTE LARYNGITIS

Upper respiratory tract infections (URTIs) are frequent complaints of singers. In particular, singers tend to suffer from laryngitis as a result of excessive voice use.[19] Acute laryngitis is defined as inflammation of the larynx and vocal fold lasting less than 3 weeks.[37] Acute laryngitis is generally viral in nature, particularly due to viruses like parainfluenza, rhinovirus, influenza, and adenovirus. Symptoms usually resolve on their own within 3 to 8 days.

It is important for physicians to be discriminating in prescribing antibiotics. This can be difficult because many patients with URTIs expect to be prescribed antibiotics, and may pressure their physicians to do so. However, antibiotics are normally not necessary, as most cases of laryngitis are of viral origin.[38] There is a vast quantity of evidence showing that antibiotics have no effect on most cases of laryngitis.[37,39,40] Furthermore, overuse of antibiotics can lead to superinfection of *Candida*.[2] The physician should educate vocalists as to why antibiotics are not useful, and seek other solutions to alleviate the patient's discomfort.

When laryngitis is bacterial in origin, species most commonly encountered with acute bacterial laryngitis are similar to those found in acute maxillary sinusitis, such as *Streptococcus pneumoniae*, *Haemophilus influenzae*, *Moraxella catarrhalis*, and *Staphylococcus aureus*.[39-41] Because of significant emergence of resistant organisms, we prefer to adapt the Allergy Health Partnership recommendations for the treatment of sinusitis. High-dose amoxicillin, normal or high-dose amoxicillin/clavulinate acid, cefuroxime, cefdinir, moxifloxacin, gatifloxacin, levofloxacin, and telithromycin are all effective antibiotic treatments. Corticosteroids can be helpful in treating the resulting inflammation, but should be used sparingly. Also, as influenza is a common cause of laryngitis, physicians can offer the singer a prophylactic influenza vaccine. However, these should not be administered before a performance, as side effects can result.

Amantadine is often prescribed to treat certain strains of the influenza virus, but this is not suggested for singers. Amantadine, which is also prescribed to treat Parkinsons's disease, has anticholinergic side effects and can induce xerostomia and xerophonia.[1] The newer viral neuramidase inhibitors (oseltamivir, zanamivir, rimantadine) have no significant drying effects and are generally more effective against the influenza virus.

TREATMENTS FOR REFLUX LARYNGITIS

Chronic laryngitis is often caused by gastroesophageal reflux disease (GERD). There are many different methods of treating acid reflux including antacids, H2-blockers, and gastric proton pump inhibitors (PPIs).[1] Aluminum-magnesium antacids are beneficial, but need to be used frequently. Calcium preparations may also be helpful, but they can eventually result in increased acid production.[2] Other commonly used antacids include phenobarbital, prochlorperazine, isopropamide, and propantheline bromide. All of these may have drying effects on the larygeal mucosa.[1,3] H2-blockers (eg, cimetidine) are quite useful in treating acid reflux. Generally, drying of the vocal mucosa is not a major side effect, but it can occur on occasion.[1,3] H2-blockers inhibit the secretion of acid from gastric parietal cells, but do little to affect the rate of acid production. Some antispasmodic drugs such as members of the belladonna alkaloid group (eg, scopolamine, atropine) have been widely prescribed for those with stomach ulcers. These, however, have an anticholinergic function and thus lead to dryness of the vocal tract.[1] Gastric proton pump inhibitors (PPIs) are a newer, very effective way of managing acid reflux, and have few adverse side effects for singers.[1,2] They have quickly become the preferred method of treatment for laryngopharyngeal reflux disease.[42] As laryngeal reflux is a more difficult disease to treat then gastroesophageal reflux disease marked by dyspepsia, most laryngologists start their patients on twice-a-day dosing. It must be emphasized that no treatment will be effective unless accompanied by a strict antireflux protocol (early dinner, elevation of the head of bed, etc).

ANALGESICS

Pain can serve an important function for the singer. Laryngeal sensation informs the singer of the degree of pressure being applied to the vibrating vocal cords.[43]

Pain in this region alerts him or her when the voice is being overstressed and helps maintain good vocal discipline. Thus, any agent that decreases proprioceptive input from the larynx and vocal folds should be discouraged.[1,44] In particular, topical anesthetics such as benzocaine, lidocaine, and analgesic throat lozenges, are potentially quite dangerous. Although use of these agents is tempting for the singer suffering from pain as a result of pharyngitis, it could cause the singer to unknowingly inflict vocal damage.[2,3]

Nonsteroidal anti-inflammatory drugs (NSAIDs) are particularly pernicious analgesics for singers. NSAIDs include common over-the-counter agents such as acetylsalicylic acid (aspirin) and ibuprofen. The anticoagulant effect of such drugs increases the risk for vocal fold hemorrhage, which can be devastating to a singer's career.[1,2,45] NSAIDs should thus be avoided, particularly before strenuous performances. If a singer absolutely must alleviate nonlaryngeal pain, acetaminophen may be a good substitute. It is not an NSAID, and therefore probably does not put the singer at risk for mucosal hemorrhage.

"LIFESTYLE" DRUGS

The stressful nature of a singer's career may cause him or her to self-medicate in a variety of ways. For one, many singers may use caffeine to help them keep up with a busy rehearsal schedule. Caffeine is a mild diuretic, and a stimulant of the central nervous system. The sympathomimetic properties of caffeine combined with its effect as a diuretic make it a potentially dehydrative agent. There is some evidence that caffeine may have detrimental effects on a singer's voice, and for this reason its use should be discouraged.[46]

Other stimulants may also have adverse effects for a singer. They can become particularly damaging when combined with raised adrenaline levels during a performance.[3] Cocaine is a stimulant that is used frequently among singers. Its use can cause serious damage to the nasal mucosa and induce vasoconstriction. It also may decrease sensorium, which can decrease voice control and lead to abusive vocal habits.[4] Amphetamines are strong adrenergic agonists, and frequently lead to vocal tract dryness.[2] "Diet pills" also often have a stimulating effect, and should be avoided.[3]

Central nervous system depressants, such as alcohol, barbiturates, and marijuana, may also have detrimental effects on a singer's voice. Any agent that inhibits a singer's sensorium can lead to poor, and potentially damaging, vocal technique.[3] Alcohol is one of the more common depressants that a singer may ingest. Alcohol intoxication results in decreased awareness, which impedes vocal discipline.[4] The effects of small amounts of alcohol, such as a glass of wine, are still debated among experts. Some maintain that because alcohol causes vasodilation, it necessarily leads to mucosal alteration, but this effect seems to vary considerably among individuals.[4]

Smoking is exceedingly damaging to the larynx. However, nicotine supplementation can have drying and stimulating effects. Antidepressants have been particularly successful in smoking cessation with performers. Bupropion is a selective blocker of central nervous system dopamine uptake. With motivated patients (which most singers are), the smoking cessation period is made significantly easier. Although many performers are concerned about any psychoactive drug affecting their stage psyche, most will find there is no effect (or even a beneficial effect).

SUMMARY

The use and misuse of medications with subtle effects may not be as important to a non-performer as it is to a singer. Minor amounts of dryness can cause a loss of the singer's passagio or high register. Undertreatment of laryngopharyngeal reflux disease can lead to disabling granulomas in a professional voice user. Forgetting to elicit use of all prescription and nonprescription drugs may allow for long-term laryngeal injury. A thorough understanding of drugs and their effect on the larynx is essential for any practitioner treating performers.

REFERENCES

1. Spiegel JR, Hawkshaw M, Sataloff RT. Voice disorders and phonosurgery I. *Otolaryngol Clin North Am.* 2000;33:771–84.

2. Thompson AR. Pharmacological agents with effects on voice. *Am J Otolaryngol.* 1995;16:12-18.

3. Lawrence VL. Common medications with laryngeal effects. *Ear Nose Throat J.* 1987;66:318-322.

4. Sataloff RT, Spiegel JR, Hawkshaw MJ. History and physical examination of patients with voice disorders. In: Rubin JS, Sataloff RT, Korovin GS, eds. *Diagnosis and Treatment of Voice Disorders.* 2nd ed. San Diego, Calif: Singular Publishing Group; 2003:137-158.

5. Wilken JA, Kane RL, Ellis AK, et al. A comparison of the effect of diphenhydramine and desloratadine on vigilance and cognitive function during treatment of ragweed-induced allergic rhinitis. *Ann Allergy Asthma Immunol.* 2003;91:375-385.

6. McMillan RM. Leukotrienes in respiratory disease. *Paediatr Respir Rev.* 2001;2:238-244.

7. Baena-Cagnani CE, Berger WE, DuBuske LM, et al. Comparative effects of desloratadine versus montelukast on asthma symptoms and use of beta 2-agonists in patients with seasonal allergic rhinitis and asthma. *Int Arch Allergy Immunol.* 2003; 130:307-313.

8. Meltzer EO, Philp G, Weinstein SF, et al. Concomitant montelukast and loratadine as treatment for seasonal allergic rhinitis: a randomized, placebo-controlled clinical trial. *J Allergy Clin Immunol.* 2000;105:917-922.

9. Verdolini K, Min Y, Titze I, et al. Biological mechanisms underlying voice changes due to dehydration. *J Speech Lang Hear Res.* 2002;45:268-281.

10. Jackson-Menaldi CA, Dzul AI, Holland RW. Hidden respiratory allergies in voice users: treatment strategies. *Logoped Phoniatr Vocol.* 2002;27:74-79.

11. Hanania NA, Chapman KR, Kesten S. Adverse effects of inhaled corticosteroids. *Amer J Med.* 1995;98:196-208.

12. Ihre E, Zetterström O, Hammarberg B. Voice problems as side effects of inhaled corticosteroids in asthma patients—a prevalence study. *J Voice.* 2004;18;403-414.

13. Roland NJ, Bhalla RK, Earis J. The local side effects of inhaled corticosteroids. *Chest.* 2004;126: 213-219.

14. Stead RJ, Cooke NJ. Adverse effects of inhaled corticosteroids. *Br Med J.* 1989;298:403-404.

15. Lavy JA, Wood G, Rubin JS, Harries M. Dysphonia associated with inhaled steroids. *J Voice.* 2000; 14:581-588.

16. Williamson IJ, Matusiewicz SP, Brown PH, Greening AP, Crompton GK. Frequency of voice problems and cough in patients using pressurized aerosol inhaled steroid preparations. *Eur Respir J.* 1995;8:590-592.

17. Toogood JH, Jennings B, Greenway RW, Chuang L. Candidiasis and dysphonia complicating beclomethasone treatment of asthma. *J Allergy Clin Immunol.* 1980;65:145-153.

18. Williams AJ, Baghat MS, Stableforth DE, Cayton RM, Shenoi PM, Skinner C. Dysphonia caused by inhaled steroids: recognition on a characteristic laryngeal abnormality. *Thorax.* 1983;38:813-821.

19. Sataloff RT. Professional singers: the science and art of clinical care. *Am J Otolaryngol.* 1981;2:262-266.

20. Verdolini K, Titze IR, Fennell A. Dependence of phonatory effort on hydration level. *J Speech Hear Res.* 1994;37:1001-1007.

21. Rhoads JM, Lowell SH, Hedgepeth EM. Hoarseness and aphonia as a side effect of tricyclic antidepressants. *Am J Psychiatry.* 1979; 136:1599-1600.

22. Lyskowski JC, Dunner FJ. Hoarseness and tricyclic antidepressants. *Am J Psyichiatry.* 1980;137:636.

23. Gates GA, Saegert J, Wilson N, Johnson L, Shepherd A, Hearne EM. The effect of β blockade on singing performance. *Ann Otol Rhinol Laryngol.* 1985; 94:570-574.

24. Damste PH. Virilization of the voice due to anabolic steroids. *Folia Phoniatr.* 1968;16:10-18.

25. Pattie MA, Murdoch BE, Theodoros D, Forbes K. Voice changes in women treated for endometriosis and related conditions: the need for comprehensive vocal assessment. *J Voice.* 1998;12:366-371.

26. Schlondorff G. Anabolic hormones and voice disorders. *Dtsch Med Wochenschr.* 1966;91:555-557.

27. Boothroyd CV, Lepre F. Permanent voice change resulting from danazol therapy. *Aust N Z J Obstet Gynaecol.* 1990;30:275-276.

28. Gerritsma EJ, Brocaar MP, Hakkesteegt MM, Birkenhäger JC. Virilization of the voice in postmenopausal women due to the anabolic cteroid nandrolone decanoate (Decadurabolin). The effects of medication for one year. *Clin Otolaryngol.* 1994;19:79-84.

29. Baker J. A report on alterations to the speaking and singing voices of four women following hormonal therapy with virilizing agents. *J Voice.* 1999;13: 496-507.

30. Talaat M, Talaat AM, Kelada I, Angelo A, Elwany S, Thabet H. Histologic and histochemical study of effects of anabolic steroids on the female larynx. *Ann Otol Rhinol Laryngol.* 1987;96:468-471.

31. Need AG, Durbridge TC, Nordin BE. Anabolic steroids in postmenopausal osteoporosis. *Wien Med Wochenschr.* 1993;143:392-395.

32. Wendler J, Siegert C, Schelhorn P, et al. The influence of Microgynon and Diane-35, two sub-fifty ovulation inhibitors, on voice function in women. *Contraception.* 1995;52:343-348.

33. Schiff M. The "pill" in otolaryngology. *Trans Am Acad Ophthalmol Otolaryngol.* 1968;72:76-84.

34. Akcam T, Bolu E, Merati A, Durmus C, Gerek M, Ozkaptan Y. Voice changes after androgen therapy for hypogonadotrophic hypogonadism. *Laryngoscope.* 2004;114:1587-1591.

35. Douglas RM, Hemila H, D'Souza R, Chalker EB, Treacy B. Vitamin C for preventing and treating the common cold. *Cochrane Database Syst Rev.* 2000;4:CD000980.

36. Van Straten M, Josling P. Preventing the common cold with a vitamin C supplement: a double-blind, placebo-controlled survey. *Adv Ther.* 2002;19: 151-159.

37. Reveiz L, Cardona AF, Ospina EG. Antibiotics for acute laryngitis in adults. *Cochrane Database Syst Rev.* 2005;1:CD004783.

38. Turnidge J. Responsible prescribing for upper respiratory tract infections. *Drugs.* 2001;16:2065-2077.

39. Schalén L, Christensen P, Eliasson I, Fex S, Kamme C, Schalén C. Inefficacy of penicillin V in acute laryngitis in adults: evaluation from results of double-blind study. *Ann Otol Rhinol Laryngol.* 1985;94:14-17.

40. Schalén L, Eliasson I, Kamme C, Schalén C. Erythromycin in acute laryngitis in adults. *Ann Otol Rhinol Laryngol.* 1993;102:209-214.

41. Hol C, Schálen C, Verduin CM, Van Dijke EE, Verhoef J, Fleer A. *Moraxella catarrhalis* in acute laryngitis: infection or colonization? *J Infect Dis.* 1996;174:636-638.

42. Koufman JA. Laryngopharyngeal reflux 2002: a new paradigm of airway disease. *Ear Nose Throat J.* 2002; 81:2-6.

43. Wyke BD. Laryngeal reflex mechanisms. *Phonation.* 1976; 528-537.

44. Proctor DF. *Breathing, Speech, and Song.* New York, NY: Springer-Verlag; 1980.

45. Neely JL, Rosen C. Vocal fold hemorrhage associated with coumadin therapy in an opera singer. *J Voice.* 2000;14:272-277.

46. Akhtar S, Wood G, Rubin JS, O'Flynn, PE, Ratcliffe P. Effect of caffeine on the vocal folds: a pilot study. *J Laryngol Otol.* 1999;113:341-345.

Chapter 15

COMPLEMENTARY AND ALTERNATIVE MEDICATIONS AND TECHNIQUES

Michael D. Seidman

Complementary and integrative medicine (CIM), also known as complementary and alternative medicine (CAM) is defined as any practice that can be used for the prevention and treatment of diseases, but not taught widely in medical schools, not generally available in hospitals, and not usually covered by health insurance. Similarly, Andrew Weil, MD, defines integrative medicine as a healing-oriented medicine that draws upon all therapeutic systems to form a comprehensive approach to the art and science of medicine.[1]

Generally speaking the amateur, semiprofessional, or professional singer often realizes benefits and accepts CIM more readily than the average population. Surow and Lovetri speculate that singers tend to be highly conscious of their bodies and frequently turn to CIM to optimize their health.[2] In their survey they found that 71% of the respondents admitted to using CIM therapies, on a fairly frequent basis. Prior to delving into the different possible CIM modalities pertinent to the singer, it is relevant to discuss the evolution of CIM.

Some of the more common and widely accepted therapies originated in Asia centuries ago; others were developed in Europe or America over the past several centuries. There are many examples of CIM therapies, as noted in Table 15-1. Conventional medicine started approximately 200 years ago, whereas alternative therapies have been present since civilization began. There are references, for example, to the healing applications of aloe vera in the Bible. During the mid-20th century, there was a rapid elimination of CIM, and it was often branded quackery or charlatanism. As a result, physicians tend to disregard practices that are not validated by double-blind, randomized, placebo-controlled studies. But clearly it is difficult if not impossible to randomize and placebo-control every type of therapeutic intervention.

In spite of the general lack of scientific research, there has been an astounding increase in the use of CIM therapies. Americans spent approximately $27 billion in 1998 and $32 billion in the year 2000 on alternative therapies. Roughly 40 to 50% of all Americans

Table 15-1. Examples of CIM Therapies

Acupuncture	Massage therapy
Alexander technique	Megavitamin therapy
Biofeedback	Naturopathy
Chiropractic	Neuromuscular therapy
Energy healing	Prayer
Feldenkrais technique	Reflexology
Folk remedies	Relaxation
Homeopathy	Remote healing
Herbal supplements	Rolfing
Hypnotherapy	Self-help groups
Imagery	Spiritual healing by others
Magnet therapy	Therapeutic touch

have tried some form of alternative therapy, according to a report in the *Journal of the American Medical Association*. Another report suggests that more than 60% of Americans are now using CIM therapies.[3]

The disturbing aspect of this is the fact that of the Americans using CIM, 70% do not tell their physicians.[4] This is quite alarming, as many of the herbal as well as some nutritional supplements can interfere with common medications, at times with potentially life-threatening effects. Increasingly, patients insist on seeing a physician who is at least open to considering CIM therapies, particularly where conventional therapies may be less effective. Currently, approximately 75% of medical schools are offering courses on alternative medicine. It is becoming increasingly clear that physicians must learn about CIM. In the best circumstances, we should utilize expertise from a variety of practitioners and collaboration between physicians and people who practice CIM is to be encouraged. Currently, this is frontier territory, but it might be the best case scenario for our patients.

CIM philosophy emphasizes prevention and wellness rather than "fixing." Generally speaking, CIM may be less costly than the use of expensive high-technology testing, surgeries, and drugs, as less invasive options typically demand less health care resources. People are beginning to ask for alternatives incorporating mental and spiritual aspects. This is based on a belief in the unity and importance of the body, mind, and spirit—essentially, these three elements cannot be separated when trying to treat someone or to maintain or improve their health. CIM professionals attempt to mobilize and enhance the healing ability inherent in each person. Furthermore, a CIM professional establishes a partnership with the patient, and treatment is directed toward the unique goals and values of each individual.

In the 17th century, the philosopher René Descartes initiated the thinking of distinct domains of human construction and the exactness of science (Figure 15-1). The pre-Descartes era shows the body, mind, and spirit as integral components of health, whereas post-Descartes these elements were separated. The conventional Western paradigm dictates that diseases are caused by internal cellular and organ dysfunction (Figure 15-2). As a result, more than 99% of all research funding in the United States is aimed at therapies focused on the body, whereas the mind and spirit are rarely investigated. Conversely, the holistic or integrative medicine paradigm (Figure 15-3) suggests that the domains of the body, mind, and spirit are inseparable and disease signals an imbalance. Optimal treatment involves addressing all domains together. Clearly, the effects of structural movement patterns, hormonal, nutritional, and genetic forces, as well as personal past, emotion, stress, and behavior patterns all play a role in the body, mind, and spirit, and should never be separated. In the holistic paradigm, it is felt that imbalances of the body, mind, and spirit are the cause of cellular and organ dysfunction. Then the real question becomes when are cellular and organ changes the result of disease rather than the cause and are both hypotheses possible?

It is becoming evident that the best practices involve providing patients with healing options. Even the most open-minded provider cannot be an expert in all therapies, or be aware of everything that is available, what the research supports, and where to refer people. Providers must be honest with patients, especially if they do not know about a treatment modality. It is important to avoid stating that something is harmful or has no evidence behind it if you have not actually investigated the subject, just as it is essential above all to do no harm.

To help singers find solutions to health problems, to provide strategies to enhance their performances, and to optimize their health, it is necessary to discuss the orchestra of therapeutic modalities available. The discussion begins with nutraceuticals and herbs, and then delves into several other potential therapeutic options.

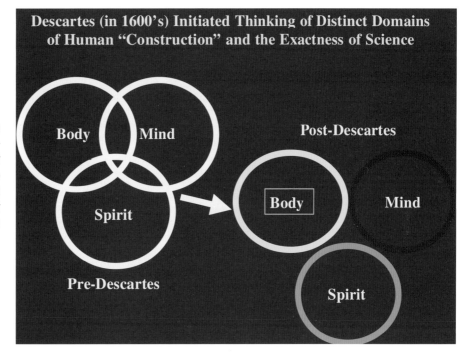

Figure 15–1. Comparison of pre- and post-Descartes thinking about the relationship of the human body, mind, and spirit. (Courtesy of Robert Levine, PhD)

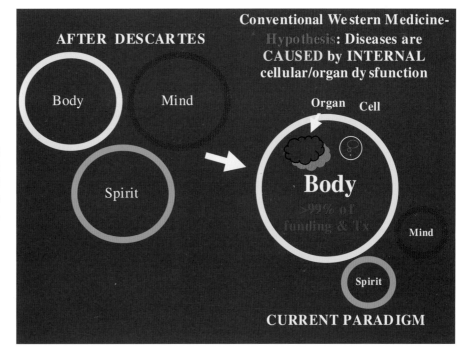

Figure 15–2. Illustration of the current paradigm of Western medicine regarding the disease process.

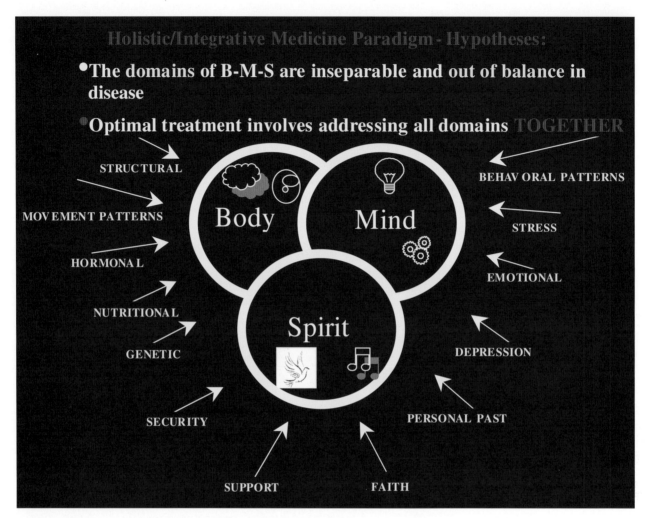

Figure 15–3. Illustration of the holistic/integrative medical paradigm of the disease process.

NUTRACEUTICALS, VITAMINS, AND HERBS

Many herbs can be used for medicinal purposes and many of them are extremely relevant to the singer. Some of the more commonly used herbs are listed in Table 15–2, where we have provided details, such as claims information, specific actions when known, contraindications, potential side effects, interactions, and dosages, when available.

There is always concern about whether a specific supplement contains precisely what the manufacturer claims. Unfortunately, there have been many examples suggesting that this is not always the case. However, herbal remedies are increasingly being sold with standardization information included on the labels. For the time being, we must take the manufacturers at their word, because this area is not regulated by the Food and Drug Administration (FDA).

One of the most reputable references with regard to the medicinal use of herbs is the Complete German Commission E. This commission provides monographs on hundreds of herbs, rating them as either positive or negative. Typically, an herb that is rated positively has reasonable scientific support and data to validate its use. An herb with a negative rating may be ineffective, unsafe, or simply not studied to the extent that sufficient information is available.

Table 15–2. Herbs Used for Medicinal Purposes

Herbal Supplement	Indications	Actions	Contraindications	Side Effects	Interactions	Dosage
Echinacea	Treatment and prevention of the common cold and flu	Immunostimulant Enhances phagocytosis	Autoimmune or chronic illness Allergy to flowers of the daisy family	Minor gastrointestinal irritation Increased urination Mild allergic reactions	Immune suppressants (ie, Neoral prednisone Imuran methotrexate	As powder extract: 300 mg cap/TID Alcohol tincture (1:5): 3–4 ml TID Juice: 203 ml TID Whole dried root: 100–200 g TID
Goldenseal	Topical antibiotic for wounds that are not healing well Mouth sores and sore throats	Strong activity against a wide variety of bacteria and fungi	Pregnancy	Gastrointestinal distress Increased nervousness		As cream, cover entire surface of the wound Tincture: swished or gargled Tea: 0.5–1g in a cup of water
Kava Kava	Mild to moderate anxiety Insomnia	Anti-anxiety Mild analgesic Muscle relaxant Anti-convulsant	Pregnancy Nursing mothers Endogenous depression	Mild gastrointestinal irritation Drowsiness Yellowish skin discoloration Balance disturbance Skin rash Enlargement of pupils	Benzodiazepine Buspirone Alcohol Barbiturates Anti-depressant Anti-psychotic	Standardized extract: 140–240 mg in 2–3 divided doses (30–70% kava-lactones)
Ginseng	Tonic Stimulant Diuretic Diabetic impotence	Physiologic effects Lower blood pressure Depress CNS activity Stimulates immune system	Coagulopathy Diabetes Insomnia Schizophrenia Cardiac disease	Bleeding Hypotension Hypoglycemia Insomnia	Medications for: Psychosis Diabetes MAO inhibitors Stimulants Coumadin Caffeine	American: Root: 0.25–0.5 po BID Asian (Panax): 0.6–3 gm 1–3 times daily

continues

Table 15-2. *continued*

Herbal Supplement	Indications	Actions	Contraindications	Side Effects	Interactions	Dosage
Gingko Biloba	Dementia Improve cognitive, sexual, and GI functions Dizziness/Tinnitus	↑ CNS blood flow Neuroprotective Free Radical ↓ capillary fragility	If the patient is on anticoagulants	Spontaneous bleeding (rare) Headache and gastrointestinal irritation	Cyclosporin SSRIs MAO inhibitors Thiazide diuretics Anticoagulant properties may induce seizures, infertility	120–480 mg/day in 2–3 divided doses
Saw Palmetto	Anti-inflammatory ↑ urinary flow ↓ symptoms of BPH	Inhibits dihydro-testosterone Diuretic Anti-androgenic	Do not take while on prescription BPH treatment	None	Caution with diuretics	160 mg BID
Pygeum Africanum	Symptoms of BPH Anti-inflammatory Diuretic ↓ cholesterol	Anti-poliferative effect on fibroblast	None reported	Nausea and abdominal pain	None known	50–200 mg stand ext/day
Guarana	Stimulant headache ↑ energy	Sympathomimetic Caffeinelike activities	Cardiac problems Renal disease HTN or hyperthyroidism	↑ heart rate HTN Anxiety Arrhythmias	Avoid other stimulants	Not specified
Feverfew	Migraine Rheumatoid arthritis	Inhibits serotonin release	Aster family allergies Avoid during pregnancies	GI upset 6–15% 1st week of use	Anticoagulants (inhib cycloxygenic)	50 mg–1.2 gm/d equivalent to 0.2–0.6
Hawthorne	Atherosclerosis Arrhythmia	Improves cardiac output and coronary blood flow	Do not use with other inotropes	Mildly sedative	Digitalis Fox Glove	160–900 mg/day

Herbal Supplement	Indications	Actions	Contraindications	Side Effects	Interactions	Dosage
Black Cohosh	Menopause Astringent Diuretic Expectorant Vertigo Tinnitus	Estrogenlike action Oxytocic Luteinizing hormone suppression Binds to estrogen receptors	None known	Occasional GI upset Nausea, headache and dizziness in high doses	None known	Extracts w/alcohol: 40–60% (v/v) corresponds to 40 mg drug
Garlic	Reduces levels of lipids in blood Prevents age-dependent vascular changes ↓ Cholesterol 10–12%	Antibacterial Antimycotic Lipid-lowering Inhibition of platelet aggregation Prolongation of bleed and clotting time Enhances fibrinolytic activity	None known	GI upset Allergic reactions Odor may pervade breath and skin	Anticoagulants Hypoglycemics	4 g fresh garlic (minced bulb and prep is taken orally)
Pulsatilla	Sedative, headaches Fluid in the ears	Antispasmodic Increases circulation Antibacterial	Avoid during pregnancy	GI upset Topically—skin irritation Mild renal and urinary tract irritation	None known	120–300 mg TID
St. John's Wort	Dizziness, Tinnitus Mild to mod depression Viral infections Wound healing	Antidepressant Weak MAOI SSRI & dopamine agonist	Avoid in pregnancy	Photosensitivity	Anti-depressants MAOI Anti-seizure meds Birth control	300 mg TID
Ma Huang	Asthma Bronchial edema (weight loss—not an approved use) Stimulant	Sympathomimetic- Bronchodilator	Cardiac problems Anxiety Hypertension Angle closure glaucoma Pheochromo-cytoma Thyrotoxicant	Hypertension, neurosis, insomnia, palpitations, hyperglycemia Death	Halothone Cardiac glycosides MAOI Guanethedine Oxytosh	15–30 mg total alkaloid or 300 mg herb/day

The herb *Echinacea* provides us with a good example of some of the issues involved in herbal remedies. *Echinacea* is a very popular herb with a reputation for combating the common cold and flulike illnesses. It is a commonly used herb by professional singers at the first sign of a sniffle, cough, or general malaise. What most people do not realize is that there are nine different subtypes of echinacea, including *Echinacea purpurea*, *Echinacea pallida*, and *Echinacea angustafolia*. Not only does each subtype have different health benefits, but those benefits vary depending on the part of the plant used. The leaf of *Echinacea purpurea,* for example, has been shown to enhance T and B cell functions, whereas the root of that same plant does not. Conversely, *Echinacea pallida* root has been shown to enhance T and B cell function but the leaf of that same plant does not. Meanwhile, *Echinacea angustafolia* is rated as a negative herb by the German Commission E. Yet while visiting numerous health food stores, there were more than 100 bottles of echinacea on the shelves and 95% of them contained *Echinacea angustafolia*![5]

Why would the market be filled with *Echinacea angustafolia* if it is a negatively rated herb? One explanation is that manufacturers are not doing their homework. Another possibility is that it is a much less expensive or more available herb. Nutritional products that contain *Echinacea purpurea* leaf and *pallida* root are to be considered, both of which have been clearly shown in scientific studies to enhance and activate T and B cell functions, to encourage phagocytosis, and to have antibacterial and antiviral properties. Unfortunately, if a study is conducted with a product made from *Echinacea angustafolia,* the results are likely to indicate that it does not work in treating cold or flu symptoms. Studies like this cast doubt on all herbal remedies.

Drug/herb interactions pose another reason for concern. *Echinacea,* for example, may interfere with Neoral, prednisone, Imuran, and methotrexate. Furthermore, consumers and physicians should understand that immunostimulants, like *Echinacea* and the herb goldenseal, should not be used for prolonged periods of time. There are also contraindications for patients who have immune disorders or severe infections, such as tuberculosis. St John's wort is a commonly used herb for mild to moderate depression, yet it can interfere with commonly used anesthetics and the results can be deadly. Thus, it is critical to learn about the potential for interactions.

The professional singer needs to be aware of the potential benefit of other supplements as well. When singers get an upper respiratory tract infection (URI), anxiety and fear set in, particularly when a show is scheduled later that day or in the next couple of days. Many professional singers turn to specific supplements. Given the plethora of choices, this paper briefly discusses only a few of the more commonly used supplements.

Ionized zinc has been demonstrated to have direct antiviral activity. In order to achieve this antiviral activity the concentration required is 0.1 mmol/L to suppress rhinovirus activity. Zinc lozenges provide approximately 4.4 mmol/L. Zinc has been shown to protect cells from damage by viral toxins, and inhibit the rhinovirus's ability to attach, enter, and infect human nasal cells. Interestingly, studies have shown both efficacy and lack of efficacy. Some of this discrepancy can be accounted for by the compounds coupled with the zinc. These additives, specifically citric and tartaric acid, mannitol, and sorbitol, are used to enhance the flavor. However, these compounds can chelate the zinc and make it ineffective.[6-12]

There is a product called Zicam that is a homeopathic gel consisting of zinc gluconate. The mechanism of action is that the zinc gel binds to viral intercellular adhesion molecule (ICAM) attachment sites, stops the spread, and inhibits viral replication. However, in some cases it may cause burning and there have been some reports of anosmia, but it is suspected that the anosmia is more than likely secondary to the upper respiratory tract infection itself (Hensley et al, unpublished data).[13]

Another product that has been noted to be extremely helpful at rapidly eradicating the common cold and flu is a proprietary formula developed by the author and marketed by Body Language Vitamin Co (http://www.bodylangvitamin.com). This product utilizes the synergistic activity of multiple herbs and supplements, including *Echinacea purpurea* leaf, *pallida* root, goldenseal, zinc, quercetin, citrus bioflavanoids, and so on. It has been shown to reduce the duration of cold and flu by 70 to 85% in 85% of users, provided it is started at the onset of symptoms (Seidman, unpublished data). The ingredients have been shown to enhance T and B cell function and phagocytosis. It, like other herbals, should not be used in patients with active autoimmune processes or patients on immunosuppressant drugs.

Uncaria tomentosa has been shown to increase T and B cell lymphocytes, and phagocyte and lymphoblast function. Its effects appear to be mediated by the activity of the constituent pentacyclic oxindole alkaloids (POAs). It has also been shown to contain quinovic acid, which reduces inflammation. There are no specific contraindications, side effects, or interactions.[14,15]

Pulsatilla (Anemone pulsatilla) acts as a sedative and an antispasmodic and can be used to treat headache, neuralgia, laryngitis, mild dizziness, and tinnitus. The herb has been demonstrated to have relaxation properties and to enhance circulation. *Pulsatilla* is not recommended for use during pregnancy. There are no known interactions although a fresh *pulsatilla* plant can cause blistering or a rash.

Aconite *(Aconitum napellus)* can be beneficial in the treatment of upper respiratory infections, influenza, facial neuralgia, arthritis, and gout. The alkaloids activate sodium channels, which have been shown to affect neural function. Aconite should not be used in conjunction with any other alkaloids such as quinine or morphine, or tryptophan. The side effects can include nausea, vomiting, dizziness, parasthesia, and palpitations.

Cordyceps sinensis enhances immunity and reduces coughing by increasing lung "chi." It acts as a bronchodilator increasing the function of natural killer and B cells. There are no specific contraindications, interactions, or side effects.[16]

Astragalus membranaceus has been known to enhance energy, by increasing resistance to disease while increasing "chi" and circulation. Additionally, it has anti inflammatory properties. It has been demonstrated to enhance the body's ability to adapt to stress, stimulates proliferation of stem cells, macrophages, and lymphocyte cells, and increases the production of interferon. Although its use is to be questioned in the presence of active autoimmune diseases, there are no significant known contraindications, side effects, or interactions.[17,18]

Ginseng *(Panax ginseng)* has been useful in the treatment of fatigue, depression, stress, sexual energy, and digestion and promotes general well-being. It is an adaptogenic stimulant that promotes secretion of adrenocorticotrophic hormome, causing a release of endorphins and enkephalins. It should not be taken during pregnancy and may interfere with anticoagulant therapy. In high doses it may cause insomnia, anxiety, and gastrointestinal upset. It should not be taken with other anticoagulants, stimulants (such as caffeine), monoamine oxidase inhibitors (MAOIs), or antipsychotics.

Goldenseal *(Hydrastis canadensis)* has been shown to be beneficial for mucosal inflammation, diarrhea and gastritis, wound healing, immune function, URI, and the flu. It is believed to act as an adaptogen (enhances body defenses) and may increase circulation. The herb should not be used during pregnancy. In high doses, it may cause nausea, vomiting, diarrhea, CNS stimulation, and respiratory failure. There are no known significant interactions. There are many more herbs that can be considered but this should provide the reader with a great start. Additionally, Table 15–2 lists additional commonly used herbs.

It is critical for health care providers to question patients specifically about the use of nutraceuticals and herbs. Proven therapeutic options should be discussed. If a viable alternative exists, it can be considered, bearing in mind, of course, that natural does not necessarily mean safe. As always, one needs to be diligent about quality control and standardization, and realize that herbal/pharmaceutical interactions do occur with some frequency. Health care professionals should also consider nutraceutical safety issues and keep an objective perspective. According to one study, the average annual mortality rates over the past 12 years show that deaths related to vitamin use occur at approximately 1 death per year and herbs cause 2 deaths per year, whereas smoking is responsible for more than 400,000 deaths per year, poor diet is linked to 300,000 deaths per year, and pharmaceutical errors contribute to more than 100,000 deaths per year.[19] Thus, it is not very likely that anyone will be harmed with nutritional or herbal therapies.

Vitamins and minerals are crucial for many different bodily functions. A number of multivitamins provide the standard vitamins and minerals, but there is really no such thing as one pill that can provide everything the body needs. Typically, it takes 4 to 10 pills a day to obtain the necessary nutrients. It is always best if the ingredients are natural and minerals are chelated. Chelating a mineral means an amino acid is bound, to the mineral. Thus, when physicians recommend Tums as a good source of calcium, this is a fallacy. Tums is calcium carbonate; the same chemical formula as stone. The absorption of calcium carbonate is approximately 2 to 4%. Thus, for my patients, I always recommended the use of a chelated calcium such as calcium glycinate, gluconate, or citrate. Furthermore, it is an added benefit if the supplement is produced in an FDA-inspected laboratory. In addition, antioxidants should have powerful molecular and cellular antioxidants that are well absorbed. Obtaining sufficient antioxidant protection could require an additional two to four pills a day.

Many nutrition experts believe that our current vitamin and mineral guidelines are too low. The recommended dietary allowances (RDA), or dietary reference intakes (DRI), were established by the Food and Nutrition Board in 1941. They are considered the best scientific judgment on nutritional allowances and are designed to meet the nutrient needs of practically all healthy people. Although the RDAs are safe and adequate nutrient levels, they are neither minimal requirements nor optimal levels. This then raises the question of whether or not we need to take supplements. There is a considerable body of evidence suggesting that the answer to this question is yes. Although conflicting results can be confusing for the general public, health care practitioners should be aware of the important role played by vitamins, minerals, and other supplements in overall health. Although the public is encouraged to adopt a healthy lifestyle, engage in stress reduction, eat a nutritious diet, and obtain adequate exercise, few people actually follow those guidelines. As a result, vitamin, mineral, and antioxidant supplements are not only necessary but recommended by an increasing number of health authorities. They play a very important role in the health and maintenance of all people and certainly professional voice users should consider some of these strategies.

Aside from nutraceuticals, many other CIM therapies warrant further discussion. Traditional Chinese medicine (TCM) encompasses both acupuncture therapy and Chinese herbal therapy. It is a system of medicine that also looks at how diet, lifestyle choices, and emotions affect a person's overall health.

ACUPUNCTURE AND CHINESE HERBAL THERAPY

Beth Kohn and Susan Jakary are well-known acupuncturists for the Center for Integrative Medicine at Henry Ford Health System. They note that TCM is based on the concept that a vital life force, or energy (called "qi," which is pronounced "chee") is what fuels all of the functions of our bodies, including respiration, digestion, elimination, and reproduction. Symptoms and chronic disease patterns reflect an imbalance in this energetic system. Traditional Chinese medicine strives to alleviate or eliminate the symptom (also called the branch manifestation) while at the same time balancing the underlying cause (called the root). This allows the body to change the course of any underlying imbalance thus giving way to alleviating chronic health issues.

The energy, or qi, moves through the body along pathways known as meridians. These meridians have names that are similar to our Western organs such as the lung, spleen, and heart meridian. Each meridian relates to certain functions and processes within the body as well as to different emotions. Each meridian also connects and relates to other meridians creating a unified system of energy within the body. One example of this is the lung meridian being closely related to respiration, health of the skin, perspiration, protection against colds and flu, and voice quality and strength. Symptoms that may reflect an imbalance in the lung meridian might include cough, hoarse voice, or laryngitis, asthma, allergies, sore throat, and the common cold to name a few. Specific acupuncture points and herbal formulas can be used to resolve the symptoms and restore balance.

Acupuncture needles are very fine, thin needles that are gently tapped into the surface of the skin. Typically, they are about 10 times thinner than conventional needles and are not considered painful when inserted. Their insertion stimulates a physiologic healing response in which endorphins and enkephalins are released into the bloodstream. The patient often senses a feeling of extreme relaxation.

Performers who need to strengthen their voice quality may find acupuncture and herbal therapies extremely effective. Chinese medicine can provide a strong foundation to support performers by protecting their voices during times when they may be more vulnerable. This may be when they are asked to perform multiples shows in a short period of time or during the cold and flu seasons. Acupuncture and herbal therapy may also be used to speed up recovery time for patients suffering from the common cold or just from the rigors of frequent voice use.

When a performer feels a sore throat or some slight fatigue signaling the onset of an upper respiratory infection (URI), they can use TCM to help prevent the progression of the illness. Chinese herbals are classically plant, mineral, or animal based and are prescribed specifically for the individual and what his or her needs are. No two patients are identical, so their acupuncture and herbal therapies are tailored to their specific needs.

Acupuncture has been demonstrated to relax and release muscle tension. It is the ease of movement by expansion and contraction of the diaphragm and surrounding external intercostals muscles that allows the lungs to inflate to capacity. In addition, it is especially beneficial to relax the muscles in the jaw, neck, shoulders, back, and abdomen. The technique of cupping is quite effective for relaxing muscles and increases circulation to these areas. Even the base of the tongue can tense, causing surrounding structures to contract, distorting voice clarity, pitch, and timbre. Lastly, acupuncture is calming and centering for the emotions. Sometimes unconscious thoughts or past emotional trauma create habitual holding patterns inside the body. Not only can this affect mental state, but could negatively affect the skeletal alignment, breathing, muscle performance, and the healthy functioning of the organ systems.

HYPNOTHERAPY AND NEUROIMMUNOPSYCHOLOGY

Donna May, a licensed hypnotherapist, notes that in her practice mind body therapies such as hypnotherapy or neurolinguistic programming (NLP) are helpful adjuncts to the professional singer. Hypnotherapy has been used for many years to facilitate relaxation and to envision a perfect performance. Many professional singers use this form of therapy. Initially, they experience several sessions with a professional hypnotherapist and then can learn to do this on their own.

It is clear that our beliefs and perceptions strongly influence behavior. You are much less likely to suc-

ceed if you are not convinced that you will. A classic example, is before Roger Bannister ran 1 mile in less than 4 minutes, it was believed to be impossible. Within the same year of Roger's landmark record, other athletes also ran the mile in less than 4 minutes because they now believed it to be possible. Similarly, Paula Radcliffe recently set a new world record by running the marathon in just under 2 hours and 16 minutes. These successes set the stage for further accomplishments. Beliefs are so powerful that they can affect our neuroimmunopsychology, and they are an invaluable asset to assist a person in achieving his or her goals.

NLP is essentially the science of how to run your brain in an optimal way to produce the result you want. An example of the power of NLP is depicted in the book, *Unlimited Power* by Anthony Robbins. In chapter 4 there is a story of one of the great musicians of the 20th century, Pablo Casals, the cellist, told by Norman Cousins, author of *Anatomy of an Illness*.[20] At 90 he was frail, arthritic, with emphysema and swollen clenched fingers. He walked with a shuffle, stooped over, his head pitched forward. Yet when he sat himself on the piano bench to play each morning, something quite miraculous happened. Casals suddenly transformed himself and went into a resourceful state, and as he did, his physiology changed to such a degree that he began to move and play producing both in his body and on the piano results that should have been possible only for a healthy, strong, flexible pianist. The story goes on to say that his fingers seemed to race above the keyboard and his entire body seemed fused with the music. "By the time he walked away from the piano, he seemed entirely different from the person who sat down to play. He stood straighter and taller and he walked without a trace of a shuffle to the breakfast table and then went out for a stroll along the beach." As Anton Chekhov said, "Man is what he believes."

NLP addresses the mind and allows the individual to form positive images that are the foothold for success. These strategies include: success strategies, modeling excellence, utilizing past successes and resources, anchoring for success, and structure and physiology body posture, breathing, facial, expression, gestures, and others.

A brief example of what a vocalist might do to harness the power of NLP is as follows: It is critical that the singer envision a past performance when they had the perfect delivery of their tonal aspects and their ability to work the crowd. It is then necessary to elicit that resourceful state of being by discovering their success strategy. What did they see, hear, say to themselves? How did they use their physiology (stand, breathe, etc)? An anchor for success could then be established and utilized for the future. By being able to put themselves in the resourceful state through anchoring, they can again achieve excellent results.

These powerful techniques can also be used to assist patients with a variety of disorders including overcoming fears and phobias, anxiety, depression, and limiting beliefs. A hypnotherapist can also utilize the above strategies by incorporating them into a hypnosis script and using the techniques with the client during hypnosis. The power of the mind is a grossly untapped area of holistic health that has real opportunity to enhance the overall outcome.

NEUROMUSCULAR THERAPY

It is important to have a brief understanding of skeletal and muscular situations that can facilitate the voice or lead to its downfall. Kyrras Conrad, an authority on the techniques of St. John neuromuscular therapy (NMT) notes that there are numerous mechanisms to support the vocalist by maximizing voice quality and endurance and by addressing vocal dysfunctions. Many of the same muscles will be treated for both wellness care and to correct abnormal or suboptimal function. Maximizing voice quality in the well person will usually involve treating all the muscles of phonation and air exchange. Vocal dysfunctions are treated by assessing the individual's particular problem and, in addition to the muscles treated in wellness care, will more specifically and thoroughly treat the muscles involved with that problem.

Voice quality, range, texture, resonance, and endurance are all affected by the tone of the associated musculature. Areas of hypertonicity are generally considered to be hypoperfused or even ischemic; ischemic areas have diminished range of motion and are believed to create trigger points. Trigger point referral sites may also develop reduced circulation, and this may manifest as pain, parasthesia, numbness, itching, and/or diminished range of motion.[21,22]

Hypertonicity of the muscles that affect the voice can occur as a result of direct trauma, such as sudden deceleration injuries, manual strangulation, and so forth; indirect trauma, such as injuries to other parts of the body that result in uneven muscle tone of the neck and shoulders; or microtrauma from repetitive use or poor posture. Practicing or performing in areas with exceedingly dry air, the presence of smoke, and so forth can also cause excessive and uneven muscle contraction.

Vocal dysfunctions are often related to muscles of the larynx, the lips, and the tongue. Movement of the tongue, resonance, and clear articulation are directly affected by the condition of the muscles of the oropharynx, nasopharynx, and laryngopharynx. The hyoglossus, palatoglossus, genioglossuss, styloglossus, the pharyngeal constrictors, palatopharyngeus, palatines, levator labii, zygomaticus, risoris, obicularis oris, buccinator, and platysma, as well as many other superficial and internal muscles, often require treatment. Endurance and air volume are also issues and are related to muscles of the thorax, such as the intercostals, pectoralis major and minor, the rhomboids, serratus anterior and posterior musculature, and the diaphragm. Mandibular range of motion is most profoundly affected by the temporalis, masseter, and medial and lateral pterygoid muscles.

Treatment strategies are developed after assessing for imbalances of muscle tone. Therapy applied to the hypertonic areas will improve circulation and allow muscles to return to normal resting length and so allow the muscles to flex and extend freely for full expression of the voice. St. John neuromuscular therapy uses several techniques such as friction, static pressure of 8- to 12-seconds duration, and trigger point therapy to externally and internally treat the bodies, origins, and insertions of all affected muscles where those muscles are entirely accessible, and treats as much as possible of those muscles to which access may be limited. Only the upper 2 to 3 inches of the pharyngeal constrictors, for example, can be treated internally in most individuals.

St. John neuromuscular therapy is a low-cost, non-invasive method to correct vocal dysfunction related to soft tissue problems and should be considered for therapy before more invasive solutions are attempted. In addition to effectively treating soft tissue pathology, this therapy will maintain good vocal health in the healthy individual as well as help perfect the voice of the vocal professional. This leads us to a brief discussion of massage therapy. Massage therapy has been demonstrated to have strong beneficial physiologic effects, including the ability to enhance immune system function[23-26] and provide a sense of relaxation and well-being. Many professional performers find benefit to the healing properties of massage.

SUMMARY

In summary, although many CIM remedies have been in existence for thousands of years, there is a general lack of randomized, double-blind, placebo-controlled studies supporting their efficacy. As a result, many health care professionals are skeptical and hesitant to recommend CIM modalities. The care of the professional voice clearly involves utilizing strategies categorized as CIM. There is tremendous public interest in alternative therapies, particularly in areas that are difficult to treat with conventional medicine. Statistics show that the amount of money being spent on CIM by the public is increasing rapidly each year. And, with increased funding now available from the NIH, preliminary research is showing that certain CIM remedies are appropriate for treating a number of acute and chronic health conditions. In view of this, it is imperative that medical professionals familiarize themselves with these options. In addition, we should be aware that modalities we may consider to be "alternative" are mainstream and accepted practices elsewhere in the world.

Because anecdotal evidence outweighs proof from clinical trials in the area of CIM, it is not always easy to determine what works and what does not. This results in products and therapies of varying quality and effectiveness.

Above all, as health care professionals, we need to remove our blinders and consider the options, without jeopardizing our patient's health. With both public interest and scientific research in CIM on the rise, our profession is certain to experience a further increase in the use of CIM therapies. For the sake of both our patients and our profession, it is essential that health care practitioners remain current in this increasingly evolving field.

REFERENCES

1. Weil Lifestyle LLC. (2005). About Dr. Weil, Available at: http://www.drweil.com/u/Page/About/. Last accessed December 2005.
2. Surow JB, Lovetri J. Alternative medical therapy use among singers: prevalence and implications for the medical care of the singer. *J Voice.* 2000; 14(3):398–409.
3. Barnes P, Powell-Griner E, McFann K, et al. Complementary and alternative medicine use among adults: United States, 2002. *CDC Advance Data Report #343.* May 27, 2004.
4. Eisenberg DM, Davis RB, Ettner SL, et al.. Trends in alternative medicine use in the United States, 1990-1997: results of a follow-up national survey. *JAMA.* 1998;280:1569–1575.
5. Blumenthal M, Busse W, Goldberg A, et al. *The Complete German Commission Monographs: Therapeutic Guide to Herbal Medicine.* Austin, Tex: American Botanical Council; 1998.
6. Korant BD, Kauer JC, Butterworth BE. Zinc ions inhibit replication of rhinoviruses. *Nature.* 1974; 12:248(449):588–590.
7. Korant BD, Butterworth BE. Inhibition by zinc of rhinovirus protein cleavage: interaction of zinc with capsid polypeptides. *J Virol.* 1976;18(1):298–306.
8. Kelly RW, Able MH. Copper and zinc inhibit the metabolism of prostaglandin by the human uterus. *Biol Reprod.* 1983;28:883–889.
9. Novick SG, Godfrey JC, Godfrey NJ, et al. How does zinc modify the common cold? Clinical observations and implications regarding mechanisms of action. *Med Hypotheses.* 1996;46(3):295–302.
10. Mossad SB, Macknin ML, Medendorp SV, et al. Zinc gluconate lozenges for treating the common cold: a randomized, double-blind, placebo-controlled study. *Ann Intern Med.* 1996;15;125(2):81–88.
11. Jackson JL, Peterson C, Lesho E. A meta-analysis of zinc salts lozenges and the common cold. *Arch Intern Med.* 1997;10;157(20):2373–2376.
12. Jackson JL, Lesho E, Peterson C. Zinc and common cold: a meta-analysis revisited. *J Nutr.* 2000; 103(Suppl S5):1512S–1515S.
13. Hirt M, Nobel S, Barron E. Zinc nasal gel for the treatment of common cold symptoms: a double-blind placebo-controlled trial. *Ear Nose Throat J.* 2000;79(10):778–780, 782.
14. Reinhard KH. *Uncaria tomentosa* (Willd.) DC: cat's claw, una de gato, or saventaro. *J Altern Complement Med.* 1999;5(2):143–151.

15. Keplinger K, Laus G, Wurm M, et al. *Uncaria tomentosa* (Willd.) DC.—ethnomedicinal use and new pharmacological, toxicological and botanical results. *J Ethnopharmacol.* 1999;64(1):23-34.

16. Li Y, Chen GZ, Jiang DZ. Effect of *Cordyceps sinensis* on erythropoiesis in mouse bone marrow. *Chin Med J (Engl).* 1993;106(4):313-316.

17. Chu DT, Wong WL, Mavligit GM. Immunotherapy with Chinese medicinal herbs, II. Reversal of cyclophosphamide-induced immune suppression by administration of fractionated *Astragalus membranaceus* in vivo. *J Clin Lab Immunol.* 1988; 25(3):125-129.

18. Zhao KS, Mancini C, Doria G. Enhancement of the immune response in mice by *Astragalus membranaceus* extracts. *Immunopharmacology.* 1990; 20(3):225-233.

19. Seidman M. Nutrition and health: fact or fantasy? Paper presented at the Annual Meeting of the American Academy of Otolaryngology-Head and Neck Surgery; September 20, 2004; Los Angeles, Calif.

20. Robbins A. *Unlimited Power.* New York, NY: Simon and Schuster; 1986:chap4.

21. Alvarez DJ, Rockwell PG. Trigger points: diagnosis and management. *Am Fam Physician.* 2002;65(4): 653-660.

22. Simons DG, Travell JG, Simons LS. *Myofascial Pain and Dysfunction: The Trigger Point Manual.* Vol I. 2nd ed. Baltimore, Md: Williams & Wilkins; 1999.

23. Zeitlin D, Keller SE, Shiflett SC, et al. Immunological effects of massage therapy during academic stress. *Psychosom Med.* 2000;62(1):83-84.

24. Birk TJ, McGrady A, MacArthur RD, et al. The effects of massage therapy alone and in combination with other complementary therapies on immune system measures and quality of life in human immunodeficiency virus. *J Altern Complem Med.* 2000;6(5):405-414.

25. Von Adrian UH. A massage for the journey: keeping leukocytes soft and silent. *Proc Natl Acad Sci USA.* 1997;13(94):4825-4827.

26. Hernandez-Reif M, Ironson G, Field T, et al. Breast cancer patients have improved immune and neuroendocrine function following massage therapy. *J Psychosom Res.* 2004, 57(1):45-52.

Part IV

Behavioral Therapies

Chapter 16

VOICE THERAPY FOR BENIGN VOCAL FOLD LESIONS AND SCAR IN SINGERS AND ACTORS

Mara Behlau
Thomas Murry

The singer depends on precise voice production and on a specific vocal quality for his or her professional subsistence. What separates singers and actors from other voice professionals is the artistic demands of the performance. As described in chapter 1, the universe of professional voice users includes clerics, teachers, lawyers, salesmen, secretaries, telemarketing agents, and stockbrokers. Although these groups of people may use their voices more than singers and actors, they do not have the artistic demands of performers. The primary distinction between singers and other voice professionals is with the artistic nature of their voices.[1] In order to identify the needs of the professional singer and actor, it is important to understand the demands of vocal quality and artistic delivery.[2] Singers as well as other professional voice users may be compared to professional athletes, who are more likely to suffer muscular injuries than the general population due to their high physical demand.[3]

> Singers, like professional athletes, need specific and often intense rehabilitation in order to return to their top performance form.

It is important to understand the concept of preferred voice in the modern life, as proposed by Behlau.[4] This requires a different dimension of vocal analysis that encompasses options of respiratory, vocal, articulatory, psychodynamic, and behavioral parameters used both by the individual and by the group in which he or she fits. The professionals may or may not be aware of these options, which are usually acquired by modeling, imitation, and training, throughout the years of their professional practice. In addition to being acquired through modeling, a professional vocal pattern or style can also be specifically trained. People who do voiceovers and singers frequently admit that they started their careers imitating a successful professional until they found their own vocal output. Those vocal choices sometimes match the professional activity in ways that become the vocal markers of the profession itself. The use of a particular voice style often allows immediate identification of the profession, for example, the voice of priests, lawyers, and newscasters. Some of the vocal options are not necessarily healthy and may lead to a potential or real risk for vocal health. For example, preparing for an audition that requires new repertoire or that requires singing and dancing may lead to habits not often used.

Expansion of repertoire for a particular show or even a particular song may result in acquired patterns not consistent with previous training.

Injuries to the singer's voice are not unusual. Singing places demands on the vocal folds and the entire vocal system that are at times excessive. Singing styles often require specific voice qualities, which may be considered as a preferred voice for a particular role. Understanding the dynamics involved is crucial to determining whether or not the changes proposed to the performer and the training program required to achieve it will be acquired without injury.

Singers acquire benign lesions and scars of vocal folds for many reasons. The diagnostic and treatment considerations for the singer go beyond the habitual references of the voice clinic. Situations for the singer and actor are very diverse and extend from the desire of having an unusual voice of success. Rock singers may have edema and leukoplakia for special effects. If not careful, however, they risk the possibility of restricted professional activity due to a vocal fold scar. Pop singers or musical theatre performers are unable to sing in tune due to scarring after surgical excision. When the singer with a scar attempts to reach certain notes, further injury is likely to occur.

> There is a preferred voice for a particular singing style, as well as a preferred voice for each singer.

The choices are not always conscious choices. Many times the required voice is simply the singer's natural voice produced in a melodious and controlled way; at other times, the required voice is adapted to meet a performance requirement. The evaluation of the dysphonia may be difficult, as no voice-related quality of life and handicap instruments are sensitive enough to measure these aspects. Besides, many singers have the ability to develop muscular compensations that mask (at least partially) real difficulties. There is even a risk of not evaluating the original problem and focusing on the secondary compensation that sometimes draws more attention.[5]

A complete analysis of the vocal problem involves the identification of factors both predisposing and contributing to the dysphonia. Individual aspects, vocal technique problems, general health, and environmental issues must be addressed. Individual factors consist of anatomo-functional predisposition, personality traits, allergies,[6] and gastroesophageal reflux.[7] General health factors are related to the use of medications,[8] and self-medication is a particular concern. Environmental factors[2] include room acoustics, sound amplification, air quality, noxious fumes and chemicals,[9,10] or other aspects related to the work environment, including rehearsal schedules, tours, and interviews.

Information obtained by observing a performance or listening to a CD may reveal aspects that are not identified in the clinical setting. For example, the posture used during singing, acting, or performing with a stage band or a large orchestra may reveal strain or excessive effort not seen in the voice clinic.

The clinician must learn to recognize that different dynamics are required for different styles and types of singing. The evaluation and treatment for each different style of singing must be accurate, objective, and timely. Care of the singer's voice must include considerations about the next auditions, number of rehearsals, and types of performances. The voice clinician must be aware of various methods, techniques, exercises, and strategies depending on the singer's needs. Some singers have already been through previous therapies that did not work or with which they were not comfortable, and new approaches may provide better results. However, the sense of urgency should not compromise the clinical sensitiveness, welcoming care, and support that the dysphonic singer needs. Artists are human beings with great susceptibility and sensitivity about their work. They react deeply to comments and observations about their art.[11]

THE SINGER'S VOICE EVALUATION

The speech-language pathologist who works with singers and actors must have knowledge about medical speech-language pathology, skills to work with a team, and specific knowledge of the vocal arts. Some general knowledge about music and the lifestyle and activities of performers is also important. However skilled the general clinical speech-language pathologist may be for treating language problems, he or she may not have the primary prerequisites for the care of singers. A voice clinician is the professional that understands his or her own responsibilities as well as those of the laryngologist, recognizing the limits of both specialists and the possibilities of the contributions of each.

The comprehensive voice evaluation begins with a detailed history, including the type and quality of singing training and the use of other voice modalities, such as teaching and liturgical. When possible, a review of voice recordings made before the current problem may be useful, as singers sometimes assign substantial importance to their last event, not recognizing the existence of earlier voice changes. The clinician should highlight the conditions surrounding the individual's present search for help and the vocal history of the singer. The contribution of specific factors that triggered the voice problem must be clarified, and other factors that may be responsible for maintaining it or for changing it since its onset must be identified. A clear understanding of the onset factors allows the singer to replace the guilt feelings associated with the problems and helps reduce the emotional overload connected to the voice disorder. Precise complaints such as "I cannot reach the A4"; "after the fourth song I notice that I lose the metal of my voice"; I notice that I sometimes sing off tune, however the others say I'm doing fine"; "I don't feel the resonance on the palate" should be specifically considered. Otherwise the patient may not adhere to the suggested recommendations or he or she may look for another clinician who will listen to and understand the importance of the specific problem.

Although the primary symptoms are usually manifested in the singing voice, the speaking voice must also be evaluated. Singing and speaking are as different as swimming the backstroke versus the butterfly. Many singers are so concerned with singing that they forget that the speaking process utilizes the same organs, but with different muscular adjustments. Moreover, while singing is usually a result of training, speaking is the result of behavioral habits acquired during a lifetime combined with emotional factors related to one's personality in the speaking situation. The clinician should always remember that most singers and actors usually talk more than they sing and talk more off stage than when acting or rehearsing.

There is no agreement on the minimum battery of tests to evaluate singers; however, ideally it should include a perceptual voice analysis, a three-point modified voice range profile (VRP), an acoustic spectrographic analysis of speaking and singing, and observations of the vocal folds during speech and singing.

The perceptual analysis of the vocal quality should be performed with several phonatory tasks. An open sustained vowel, such as "a" like in "accent" or "e" like in "egg," should be used to evaluate the sound resource characteristics and connected speech. An evaluation of voice quality, tune matching, and register changes should also be included. Clinician rating scales may also be used, such as GRBAS[12] or CAPE-V[13] (see Appendix 16–1). However, neither scale fully addresses the singer's needs. The CAPE-V enables a more comprehensive description of voice quality as it relates to severity and to the number of deviated vocal parameters.

The Voice Range Profile (VRP) is commonly employed in Europe but rarely in other places, probably due to its difficulty and the amount of time it takes to complete. However the 3-dimensional VRP graph consisting of the mean, lowest, and highest fundamental frequency and minimum and maximum loudness helps to analyze the singer's vocal pliability (see chapter 9).

The acoustic analysis by the extraction of measures of fundamental frequency, jitter, shimmer, and noise measures may not be reliable in some situations because of irregularity in the acoustic signal.[14] Nevertheless, the descriptive spectrographic analysis is greatly valued and serves as a powerful visual feedback for the singer.

The stroboscopic evaluation,[15] and particularly the phonoscopic analysis[16] is essential to the singer, not only to establish the diagnosis, but also to show small deviations that may have been overlooked by other less comprehensive evaluations. During the phonoscopic examination, the clinician obtains information about the laryngeal behavior during high and low pitch, soft and loud volume, whisper and sound, intermittent voice production, and so on.

Investigation of the impact of the singer's dysphonia on his or her professional activities can be done by means of a set of questions checking on rehearsal and show cancellations, contract breaks, reduction of singing activities, increase of warm-up time, and fatigue after a performance. The use of established instruments may help in this task.[17-22] No specific protocols to evaluate singers have been validated to do this; however, as one spends more time with singers and actors, a standard set of questions usually evolves.

To summarize the evaluation, it is interesting to note that there is generally no direct relationship between the size of the lesion and the vocal deviation or between what is perceptually observed and acoustically measured or between the visual analysis of the vocal folds and the vocal output. Most significantly, there is little or no relationship between the dysphonia impact evaluation and self-perceived severity.

THE SINGER'S VOCAL REHABILITATION PROGRAM

> Voice therapy is the primary management strategy for the treatment of benign laryngeal lesions in singers because of its conservative nature and because it potentially lowers the risk for future problems.

The ideal situation for most singers with a vocal injury is to take part in a voice therapy program that includes vocal education, psychodynamics and voice training with the help of a singing specialist.[23] There are major differences among singers, however, in voice training and vocal rehabilitation (see chapter 6). It is necessary to differentiate the vocal intervention with a short-term purpose, such as placing the voice on a CD track in 2 days or performing in a show the next day, from interventions with long-term purposes, such as helping a rock singer to find alternative muscular adjustments in order to have a less aggressive voice production. The behavioral model can be used for most singers' problems. The medical model may be used in certain cases. In this model, the patient plays a more passive role initially. He or she must be active in voice rehabilitation.[24] Some lesions can be reabsorbed and some voices can definitively improve even in the presence of a lesion. The plasticity of the voice can be checked to give a more precise evaluation on the benefit of vocal rehabilitation.[25]

Whenever possible, the vocal education, psychodynamic, and training tripod should be employed.[26] Vocal education and vocal hygiene guidelines must be viable and include alternative strategies to change maladaptive habits. The clinician must be realistic and understand that it is easier to execute a series of exercises than to comply with changes in habits or behavior. Psychodynamic therapy goes beyond analysis of the emotions. However, analysis of the emotional impact of the deviated singing voice to the public may help to define schedule, rehearsal, and shows issues.

Vocal training options are wide-ranging[27] and can either include more schematic and predefined treatment, such as vocal function exercises,[28] confidential voice therapy,[29] and the Lessac-Madsen resonance method[30,31] or adapted exercises.[26,32] However, due to the urgent characteristic of the management of these professionals, varied exercises are usually employed and are combined and modified according to the pathophysiology of the condition, the reported complaint, and the observed vocal deviation, which represents a combination of philosophic, physiologic, and symptomatologic education and counseling. An eclectic approach described by Behlau[26] consists of the seven categories for the treatment of dysphonia shown in Table 16–1.

Many singers succeed very well with an expedient treatment focused on their complaint and diagnostic findings. Others will have recurrent lesions that must be followed up for a long period of time. The majority do not accept a surgical procedure, although it may ultimately be the best treatment. Even then, the singer can benefit from voice rehabilitation.

Table 16–1. The Seven Categories of Treatment for Dysphonia

1. Body Method
2. Speech Organs Method
3. Auditory Method
4. Speech Method
5. Facilitating Sounds Method
6. Phonatory Competence Method
7. Voice Activation Method

BENIGN VOCAL FOLD LESIONS AND VOCAL FOLD SCARS IN CLASSICAL AND COMMERCIAL CONTEMPORARY MUSIC (CCM) SINGERS

The main benign vocal fold lesions seen in singers and actors are: nodules, cysts, polyps, Reinke's edema, and leukoplakia. In addition, a particular challenging condition is the vocal fold scar, which usually has an iatrogenic nature and can bring devastating consequences to the singer's life. Figure 16–1 shows a vocal fold scar in a 31-year-old female singer who developed a voice problem while rehearsing for a CD.

Diagnostic accuracy and a detailed evaluation of vocal behavior will allow specific treatment planning. However clear the relationship between a certain causal factor and the vocal deviation may be (for instance, gastroesophageal reflux and hoarse voice with limited singing range), a complete evaluation is indispensable, because the co-occurrence of several events is very common. More often, the voice disorder is not related to one factor, event, or time period. Voices that do not change with trial therapy have reduced possibilities for voice rehabilitation. Many therapeutic strategies may be utilized, such as changing the vocal quality by modifying the respiratory pattern, glottic closure, resonance, and articulation. Voice monitoring may also be employed, for example, visual monitoring using laryngeal or spectrographic instrumentation, auditory monitoring via auditory feedback, or vocal amplification and proprioceptive monitoring, such as identification of regions of tension or muscular biofeedback.

Figure 16–1. Vocal fold scar with sulcus on the left vocal fold of a CCM singer.

In this chapter, two categories of singers are described, classical and commercial contemporary.[33] This categorization may be simplistic and overlapping, but it facilitates understanding the major differences found between the two groups. Although there may be exceptions and singers may not fit in either category, for comparison we can generalize two different profiles.

Classical singers usually have a long history of singing classes, greater knowledge of vocal production, and systematic practice and training. They look for help early when having a voice problem as even minor deviations in the vocal quality can compromise a performance. They usually do not smoke or consume significant amounts of alcohol. They do not sing with amplification and rarely use sound technology resources except in the recording studio. Classical singers are initially more responsive to suggestions made than commercial contemporary singers as they are used to following vocal practice schedules and specific singing exercises.

In contrast, the commercial contemporary singers typically have a short history of singing lessons or no professional voice training. They may not appreciate the voice production mechanism as readily as a classical singer. In fact, some singers even believe that singing classes and vocal knowledge may hinder voice spontaneity. Whether this idea evolves from colleagues or is just due to their repertoire is uncertain, but untrained singers have a less systematic approach to vocal warm-up and rehearsal and generally take longer to look for help. This may be because small deviations in their vocal repertoire may not compromise performances but actually add to their appeal. For some singers, voice modification or stylistic changes are, at least in part, accepted in the singing styles of commercial contemporary singers. There is a greater likelihood that they smoke and drink alcohol, even during performances (one can recall classic videos of cabaret singers with a cigarette). They sing with a microphone and with sound technology that can minimize some vocal deviations. Contemporary singers tend to be less adherent to the suggestions made due to a more unstable schedule and irregular life habits. They often sing in more than a single style and they feel that experimentation with styles may actually increase their popularity.

A review of 30 singers classified according to their singing style, recently seen by both authors, is presented in Tables 16–2 and 16–3.

Table 16–2. Review of 15 Consecutive CCM Singers Presenting with Voice Complaints

Contemporary Singer	Style and Training	Complaint	Type of Lesion	Management	Outcome
1. Female, 36y-old Nonsmoker Allergy	Pop singer 4 years classical training	1½-year vocal complaint Local show	VF nodules Similar episode 6 years ago	Vocal rehabilitation High compliance	Dismissed Reabsorption of lesion and adapted voice
2. Male, 34y-old Smoker	Pop singer No singing training	2-year vocal complaint Local show	VF polyp	Vocal rehabilitation Noncompliant Refused surgery	Follow-up Lesion with better voice, but fatigue
3. Female, 32y-old Smoker	Gospel singer 2 years classical training	1-year vocal complaint Recording CD	Epidermoid cyst + mucosal bridge	Vocal rehabilitation Moderate compliance	Follow-up Lesion with better voice and less fatigue
4. Female, 28y-old Nonsmoker GE reflux	Gospel singer No singing training	1-month vocal complaint After a 4-day festival	Hemorrhagic polyp	Surgery and vocal rehabilitation pre and post-op	Dismissed No lesion and adapted voice
5. Female, 34y-old Nonsmoker	Latin music (salsa and mambo) singer + musical theatre Irregular 10 years classical training	Vocal complaint after 1 month intense rehearsals	VF nodules	Vocal rehabilitation High compliance	Dismissed Reabsorption of lesion and better voice
6. Male, 42y-old Smoking GE reflux	Brazilian pop music No singing training	1½-year vocal complaint Touring with show	Leukoplakia and edema	Vocal rehabilitation Surgery programmed High compliance	Follow up Lesion but better voice and less fatigue
7. Male, 43y-old Smoker	Brazilian country music No singing training	2-year vocal complaint Several similar episodes during past 15 years Touring with show	Epidermoid cyst	Refused surgery Vocal rehabilitation Low compliance	Follow up Lesion and some vocal improvement (did not cancel shows)
8. Male, 29y-old Smoker	Rap singer No singing training	1-year vocal complaint Touring with show	Leukoplakia and edema	Vocal rehabilitation Low compliance	Abandoned Lesion and vocal improvement

Contemporary Singer	Style and Training	Complaint	Type of Lesion	Management	Outcome
9. Male, 31y-old Smoker Reflux	Heavy rock singer Pop and rock training	6-month vocal complaint Preparing for recording CD	Edema	Vocal rehabilitation High compliance	Dismissed No lesion and adapted voice, no fatigue
10. Female, 39y-old Nonsmoker	Romantic singer No training	8-month vocal complaint Recording CD Previous episode 3 years ago	Epidermoid cyst	Vocal rehabilitation	Dismissed Lesion but adapted voice
11. Female, 16y-old Nonsmoker	Broadway shows 1 year training	3 months Can't produce high notes New teacher 4 months ago	Bilateral VF. lesions Vocal nodules	Voice therapy 6 visits New singing teacher Moderate compliance	Dismissed Nodules reduced but not completely Began show rehearsal
12. Male, 34 y-old Non Smoker Reflux	Broadway show and pop singer 8 years lessons B.A. Music	1½ years range reduced since recording in a studio	Right VF stiff Possibly old hemorrhage	4 sessions voice therapy surgery Epidermal cyst Voice therapy post-op High compliance	Full voice use 6 months later after voice therapy and singing lessons
13. Male, 28y-old Nonsmoker Reflux	Pop singer No training	1-year complaint Sings in rock band	Granuloma Edema	Reflux therapy Voice therapy Singing teacher	Dismissed Edema No granuloma Continue performing
14. Female, 24y-old Nonsmoker	Broadway show singer 6 years classical training	4-month complaint After singing sick	Vocal polyp Reactive lesion	Voice therapy Refused surgery High compliance	Polyp remains No reactive lesion Dismissed to new singing teacher
15. Female, 31 y-old Past history of smoking Moderately obese	Pop singer 8 years classical training M.A. Music Education	3-month complaint after making new CD	Bilateral VF nodules Reflux	Voice therapy Stop singing 6 weeks Moderate compliance	6 sessions—stopped Returned 4 months later 6 additional sessions Weight loss—mild edema

continues

Table 16-3. A Review of 15 Consecutive Classical Singers Presenting with Voice Complaints

Classical Singer	Style and Training	Complaint	Type of Lesion	Management	Outcome
1. Female, 49y-old Nonsmoker	Dramatic soprano + Brazilian pop (crossover) 33 years classical training	1-week vocal complaint Wagner Festival	VVFF edema Previous episode of VF glandular cyst, removed by surgery 15 years ago	Vocal rehabilitation High compliance	Dismissed Reabsorption of lesion and adapted voice
2. Female, 34y-old Nonsmoker GE reflux + stomach polyp	Lyrical soprano + choral singing 16 years classical training	6-month vocal complaint During choral singing	VVFF edema	Vocal rehabilitation High compliance Stomach polyp removal	Dismissed Adapted voice
3. Female, 28y-old Nonsmoker	Lyrical soprano 3 years classical training	2-month vocal complaint Post-touring with concert	Edematous VVFF nodules	Vocal rehabilitation Moderate compliance	Dismissed Reduced lesion with adapted voice
4. Male, 42y-old Nonsmoker GE reflux	Baritone + choral director 13 years classical training	1-month vocal complaint Post-chorus festival	Edema + VVFF hemorrhage	Vocal rest and vocal rehabilitation	Dismissed No lesion and adapted voice
5. Male, 39y-old Smoker GE Reflux	Tenor + choral singing 11 years classical training	Vocal complaint after 2 months intense rehearsals	Leukoplakia	Vocal rehabilitation Moderate compliance	Follow up Reduced lesion and better voice
6. Female, 46y-old Nonsmoker GE reflux	Lyrical soprano + Brazilian pop (crossover) 20 years classical training	3-month vocal complaint During pop music CD recording	Epidermoid cyst	Vocal rehabilitation High compliance	Dismissed Lesion but better voice
7. Female, 37y-old Nonsmoker	Lyrical soprano 10 years classical training	4-month vocal complaint	VVFF nodules	Vocal rehabilitation High compliance	Dismissed Lesion reabsorbed
8. Male, 39y-old Nonsmoker GE reflux	Baritone 17 years classical training	2-week vocal complaint After concert abroad	VF polyp	Microsurgery + pre and post-op vocal rehabilitation High compliance	Dismissed Lesion removed and adapted voice

Classical Singer	Style and Training	Complaint	Type of Lesion	Management	Outcome
9. Female, 26y-old Nonsmoker	Soprano Chamber music 1 year classical training	2-year vocal complaint	VVFF nodules	Vocal rehabilitation High compliance	Dismissed No lesion and better voice
10. Female, 25y-old Nonsmoker	Lyrical soprano + choral singing + wedding singer 2 years classical training	6-month vocal complaint After tight agenda	VF nodules	Vocal rehabilitation Moderate compliance	Follow up Lesion but better voice
11. Female, 21y-old Nonsmoker	Lyrical soprano 4 years classical training	9-month complaint after change of teachers	VF polyp reactive lesion	Vocal hygiene Voice rest modified High compliance	Reduced edema Normal voice
12. Female, 31y-old Nonsmoker	Soprano 18 years classical training	3 months after extensive auditions	Bilateral edema	Vocal hygiene Voice rest modified High compliance	Reduced edema Normal voice
13. Male, 18y-old Nonsmoker	Tenor 3 years classical training	1-year complaint after school show	Unilateral lesion	Voice therapy Microsurgery	Dismissed No lesion Voice improved after 6 months
14. Female, 27y-old Nonsmoker	Coloratura soprano 11 years classical training	2 years narrowing range	No lesion Strained speaking voice	Voice therapy New singing teacher Moderate compliance	Dismissed to singing teacher after 6 sessions of voice therapy
15. Female, 37y-old Nonsmoker	Soprano—University faculty 19 years classical training	12 months weak upper range	Unilateral VF paresis LPR	Voice therapy	Reduced performance schedule Continue teaching

Vocal Nodules

Vocal nodules (see Figure 16–2) in classical singers are predominantly seen in females. They occur in young women 25 to 35 years of age. They are bilateral lesions and symmetric in position although they can be asymmetric in size. Perhaps, vocal nodules are the most common laryngeal lesions in young female singers, just as they are in nonsingers.[34] Vocal nodules occur in sopranos and sometimes represent only an adaptation of the system to high mechanical demands. In many cases, there is neither a vocal complaint nor apparent deviation of the speaking and singing voice. Others, however, complain of loss of pitch range or excess breath at low frequencies.

Vocal nodules associated with a vocal complaint may occur in female classical singers at the beginning of their careers or after singing demanding roles. Vocal nodules in those conditions are likely to be edematous and respond very well to voice treatment. The voice of the patient with vocal nodules is generally rough with varied degrees of breathiness, a probable frequency change to a lower pitch, and the loss of high notes in the vocal range. In these patients, a program of vocal conservation may be used to reach an immediate effect that is short lasting, with voice use limited to essential situations to speed up the lesion recovery.

Vocal nodules in commercial singers may occur at the beginning of their careers; however, they usually report a long history of dysphonia with fluctuating vocal quality. A particular event may represent the reason for medical consultation.

Vocal nodules in these patients can be either edematous or fibrotic with involvement of the laryngeal vestibule and tension in the extrinsic laryngeal musculature. Those lesions may not always respond positively to voice treatment. It may be more difficult to make these singers sensitive to a program of vocal conservation.

In addition to vocal instruction and conservative voice use, there are three main avenues of management: (1) confidential voice therapy, (2) resonance therapy, and (3) varied exercises of tongue, lips, and tongue-lip trills. The confidential voice therapy may be employed as an initial strategy of treatment when there is enough time to do so. Resonant voice therapy and/or varied vocal exercises may be added later. Environmental or schedule changes, if possible, should be immediately considered to maintain maximum vocal hygiene.

Vocal Fold Cysts

Vocal fold cysts are significantly different from vocal nodules in terms of diagnosis and treatment. Cysts may be either unilateral or bilateral. In case of bilateral cysts, the diagnosis is more difficult to establish. Vocal fold cysts occur in both sexes and all ages. They can be associated with edema, contralateral reaction (nodular lesions), and with other benign lesions such as polyps and leukoplakia. Cysts may be either epidermoid or glandular and the latter have easier outcome, with less chance of postoperative dysphonia. Singers with cysts may have profoundly deviated voices, depending on the location and the adherence of the cyst to the vocal ligament. The occurrence of cysts in popular singers seems to be more common than in classical singers. It may be that classical singers have a great need of a superior vocal quality and therefore seek help sooner. The nonclassical singer, on the other hand, often tolerates minor deviations in voice quality allowing structural changes to develop.

Figure 16–2. Vocal nodules seen in a young female singer.

> The treatment for vocal fold cysts is voice therapy prior to and after surgery.

Exophytic cysts surrounded by flexible mucosa are lesions of relatively easy surgical management. Vocal fold cysts that are subepithelial are more difficult to treat surgically and behaviorally. They can potentially produce scars, causing significant dysphonia that is difficult to reduce with any kind of treatment. The singer's voice with a cyst can vary, but roughness and tension are the most common elements.

Vocal rehabilitation should be directed to the reduction of secondary lesions and to the search for a vocal balance as cysts do not reduce with exercises. Facilitating sounds and varied exercises that make the mucosal wave more flexible (such as tongue and lip trill with scales, nasal sounds, and voiced fricatives) have a positive response. Laryngeal manipulation exercises to reduce tension in the neck, throat, larynx, and shoulders are often suggested. Surgery must be carefully planned[25,35-37] and vocal rehabilitation after surgery is mandatory to optimize results.[38,39]

Vocal Fold Polyps

Vocal polyps are generally unilateral lesions (10% of bilateral presentation), and are more characteristic of the male sex, occurring at any age. A change in voice quality is evident, with roughness and fundamental frequency bifurcation. Singers may note a loss of high frequency especially at pianissimo. Polyps may be associated with a history of recent dysphonia, intense phonotrauma, nonhabitual violent physical activity such as an extensive recording session, cheering at a football game,[40] gastroesophageal reflux conditions,[7,41] and use of the voice in noisy environments.[42]

The occurrence of polyps in classical singers is lower than in CCM singers. Popular singers, particularly in the most vocally aggressive styles such as heavy rock and gospel music singers, may reflect a tissue response to excessive glottic compression. The presence of a polyp may help the singer to compose his or her image up to the moment that vocal fatigue, limitation of vocal range, and loss of tune control take the singer to the voice clinic. Although the indicated approach is usually surgical removal, there are anecdotal reports of progress with voice therapy. Voice rehabilitation may reduce the size and shape of the polyp resulting in an acceptable voice for a pop singer.

Rehabilitation options include tongue and lip trill associated to musical scales to improve vocal fold flexibility and to provide a better distribution of the impact during voice production. Control of vocal attack and a better use of resonance may also be tried, especially in the speaking voice. Digital manipulation of the larynx and postural change exercises (with movements of head and neck) may offer tension relief. It should be pointed out that changes that modify or diminish the vocal image may be rejected by the singer.

Reinke's Edema

Reinke's edema is a superficial and diffuse tissue change, which can be either unilateral or bilateral and symmetric or not. It generally occurs in singers over 45 years of age and it is strongly related to smoking,[43] gastroesophageal reflux,[41] and hormonal problems in women.[44] The occurrence in classical singers is rare due to good vocal hygiene, no smoking, and good vocal education. The voice is typically low and may interfere in the identification of sex; the history is quite long and the vocal change is usually reported to be slowly progressive over a long period of time.

Reinke's edema is common in commercial singers, such as in night club, jazz, R&B, and soul music singers. The low voice may be considered a positive differential feature for the singer, who is also going to reject any treatment that compromises his or her vocal signature. Nevertheless, signs and symptoms of fatigue and lack of pitch and loudness control may make the singer look for assistance. It is interesting to note that, even after surgical removal of the lesion, there is a partial return of the edema about 2 to 3 months later[45] and, thus, the voice remains low (but not as low as before treatment), with easier vocal production. Patients must be properly instructed, and if the indication of treatment is surgery, voice education and preoperatory intervention should be carried out to optimize the results after surgery.[46] The options of voice therapy include tongue and lips trills, stretching and shortening of vocal folds exercises, vocal tract semioccluded exercises, and massage on the neck region when the extrinsic musculature is involved. For the postoperative phase of treatment, trills and musical scales will offer the recovery of the high regions of the voice range.

Leukoplakia

Leukoplakia is a condition in which white lesions are seen on one or both vocal folds. The organic causes include smoking, alcohol consumption, gastroesophageal reflux, and genetic predisposition. Leukoplakia is more frequently found in males and less likely to occur in women. When the leukoplakia is diffuse with ample and shallow lesions and nondefinite border on both vocal folds, it may represent an irritation response due to phonotrauma or gastroesophageal reflux[47]; in those cases, vocal rehabilitation should be tried instead of surgery. Classical singers may present with leukoplakia that is often associated with gastroesophageal reflux[41] or caused by genetic predisposition. On the other hand, for most people and popular singers, the lesion is probably due to the influence of smoking,[48] alcohol, and vocal behavior.[49] The voice is rough with fluctuating deviation and greater severity due to the lesion rigidity. Moreover, strained vocal quality is frequently present. Singers with leukoplakia may suffer great disarray in their vocal image and usually look for immediate assistance. However, when leukoplakia is associated with Reinke's edema, it may compose and characterize the singer's voice.

> Of all benign laryngeal lesions, leukoplakia is the one that deserves greater attention as far as the risk to develop a cancer is concerned.

Concerns about health should come before any consideration of vocal style and preference. Thus, surgical biopsy is usually the first choice, especially in patients who smoke. Vocal rehabilitation following surgery may be required. Redistribution of the phonatory impact along the vocal folds with exercises helps to reduce glottal attack and increase respiratory-phonatory control.

Vocal Fold Scar

Vocal fold scars usually have an iatrogenic nature,[50] due to either an undesirable consequence of benign lesion removal or traumas during intubation or extubation of other surgery. They may also be a result of recurrent laryngitis or a residual consequence of an acute vocal trauma. Scars represent buildup of rigid tissue, whose consequences may be career-threatening to a singer. The vocal quality may be polyphonic, with breathiness, strain, fundamental frequency bifurcation, frequency breaks, voice breaks, and evident phonatory effort. There may be vocal compensatory mechanisms that include ventricular phonation, compensatory nasal resonance, lifted rib cage, and increased subglottic pressure. There is no ideal treatment. Medication, surgical modification, or voice rehabilitation are usually attempted. Some case reports suggest good long-term results with voice rehabilitation. The treatment regimen differs from that employed for benign lesions. The management of vocal fold scars may last longer than 1 year, with periodic vocal and laryngological follow-up. Improvement may be gradual, which demands careful documentation in order to observe the small changes that occur over time. Use of the Voice Handicap Index may be the best guide to changes that occur.

The rationale for voice rehabilitation for vocal fold scars can be summarized as follows:

1. Initially, there should be an attempt to separate what is compensatory or secondary to the scar from the original deviation itself. To do that, supraglottic and vocal tract adjustments should be addressed, reducing excessive extrinsic muscular activity that may include high larynx, mandibular stiffness, tongue displacement, and body posture deviation.
2. Voice assessment should evaluate whether the main complaint is related to the vocal quality deviation, fatigue, or lack of constant and acceptable phonation.
3. If the problem resides in voice quality changes, all possible mechanisms that lead to the voice previously obtained should be tried. If changes in the source are not possible, the manipulation of the tract (resonance) is indicated as an attempt to get closer to a desired vocal quality.
4. If the vocal endurance is the main problem, glottic closure must be re-evaluated endoscopically. An extensive closed phase is often responsible for vocal fatigue. Treatment to reduce vocal fatigue can be done with vocal function exercises[28] chant talk, vocal tract semioccluded exercises such as glottal stability—hand over mouth or finger-kazoo, and maximum phonation time exercises with vocal quality control.

5. If glottic phonation/sonority is acceptable, a widening of the dynamic vocal range should be pursued using variation of pitch and loudness exercises and maximum phonation time exercises using voice quality control.

6. If there is not enough glottic tone in the voice, treatment with phonation triggering should be specifically carried out by means of short phonatory bursts. To achieve enough sonority, the selected exercises must be intensely repeated. Initially, the volume of the voice may be increased slightly to help phonation during the first few days. Some of the indicated exercises are the sequential repetition of a nasal sound (eg, "m-m-m-m" or "n-n-n-n-n") or

a voiced fricative (eg, "z-z-z-z"). These sounds must be short, produced in a series, on an average of 6 to 8 times a day. As soon as sonority/phonation is produced for at least 50% of the voice production, the individual must go back to his or her habitual loudness. When sonority/phonation is constant, a widening of the dynamic vocal range should proceed.

Although the vocal rehabilitation of vocal fold scars has not been submitted to controlled clinical research yet, there are reports in the literature that the intervention may last up to a year.[26, 37]

An example of voice quality change with vocal rehabilitation is shown in Figure 16–3A and 16–3B.

Figure 16–3. Postsurgical scar in a 46-year-old female teacher after removal of bilateral vocal fold cysts. **A.** Before vocal rehabilitation: Spectrographic analysis (narrow band filter, 45 Hz) of the sustained vowel æ, as in apple. Notice effort to initiate phonation, instability of vocal quality, and fundamental frequency bifurcation on the trace (presence of subharmonic), high fundamental frequency (from 255 Hz to 276 Hz), and reduced maximum phonation time (4.83). **B.** After vocal rehabilitation: Spectrographic analysis (narrow band filter, 45 Hz) of the sustained vowel æ, as in apple, after 4 months of intensive vocal rehabilitation. Notice instability at glottal attack but a better stability of trace, a lower fundamental frequency (212 Hz), and a larger maximum phonation time (7.04).

Following use of exercises such as nasal prolongations and fricative buzz using the /z/ onset of phonation and maintenance of stability can be seen. Both voice quality and duration of phonation improved in this patient.

SUMMARY

Vocal rehabilitation is the most important treatment modality for benign lesions of the vocal folds in singers. Although surgery is indicated in some cases, voice therapy which begins as trial therapy may be the primary rehabilitation program for many singers. Awareness of the preferred voice for the musical style and the desired voice for the singer is essential for the proper management of performers. A clear and projected vocal quality is not necessarily desired by heavy rock and gospel singers. The voice clinician should consider the singer's preferred style and respect personal options, when vocal health and career longevity are not compromised.[51] The voice specialist clinician combines his or her medical knowledge with an understanding of the artistic realm of the singer.

REFERENCES

1. Fussi F, Magnani S. *L'arte vocal. Fisiopatologia ed educazione della voce artistica*. Itália: Omega; 1994.
2. Vilkman E. Voice problems at work: a challenge for occupational safety and health arrangement. *Folia Phoniatr Logop*. 2000;52:120–125.
3. Stemple J. Management of the professional voice. In: Stemple J., ed. *Voice Therapy. Clinical Studies*. St. Louis, Mo: Mosby; 1993:155–171.
4. Behlau M. Vozes preferidas: considerações sobre opções vocais nas profissões. *Fono Atual*. 2001;4: 10–14.
5. Hsiung MW, Hsiao YC. The characteristic features of muscle tension dysphonia before and after surgery in benign lesions of the vocal fold. *ORL J Otorhinolaryngol Relat Spec*. 2004;66:246–254.
6. Cohn JR, Spiegel JR, Hawkshaw M, Sataloff RT. Allergy. In: Sataloff RT. *Professional Voice: The Science and Art of Clinical Care*. 2nd ed. San Diego, Calif: Singular Publishing Group; 1997:369–374.
7. Sataloff RT, Castell DO, Sataloff DM, Spiegel JS, Hawkshaw M. Reflux and other gastroenterologic conditions that may affect the voice. In: Sataloff RT. *Professional Voice: The Science and Art of Clinical Care*. 2nd ed. San Diego, Calif: Singular Publishing Group; 1997:319–329.
8. Spiegel JR, Hawkshaw M, Sataloff RT. Dysphonia related to medical therapy. *Otolaryngol Clin North Am*. 2000; 33:771–784.
9. Herman Jr, Rossol M. Artificial fogs and smokes. In: Sataloff RT. *Professional Voice: The Science and Art of Clinical Care*. 2nd ed. San Diego, Calif: Singular Publishing Group; 1997:413–427.
10. Williams NR. Occupational voice disorders due to workplace exposure to irritants—a review of the literature. *Occup Med (Lond)*. 2002;52:99–101.
11. Sapir S, Mathers-Schmidt B, Larson GW. Singers' and non-singers' vocal health, vocal behaviors, and attitudes towards voice and singing: indirect findings from a questionnaire. *Eur J Disord Commun*. 1996;31:193–209.
12. Hirano, M. *Clinical Examination of Voice*. New York, NY: Springer-Verlag; 1981:81–84.
13. American Speech-Language Hearing Association. (ASHA). 2003. *Consensus Auditory-Perceptual Evaluation of Voice (CAPE-V)*. 2003 document text available from: http://www.asha.org.
14. Titze I. Workshop on acoustic voice analysis. Iowa City, Ia: National Center for Voice and Speech; 1995.
15. Elias ME, Sataloff RT, Rosen DC, Heuer RJ, Spiegel JR. Normal strobovideolaryngoscopy: variability in healthy singers. *J Voice*. 1997;11:104–107.
16. Leonard R, Kendall K. Phonoscopy. a valuable tool for otolaryngologists and speech-language pathologists. *Laryngoscope*. 2001;111:1760–1766.
17. Sataloff RT. Voice and speech impairment and disability.In: Sataloff RT. *Professional Voice. The Science and Art of Clinical Care*. 2nd ed. San Diego, Calif: Singular Publishing Group; 1997:795–800.
18. Jacobson BH, Johnson A, Grywalski C, Silbergleit A, Jacobson G, Benninger M, Newman CW. The voice handicap index (VHI): development and validation. *Am J Speech Lang Pathol*. 1997;6:66–70.
19. Hogikyan ND, Sethuraman G. Validation of an instrument to measure voice-related quality of life (V-RQOL). *J Voice*. 1999;13:557–569.
20. Benninger M, Sataloff RT. The evaluation of outcomes and quality of life in individuals with voice disorders. *J Singing*. 1999;56:34–43.
21. Murry T, Rosen, C. Voice handicap index in singers. *J Voice*. 2000;14:370–377.

22. Ma EP-M, Yiu EM-L. Voice activity and participation profile: assessing the impact of voice disorders on daily activities. *J Speech Lang Hear Res.* 2001;44: 511-524.

23. Emerich K, Baroody M, Carrol L, Sataloff R. The singing voice specialist. In: Sataloff RT. *Professional Voice: The Science and Art of Clinical Care.* 2nd ed. San Diego, Calif: Singular Publishing Group; 1997:735-754.

24. Stone Jr RE. The speech-language pathologist's role in the management of the professional voice. In: Benninger MS, Jacobson BH, Johnson AF, eds. *Vocal Arts Medicine: The Care and Prevention of Professional Voice Disorders.* New York, NY: Thieme; 1994:291-317.

25. Dejonckere PH, Lebacq J. Plasticity of voice quality: a prognostic factor for outcome of voice therapy? *J Voice.* 2001;15:251-256.

26. Behlau M, Madazio G, Feijo D, Azevedo R, Gielow I, Rehder MI. Aperfeiçoamento vocal e tratamento fonoaudiológico das disfonias. In: Behlau M, ed. *Voz. O livro do especialista.* vol 2. Rio de Janeiro, Brazil: Revinter; 2005:409-564.

27. National Center for Voice and Speech. *A Vocologist's Guide: Voice Therapy & Training.* Iowa City, Ia: Author; 1994.

28. Stemple J, Lee L, D'Amico B, Pickup B. Efficacy of vocal function exercises in the practice regiment of singers. *J Voice.* 1994;3:271-278.

29. Colton R, Casper J. *Understanding Voice Problems: A Physiological Perspective for Diagnosis and Treatment.* Baltimore, Md: Williams & Wilkins; 1990.

30. Lessac A. *The Use and Training of the Human Voice: A Biodynamic Approach to Vocal Life.* Mountain View, Calif: Mayfield; 1997.

31. Verdolini K, Druker DG, Palmer PM, Samawi H. Laryngeal adduction in resonant voice. *J Voice.* 1998;12:315-327.

32. Casper J, Murry T. Voice therapy methods in dysphonia. *Otol Clin North Am.* 2000;33:983-1002.

33. Lovertri JL, Weekly EM. Contemporary commercial music (CCM) survey: who's teaching what in non-classic music. *J Voice.* 2003;17:207-215.

34. Herrington-Hall BL, Lee L, Stemple J, Nieme KR, McHone MM. Description of laryngeal pathologies by age, sex and occupation in a treatment-seeking sample. *J Speech Hear Disord.* 1998;53:57-64.

35. Bastian RW. Vocal fold microsurgery in singers. *J Voice.* 1996;10:389-404.

36. Sataloff RT. *Professional Voice. The Science and Art of Clinical Care.* 2nd ed. San Diego, Calif: Singular Publishing Group; 1997.

37. Zeitels SM, Hillman RE, Desloge R, Mauri M, Doyle PB. Phonomicrosurgery in singers and performing artists: treatment outcomes, management theories and future directions. *Ann Otol Rhinol Laryngol Suppl.* 2002;190:21-40.

38. Casper J, Behlau M. Vocal rehabilitation before and following phonosurgery. In: *Proceedings of 25th World Congress of the International Association for Logopedics and Phoniatrics.* Montreal, Canada: IALP; 2001:361.

39. Murry T. Pre- and postoperative phonotherapy. *J Singing.* 2001; 57:39-42.

40. Roch JB, Cornut G, Bouchayer M. Mode d'apparition des polypes des cordes vocales. *Rev Laryngol Otol Rhinol (Bordeaux).* 1989;110:389-390.

41. Koufmann J. Gastroesophageal reflux and voice disorders. In: Rubin JS, Sataloff RT, Korovin G, Gould WJ. *Diagnosis and Treatment of Voice Disorders.* New York, NY: Igaku-Shoin; 1995:161-175.

42. Rontal E, Rontal M, Jacob HJ, Rolnick MI. Vocal cord dysfunction—an industrial health hazard. *Ann Otol Rhinol Laryngol.* 1979;88:818-821.

43. Matsuo K, Kamimura M, Hirano M. Polypoid vocal folds: a ten year review of 191 patients. *Auris Nasus Larynx.* 1983;10(suppl):37-45.

44. Abitbol J, Abitbol B, Abitbol P. Sex hormones and the female voice. *J Voice.* 1999;13:424-446.

45. Bouchayer M, Cornut, G. *Phonosurgery for Benign Vocal Fold Lesions* [videotextbook]. Gibraltar: The 3 Ears; 1994.

46. Koufman J, Blalock PD. Is voice rest never indicated? *J Voice.* 1989;3:87-91.

47. Gadelha ME, Pontes P, Guidugli J, Gregorio LC. Morphological aspects of vocal fold leukoplakias. Correlation with histopathological classification. In: Isshiki N, ed. *Proceedings 3rd International Symposium of Phonosurgery.* Kyoto, Japan: International Association of Phonosurgeons; 1994.

48. Gillis YM, Incze J, Strong MS, Vaughan CW, Simpson GT. Natural history and management of keratosis, atypia, carcinoma in situ, and microinvasive cancer of the larynx. *Am J Surg.* 1983;146: 512-516.

49. Perrin C, Long FX, Mariel P, Barthelme A, Prokopik JD. Leucoplasies et dysplasies des cordes vocales. *J Français d'Oto-rhino-laryngol (Audiophonl Chir).* 1983;32:487-491.

50. Rosen, D. Vocal fold scar: evaluation and treatment. *Otolaryngol Clin North Am.* 2000;33:1081-1086.

51. Miller R. Voice skill and vocal longevity. *J Singing.* 1998; 54:35-37.

Consensus Auditory-Perceptual Evaluation of Voice (CAPE-V)[13]

Name: _____   **Date:**_____

The following parameters of voice quality will be rated upon completion of the following tasks:
1. Sustained vowels, /a/ and /i/ for 3-5 seconds duration each.
2. Sentence production:
    a. The blue spot is on the key again.   d. We eat eggs every Easter.
    b. How hard did he hit him?   e. My mama makes lemon muffins.
    c. We were away a year ago.   f. Peter will keep at the peak.
3. Spontaneous speech in response to: "Tell me about your voice problem." or "Tell me how your voice is functioning."

> **Legend:** C = Consistent   I = Intermittent
> MI = Mildly Deviant
> MO =Moderately Deviant
> SE = Severely Deviant

SCORE

Overall Severity _____ C I ___/100
     MI   MO   SE

Roughness _____ C I ___/100
     MI   MO   SE

Breathiness _____ C I ___/100
     MI   MO   SE

Strain _____ C I ___/100
     MI   MO   SE

Pitch (Indicate the nature of the abnormality): _____
_____ C I ___/100
     MI   MO   SE

Loudness (Indicate the nature of the abnormality): _____
_____ C I ___/100
     MI   MO   SE

_____ _____ C I ___/100
     MI   MO   SE

_____ _____ C I ___/100
     MI   MO   SE

COMMENTS ABOUT RESONANCE: NORMAL   OTHER (Provide description):_____

ADDITIONAL FEATURES (for example, diplophonia, fry, falsetto, asthenia, aphonia, pitch instability, tremor, wet/gurgly, or other relevant terms):

Clinician:_____

Chapter 17

STRATEGIES FOR DEALING WITH VOCAL TENSION

Janet Madelle Feindel

As a young acting student, studying at the Royal Academy of Dramatic Art, in London, England, I was fortunate enough to witness two performances by an actor named Michael Pennington at the Royal Shakespeare Company. He played the role of Berowne in Shakespeare's *Love's Labours Lost* and the Duke in *Measure for Measure*. In the first instance, I was seated in the uppermost balcony and in the other, the middle orchestra. In each case, I experienced this actor's voice as if he were sitting next to me, speaking in my ear in spite of the fact the theater seated over a thousand people. His voice effortlessly revealed the nuances of the character. In May 2003, I attended the New York City Broadway production of Eugene O'Neill's *Long Day's Journey Into Night* at the Plymouth Theater. Vanessa Redgrave played Mary Tyrone. Ms. Redgrave's voice emitted from her whole being and exposed the character's innermost thoughts and emotions. She connected the thought with the breath and her intention in her portrayal in a seemingly effortless and translucent manner; in the same way a dancer makes the *jeté* look easy. This ease of speaking takes huge talent and years of practice.

HEALTHY, EXPRESSIVE, AND EFFECTIVE VOICE USAGE

An important premise frequently overlooked by actors and directors is that healthy voice usage is expressive voice usage. People often mistake phony emotion, or what Patsy Rodenburg refers to as "bluff acting," for a genuine relationship to the text.

The voice mechanism should be free enough to reflect the needs of the character. The actor's psychophysical awareness should be such that the actor's voice and body respond to the thought with spontaneous changes in the pitch, rhythm, dynamic, and tonal variety, rather than following a prescribed approach. Tension impedes this possibility, creating a multitude of vocal tension issues.

As part of the curriculum at Carnegie Mellon's School of Drama, students learn to identify healthy, effective, and expressive voice usage and unhealthy, ineffective, and inexpressive voice usage. This is done through discussion and examples of film and stage acting. To identify healthy voice usage, all the following characteristics should be evident:

- Physical ease.
- Clear unobstructed tone.
- Resonant sound; that is, the sense that the actor fully embodies the voice and one has the sense as stated earlier that the voice emits from the whole body, not just the mouth.
- A sense of release as the person expresses heightened emotions rather than a sense of constriction and pulling down in the body.
- A precise relationship with the thoughts and intentions that the actor wishes to communicate, resulting in clear crisp articulation that does not sound affected but yet is vigorous. The actor uses the language to fully carve out the ideas to impact another human being.
- The person is "in his or her back," which means the person is supporting the voice with the use of the back part of the rib case and, hence, utilizing the full capacity of the diaphragm as opposed to squeezing and "pulling down" on the release of breath and thought.

The rib swing is a useful way for performers to think about the breath support. Too often the actor squeezes from the diaphragm, pushing the ribs together, which actually causes constriction in the shoulder, neck, jaw, and larynx areas, hence weakening support rather than aiding it. This habit also tends to produce a forced sound rather than a free sound, because the actor is attempting to find power through pushing rather than release. It is also important to remember that the diaphragm is not a pouch below the sternum but extends across the whole torso, like a flexible parachutelike drum.

To identify unhealthy voice usage, some or all of these characteristics will be evident:

- Tension around the neck, face, and shoulder muscles.
- Poor alignment; that is, the neck pushing out or the chin pulling too far to the chest.

- Unbalanced breath support, which is either a too breathy and "off voice" vocal quality or not enough breath support for the effort of the sound, causing a hoarse, forced, and/or crackling sound.
- A tendency to pull down and tighten when speaking, pushing the words and ideas out, with extra tension at the ends of lines "squeezing the meaning out" rather than letting them release effortlessly.
- At times, an overemphasis on articulation rules, with the actor "playing the voice" rather than playing the scene, thereby obscuring the meaning rather than integrating clear articulation to communicate ideas with clarity.

TRAINING

The physical aspects of voice training follow a progression much like the training of an athlete, with exercises to develop vocal flexibility, stamina, and strength similar to exercises used in singing training. Voice training also involves aspects of movement and alignment or postural awareness (such as the Alexander technique), because muscular tension constricts sound vibration and full expression in the actor.[1]

> As a trainer of the speaking voice for actors, I strive to teach students to achieve the same vocal freedom and expression Michael Pennington and Vanessa Redgrave demonstrated.

Voice training differs from the training of the athlete, however, in an important aspect. The actor needs to coordinate the physical aspects of the training with the impulse of the thought, the imagination, the intention of the character as written, and the need to communicate to affect another on stage. All the aspects of speaking voice training must therefore be connected to the speaking of text, as the actor needs to incorporate the principles of voice into his acting, finding the "ladder of the thought."[2]

This delicate interplay of goals challenges voice/speech trainer and student alike: making these connections becomes a unique process in many respects. The vocal mechanism involves all facets of the individual: psychological, physiologic, spiritual, as well as anatomic. The study of the speaking voice becomes intensely personal in many respects, even more than other aspects of actor training such as movement and facial expressions. The teacher provides a map but the actor takes the internal journey. The physical voice in its ease, dynamic, and flexibility reflects the inner workings of the individual, what Cicely Berry refers to as "That Secret Voice."[3] This personal aspect of voice makes it important to create a positive, supportive atmosphere while still maintaining a sense of purpose and discipline in both teaching and coaching situations. Training of the voice may, therefore, incorporate personal writing and therapeutic techniques as tools to open up the full range of the actor's vocal experience both in the practical and in the metaphorical sense. Addressing vocal tension requires a solid understanding of vocal mechanics and sensitivity to acting concerns as well as the emotional make-up of the actor.

CHANGING HABITS: ALIGNMENT AND THE ALEXANDER TECHNIQUE

Voice development involves changing habits. Tensions in the voice often stem from habits established in early life so that the elimination of such tensions is not something that happens overnight. Often students have breakthroughs and can deliver a whole speech with considerable freedom, but the real challenge is the ability to sustain that freedom over the course of a month of performances. However, habits persist and the unconscious resists change. Often, when change in the voice occurs the habit seems to rear its head even more stubbornly than before. So the old adage "three steps forward, two steps behind" definitely applies to the learning curve in voice training. It takes hours of practice and acceptance of the emotional self to allow full vocal freedom precisely because the voice reflects our emotional landscape. This is where the application of the principles of the Alexander technique proves useful because the principles address habitual response.

Alignment refers to the way an actor stands and moves, allowing for maximum ease and appropriate breath support. On a deeper level, alignment refers to the delicate interplay of the actor's thought, breath, and movement impulses. The actor needs to move with ease, finding the most flexibility without excess tension. If an actor plays Richard III, requiring uneven carriage, he or she must still find an inner kinesthetic freedom within the posture that allows the actor the vocal relaxation necessary to deliver heightened text for 3 hours. If the actor does not achieve this balance, the posture itself can create the potential for vocal tension and possible vocal damage. The incorporation of proper alignment, as part of training the voice, provides a challenging task for the actor.

The Alexander technique deals specifically with the alignment principles developed by Frederick Mathias Alexander, born in Australia in 1869. He specialized in "recitations" of Shakespeare. When he began performing, he continually lost his voice. When he was unable to find a medical remedy, he studied his movement patterns in front of a mirror for a decade. Alexander analyzed the "habits" that were causing the vocal misuse. He noticed the following as he began to recite:

1. He tightened his neck muscles;
2. This caused his chin to lower;
3. This resulted in his larynx tightening and pulling down; and
4. His breath support became shallow.

He discovered that he was not able to stop these habits at will. What he was able to do, however, was prevent pulling back his head, which resulted in the disappearance of the other two habits. As he began to master this new approach, his hoarseness discontinued.

He began to understand that patterns of use were not just physical but involved mental conceptions as well. He coined the idea of "inhibition" from these observations. Before he started a habitual movement, he stopped and "inhibited" the tense habit before it began. He then gave himself new thought directions related to the movement: let the neck be free, to allow the head to go forward and up, and to allow the back to lengthen and widen. He named these the "means whereby."[4]

Voice training involves changing habits. The Alexander technique helps enormously to effect that change. Most respected acting schools include the Alexander technique in the core curriculum. Sessions are individual and/or group classes. The student is taken through a series of "procedures" exploring "positions of maximum mechanical advantage." These involve getting in and out of a chair, using the movement as a way to discover and apply the principle of inhibition. Teachers of the Alexander technique also teach "constructive rest" done on the floor or on a massage table. (See the end of the chapter for a description of constructive rest and other resource material on the Alexander technique.) The student can often make more sense of the principles in a lying down position then apply these principles in standing activity. The teacher guides with gentle touch, directing the student to become more aware of her or his habitual tensions and how "inhibiting" (or "stopping to observe") the habitual response can help the student bypass these tensions. The important component here involves the fact that the teacher must also utilize and incorporate the principles of the directions in order that the teacher's touch can guide the student.

Voice and speech trainers have the ability to diagnose what is not working effectively. It is much more challenging to actually give the student constructive ways to improve his or her voice. One of the challenges of voice work involves guiding the student to consciousness about one's habits while eschewing self-consciousness, which is the enemy of all good acting. Voice training involves awareness of habits and looking for ways to release tension to allow the organic freedom of the voice to emerge. To achieve this, effective voice training takes about 3 to 4 years to build a foundation and as much as 10 years to master. Any good actor, worth his or her salt, will continue voice work throughout his or her career.

THE PSYCHOPHYSICAL CONNECTION: VOICE IS MORE THAN JUST A SOUND

The overall psychology of the individual is extremely important in tackling any vocal tension issue, as voice tension is generally a symptom of the individual's tension. If at all possible, it is generally more effective to address any issue by guiding the actor to a deeper understanding and kinesthetic relationship to language. Once this is addressed at least to some extent, dealing with more specific manifestations of tension, such as soft palate tightness, jaw tightness, tension in the shoulder and neck muscles, poor articulation, and so forth, will prove easier. That said, every individual is different and one needs not only good diagnostic skills but also many approaches at one's fingertips as well as flexibility. Each person responds differently and even the same person responds differently at different times. The process involves exploration, and the journey is not necessarily logical. This is why the interdisciplinary approach to dealing with vocal issues proves so effective. Sometimes one must start where one observes the problem and then attempt, with the collaboration of the actor, to unravel what the source of the issue is. When a massage therapist finds a tension spot, sometimes it is harmful to massage that spot immediately. It is more effective to tend to the muscles around the knotted muscle first. The same is true in voice work. Sometimes tackling the issue head-on only causes self-consciousness in the actor and compounds the problem. It can prove useful to take a different tack all together and then this can lead to an indirect solution to the immediate problem.

Some tension issues may only involve a minor technical adjustment or change of perception. For example, the actor's first response to moving into a bigger space often is to shout when, in fact, shouting creates the exact opposite to the desired effect. The text becomes less clear and the actor more difficult to understand. The adjustment that does have to happen, however, is that the actor must perceptually *include* the entire audience and speak more clearly. Then the voice will carry. The ability of the voice to carry stems from the actor's thought, rather than the actor consciously pushing for volume. The paradox is that when the actor listens to him or herself, attempting to modify the sound, volume, or pitch in some way, it creates a disconnect between the actor's natural impulse to the language and results in less volume and a less convincing performance.

From 1994 to 1999, I served as Voice and Dialect Coach at the Canadian Stage Company's Dream in High Park, in Toronto, Canada. The Canadian Stage Company in Toronto produces an outdoor Shakespeare program every summer. When the company moved to the outdoor space, the actors became nervous and began shouting the text, which made it unintelligible. The vocal coach asked the actors to work in partners, one actor speaking the text on the stage and the other moving gradually farther and farther toward the back of the audience space. The goal was to let the actor on stage know when he or she was being clear and heard and when not. What invariably happened was that as the partner got farther away, into the house, the actor on stage would begin to push and the partner in the audience would communicate that he could not understand the actor on stage. This would go on until the actor on stage was guided or discovered the necessary adjustment on his or her own, to speak slightly more slowly, using the consonants more and let "the thought propel the sound," that is, striving to communicate the text as clearly as possible, including the large row of the amphitheater. When they regained their composure by putting their attention back onto the thought and clarity of the ideas, speaking slightly more slowly, and using their consonants more crisply, the actors would regain intelligibility and the ability to fill the space. Until each partner experienced this exercise, it was difficult for the actors to believe that the effort was in the clarity of the thought, rather than physically pushing the sound out.

Technique involves a balance of technical freedom, a "clear channel" and the psychokinesthetic mechanism's ability to respond spontaneously to the thought and to the requirement of the space. Therefore, if the space is larger, and the actor includes this fact into his or her awareness, the voice will naturally fill the space, as an extension of the thought. Pushing for volume, on the other hand, will not have the desired effect but result in garbled text.

One cannot separate the person from the voice; the voice reflects the person's intention, need, and thought. Tension in the voice, unless caused by some malfunction, generally reflects tension in the person or at least a lack of thorough understanding of the text. Unless one fully takes into account the specifics of each thought, one cannot realize his or her vocal potential. It is not enough to free the sound, but the actor must sculpt the ideas with precision, commitment, and a full kinesthetic relationship to the language. This is one of the most important issues in tackling voice tension.

GETTING THE WHOLE PICTURE AS A COACH

Effectively addressing vocal issues involves awareness of the psychology of the actor and the interplay between the director's vision and the actor's execution of that vision or at least how the actor perceives the director's vision. The coach needs to discern the vocal mechanics that interfere with vocal ease of delivery. One must bear in mind that dealing with the actor's voice is an extremely individual process; therefore, no one exercise works identically in each instance. One has to diagnose the difficulty based on the sound, the physical manifestation of tension and then analyze how this impacts the acting process. The process can prove quite complex.

The actor is, ideally, the best judge of when vocal tension occurs; however, occasionally the actor denies the problem. When actors develop voice problems, there is loss to the theaters in terms of time and money as well as the inconvenience of rescheduling performances or rehearsing an understudy. Unfortunately, some directors communicate in a way that can inadvertently create vocal tension as well.

Certain psychological limitations at times do not allow an actor to admit and to deal with vocal problems, even though these issues are clearly causing the actor professional difficulty.

In the context of a production, vocal problems emerge in a variety of ways. The audience may complain of not "hearing the actor." In reality, this usually means not "understanding" the actor rather than the actor not being loud enough, as described in the previous section. Sometimes actors are too low, often because the scene requires delicacy and an intimate sentiment, but the actor needs to share that with the audience. Or an actor plays the role with a dialect so strong that the actor cannot be understood because he or she focuses more on the dialect than on the character's intentions. Or the actor speaks with so much hoarseness that it is unpleasant to listen to and becomes distracting to the audience. Or an actor screams without proper support, going for a generalized emotion, rather than a specific intention. All these situations are recipes for vocal fatigue, misuse or—worst-case scenario—vocal injury, the most common of which being the occurrence of vocal nodules.

As a coach, one has to comprehend the goals of both the director and the actor. Sometimes the director asks for something but due to lack of vocal understanding does not know how to guide the actor to it in a vocally healthy way. Actors are under tremendous pressure to produce results. When a director asks for a particular effect, the actor tends to attempt without any regard for the healthiest way to achieve it. The freelance nature of the actor's work creates a tension in itself and the actor is always on display, frequently wondering where and when the next contract for employment will come. This can create in the actor a need to please the director and, therefore, a pressure to perform whatever is requested of the actor, sometimes to his or her detriment. Often, in attempting to go for a result requested by the director, the actor forgets to maintain and incorporate the principles of healthy voice use and alignment. Considering these factors, anyone working with the actor on vocal issues needs to understand the pressures the actor is under, the vision of the director, and the needs of the overall production.

APPLYING THE PRINCIPLES OF THE ALEXANDER TECHNIQUE

The Alexander principles help actors enormously. An actor can learn to "inhibit" or "stop" the tension habit and thereby free his or her performance. Alexander used the word "inhibition," which in some respects is a little unfortunate in acting training, as it evokes the idea of repression, which does not help the actor. This is not the way in which Alexander meant it, however. He meant that by stopping, we then have the opportunity to make a choice to do something different. This allows us to stop the offending habit long enough to figure out ways to prevent it. The most obvious benefit is that once the actor frees her or his head, neck, and torso relationship, this minimizes tension in the neck muscles, which allows the larynx to function more effectively.

Many of the principles of voice training do include the idea of "inhibition" or "stop" (though the voice teacher may not necessarily refer to the idea in quite the same way). Alexander found if he concentrated on the end result, his habitual tension returned. However, if he focused on the steps to get there, "the means

whereby," he was able to perform the given task without the tension returning. In so doing, the Alexander technique trains the mind to bypass its initial response to specific stimuli.

The Alexander technique should be integrated with all aspects of both directing and acting training. The actor should be blocked in ways that allow for proper alignment and easy breath support. If an awkward position is unavoidable, the actor wants to think of the neck lengthening and the shoulders releasing (not pushing) apart as much as possible. The position itself may look constricted but the job of the artist is to find an inner release in that position. The actor should search for the most efficient movement, using the least amount of tension possible. The beauty of the Alexander technique is that the principles can be applied to any position.

In a production of *Uncle Vanya*, directed by a well-known European director, the final scene was dramatically weakened by the director and actor not understanding the Alexander principles of alignment and body mechanics. The final scene in which Sonya speaks so eloquently about life's purpose was all but lost on the audience because the poor actress was so collapsed on the table, one could barely hear or understand her, due to her lack of breath support and positioning of her neck, causing constriction in the larynx. Had she only moved forward from the hip joints, thereby keeping her back open, which would have allowed her to use the swing of her back ribs and give her the support she needed, we would have experienced the extraordinary moving quality of this monologue, and been given the same physical impression. If only both director and actor had received training in the voice and the Alexander technique and applied this knowledge in that setting!

The idea of not "end gaining" that Alexander spoke of plays an important part in the development of character within a play. An actress playing Blanche in *Streetcar Named Desire*, for example, has to play her objective strongly to arrive at the end of the play in the appropriate emotional state. If she focuses on achieving the emotional state during the course of the play, her performance appears forced and unbelievable. Through text analysis, she explores her objectives and plays those thoroughly. When the character does not achieve her goals (ie, Mitch does not marry Blanche and she has no route to survival), Blanche finds herself desperately attempting to make her situation more tolerable. She fights against the obstacles presented to her, which creates the appropriate emotional response. This is the equivalent of the "means whereby" in the Alexander technique sense; she does not attempt to create an emotional response but it stems from her not achieving her goal.

> In a workshop with Cicely Berry, O.B.E., Voice Director of the Royal Shakespeare Company, England, and Andrew Wade, Voice Coach at the Guthrie Theatre and formerly Head of Voice at the RSC, the following occurred: A woman delivered a piece of text, a performance which might be described as histrionic. It was extremely tight vocally, overemotional, forced, and difficult to listen to. Berry asked the actress to pick up all the shoes (of the participants in the workshop) in the room, sequentially. The actress walked around the room, picking up the shoes, putting them into a pile, as she spoke her text. The actress's vocal delivery suddenly became like quicksilver and her delivery animated, charming, and engaging; all this while she was organizing the shoes. Her voice resonated with ease and full support as she utilized her full range.

What happened? The task of putting the shoes in order took her attention off the end result, that is, "inhibited" her habitual response to the delivery of text, and allowed her to discover the inherent freedom within the energy of the text. One might say she got out of the way of the text, letting it play her. Instead of imposing her own preconceived idea of the way the text should play and manipulating her delivery, she found a more intuitive connection to the language. By taking the attention off the result, ironically, the outcome proved far more interesting to the listener. There exist many similar exercises to "take the weight off the text."

During rehearsals of *Love's Labours Lost,* directed by Robin Phillips at the Stratford Festival in 1979, the following occurred. The scene was going reasonably well, but the actresses involved were becoming overly concerned with the language, which was causing a heaviness and self-consciousness in delivery. Mr. Phillips asked the actresses to repeat the scene and mime pinning their hair up with bobby pins at the same time. The scene became quite lively, more animated but in a relaxed, rather than pushed, way. The voices became freer and more expressive as the relationships of the characters became more playful. This simple exercise enabled the actresses to "take the weight off the words" and find a more natural delivery of the lines as well as a lighter approach to the scene. The act of miming pinning up the hair "inhibited" the habitual tendency to "push" the meaning out of the text and the voice, rather than allow them to flow naturally.

"YOU'VE GOT TO BELIEVE THEY CAN DO IT"

The Hidden "s"

An excellent bit of guidance is from Cecily Berry, who said, "You've got to believe they can do it." Invariably, this idea relaxes the actor and sometimes literally in the next minute the actor will actually achieve the very thing that overcomes the problem. If the actor does not achieve it immediately, often he or she masters the specific challenge by the next tutorial or class.

> While coaching at the Stratford Festival in Canada, the director of one of the productions expressed concern about a particular actor because of his sibilant "s," an "s" that hisses and catches our ear more than one would like. I was searching for a solution that would help this soft-spoken young man. We worked with traditional ways to "fix" the "s," with mild success: working on tongue placement, reading drills, and so on.
>
> The sibilant "s" in the case of this man was the result of faulty support

and what seemed to me a kind of vocal mannerism. My instinct told me a clue was missing but I did not know what. Finally, I asked him if English was the mother tongue of his parents. He told me they were Serbian. This was during the war in former Yugoslavia. I asked him to imitate his father. The actor then spoke with a thick Serbian accent and his voice became strong and full and his delivery extremely clear. Then I asked him then to speak his Shakespeare text in that same accent and again, the voice was full, strong and the sibilant "s" was completely gone. Then I asked him to speak the text again, with his father's "voice" but without the Serbian accent. He managed to speak the text clearly, with full voice and the "s" issue was completely nonexistent. Clearly, the "s" issue was a byproduct of an overall voice use issue. The man had seemingly cut himself off from his roots in some way, causing a lack of overall support in his speaking. This lack of support impacted him both physically and psychologically, creating a disconnect that resulted in a breathiness and the sibilant "s." The traditional exercises had not effectively solved this actor's sibilant "s" problem, because it was merely a symptom of a more complex issue.

Sometimes in the training of an actor, teachers insist that the tongue placement for the "s" be at the alveolar ridge. In point of fact, everyone has a differently shaped mouth and sometimes this tongue placement does not work. Rather, placing the front of the tongue against the back of the lower front teeth is more effective in some cases. It is important to make sure the individual actor knows where he or she should say an "s" or a "z." Voiced sounds (ie, d, n, l, r, ch, g, dg, etc) preceding "s" generally require the sound "z," whereas unvoiced sounds (ie, t, st, b, k, etc) require an "s" sound. One challenge in dealing with

articulation issues such as the production of "s" or "z," is that the poor actor can become so focused on the production of the s or z, that the rest of the vocal process comes to a halt, producing tension in the neck and shoulders, jaw, tongue root, and the rest. The actor must include physical ease and breath support when dealing with articulation issues.

A similar example came up at Stratford with an actor of Asian descent. It was assumed that the young actor could never master Shakespeare, that "it just wasn't in him." The young actor came to tutorial quite distraught, as he had been getting negative feedback about his voice use, not to mention the unspoken feedback about his perceived inability with Shakespeare. He was also told that he spoke Shakespeare in a "monotonous" way. During the tutorial, this young man explored speaking text, soft palate exercises, and breath support. Although he made minor improvements, nothing really made much of an impact. Finally, he was asked to speak the text in Chinese, his mother tongue. It was fascinating to hear his use of rhythm and language and how much richer the text was, even to the non-Chinese listener. It became apparent that many of the sounds had a rather nasal twang, and that many of the Chinese sounds used the palate in the dropped position rather than the lifted position that the majority of English sounds require. Part of the "monotonous" quality to his speaking of Shakespeare in English had to do with the fact that his soft palate took on a fixed position when he spoke, which did not allow for the normal flexibility and responsiveness. The young man then worked on loosening the soft palate, speaking the text with the yawn, and speaking the text first in Chinese-Mandarin and then again in English, singing the text in Chinese and then singing the text in English. The switching back and forth from Chinese to English was the key. This enabled him to eventually find the same freedom he had discovered in the exercises and incorporate this freedom into the speaking of the text so that that. over time, having identified the habit of what he was doing, he was able to approach the English text with the appropriate ease and flexibility necessary to allow the natural rhythm of the text. The older habit, completely appropriate for Chinese, had to be halted internally to allow him to develop a new relationship to the language.

What is important in both these examples, however, is the fact that once the coach acknowledged the actor's heritage as part of the vocal process, the actor managed to find a stronger commitment to the text; to use his full self in approaching the text, which enabled him to find his full voice. This is one of the most important issues in tackling voice tension. It is rarely a simple case of addressing the muscle in and of itself, but must be coupled with an understanding of the psychological components to achieve any level of success.

SIMPLE EXPLORATIONS TO HELP ELIMINATE VOCAL TENSION

Here are some simple exercises designed to address particular issues. With all these exercises, the approach should be one of exploration rather than going for an end result. Each individual responds slightly differently and if one exploration does not work, one should just go on to another. There is no right or wrong, just a chance to look at the vocal experience from another angle, which generally opens up new possibilities. Any sense of judgment creates further tension, so the coach must "believe the actor can do it." This will communicate unconsciously to the actor and create a more positive and productive working environment.

Tension in the Tongue Root

This results when someone is "driving the sound" by tightening the root of the tongue, attempting to find power by pushing with the back of the tongue and the tongue area below the chin. Generally, this habit is compensating for lack of appropriate support and an effort to achieve something within a performance.

Sit in a relaxed, upright position. Release the tongue out so that the outline of the tongue meets the outline of the lower lip. If the tongue won't rest comfortably in this position, gently hold the tongue. One should make sure the tongue is not being pressed down with too much force nor that the jaw is tightening to help out the situation. Then speak the text, slightly slower than usual, making sure to convey meaning clearly. After speaking a section of text in this fashion, which feels ridiculous, slide the tongue back into the mouth and speak the text again. Often the text will become clearer and the vocal tone richer because the exercise

gives the tongue root and jaw an opportunity to relax. Because one has to take the text more slowly, the breath support improves, as does the clarity of the thought.

Tension in the Jaw

Massage the jaw hinge gently. Then, with clean fingers, place forefingers gently between the upper and lower back molars, as one speaks the text. Then remove the fingers, but continue to keep the same space between the teeth as one speaks. Generally, one finds a fuller, easy sound by simply opening the jaw in a more relaxed fashion.

Another approach to alleviate jaw tension is to rub the hands together, place them on the jaw hinges, and then tilt the head over to one side, resting the head in one hand and then massaging the opposite jaw hinge. Then come back to center, with both hands on the jaw hinges and tilt over to the other side and massage the hinge of the other jaw. Come back to center and notice if the jaw muscles have relaxed.

Tight Soft Palate and Nasality

If the text sounds pitched and with an overbalance of nasal resonance, the problem is usually a dropped soft palate. There are a number of soft palate exercises but the simplest is to count from one to ten on a wide yawn then take the text on a yawn, so the actor can get the sense of the space inside the mouth. Then the actor speaks the text again, without actually yawning but allowing the sensation of yawning to inform the delivery. The actor generally discovers more sense of space in the mouth and a better balance of the nasal and mask resonators because of the lift of the soft palate.

Dealing with a Raspy Sound

If the actor tends to use too much force in speaking, resulting in a raspy, forced sound, then having the actor imagining the sound out the back of the neck is useful. In groups, partners can work together, putting a hand gently on the back of the neck and having the actor sigh a "huh" into the hand. This generally takes the pressure off the larynx by putting the attention elsewhere. One can also successfully apply the same idea to text. Moving down the body, an actor can put his or her hand at the back of the neck and sigh "huh" into the hand. The hand should pick up sound vibrations. If the actor is pushing vocally too much, the vibrations will be less. So, the more the actor releases with ease, the greater the sound vibrations. This is useful when actors are experiencing laryngeal pushing and tightening of the muscles around the larynx. Similarly, the actor can "kinesense" (sense kinesthetically) the sound moving out the skull. The hand can be placed on the skull and the actor can become aware of sound vibrations in the head. These can also be done as partner exercises.

If the actor tends to vocally push, it can be quite useful to a performer to conduct an activity while speaking the text. For example, if the actor puts away books, or wipes the blackboard, this can often take the pressure off the words and allow the actor more vocal ease.

Improving Support

In dealing with support, the most important thing is the movement of the intercostal muscles. This is the only effort required in breathing, while other efforts interfere with effective breath support. Attempting to suck in a big breath generally tightens the upper chest muscles, impedes free flow of sound and is counterproductive. It is important for actors to understand the anatomy of the diaphragm because too many people have an inaccurate picture of exactly what it is and what it does. One must remember the diaphragm extends around the full circumference of the lower ribs and expands and drops like a drum, causing a vacuum, which draws in the breath and releases up as the ribs contract on the release of breath. The main focus of the actor should always be on allowing the ribs to swing out, rather than contracting in. Putting emphasis on contracting the ribs in toward the body on the release of breath and sound creates a tendency to pull down and constrict the shoulder and neck muscles, resulting in tension around the larynx.

Lie on the floor, in fetal position, with the upper arm over the head and the lower arm under the head, so the neck is not crunched. Have a partner start at the top of the ribs closest to the ceiling, up beyond the collarbone and say, "These are your ribs." The partner moves all the way down, piece by piece saying, "These are your ribs" all the way down to the lower ribs. Then the first person sits up and compares the rib freedom of each side. In most cases, the individual will experience much more awareness of the full extent of the rib case and the movement of the ribs on the side just worked with. Then one can repeat the same thing on the other side. This exercise also helps to sense the differentiation between the ribs and the shoulder girdle. Many actors squeeze the upper arms to the upper ribs and this constricts support. The elbows and ribs are enemies and like a little space between them.

It is important to remind actors that the spine lengthens on the outtake of breath, which in a way seems counterintuitive. However, if the actor can work with that image, some wonderful things can happen. Instead of the typical pull down, tighten, and squeeze for "power" ("bluff acting"), the actor can find the length and width in the release of the thought, thereby eschewing the typical squeeze actors often resort to, which does nothing but create vocal tension and unbelievable acting "moments." The squeeze obstructs free expression because it tightens the breathing mechanism and pulls everything inside, rather than sharing it out. Actors can explore finding the ease of full expression if they really let it release and sense the length as they release the text. The bigger the stakes, the more release the actor needs.

An actor can move one arm pointing toward the ceiling and the other to the side as she or he speaks the text, so as to remind her or himself of length and width. Then repeat this, imagining one is moving the arms and notice if one has more sense of ease.

If the actor is having difficulty finding appropriate support, ask the actor to lift the arms out to the side, with each intake of breath and then, while speaking the text, take the arms back down to the sides of the body. This usually helps the actor to engage the back area of the ribs and opens up the support. Sometimes the actor, if open to something playful, can imagine angel wings and move the arms in this manner while speaking the text.

If an actor does not seem to be embodying the text, then here are a few ideas to help the actor "get into his or her back." The actor can imagine one is wearing a sound cape, and that the sound and ideas of the voice are moving through the cape. The actor can speak to someone, picturing the person behind him or her, imagining a mouth in the back, as if one is speaking from one's back. If the actor doesn't click with the mouth image, then even just speaking to someone behind can help the actor use his or her full breath support and gain a fuller kinesthetic awareness.

Tension in the Neck and Shoulder Areas

A simple Alexander idea is to practice text, pretending one has a second head on top of one's real head. One immediately finds length and width and more ease in the speaking of the text. A guided body check can prove useful as well:

Sense the width of the back,

The distance between the eyebrows and the back skull,

The occipital joint, sense the head moving up and away from the body,

The distance between the shoulder blades,

The back of the arms,

The backs of the legs,

Sense the sitting bones,

The soles of the feet on the floor,

The distance between the ankles and the toes.

This helps ground the actor, reminding him or her of the full body connection, which in turn aids the release of tension around the neck, jaw, and shoulders. Addressing the overall psychophysical use generally makes addressing any specific tension areas, such as jaw tension, neck tension, soft palate inflexibility, and so forth, much easier.

Constructive Rest

Lie on the floor or a table, with the knees up toward the ceiling, feet flat on the ground, with a book under the head. The book should allow the neck to lengthen so that the neck is not overly arched or the head so high that the chin is pressing down on the larynx. One then thinks in a number of directions—out through the top of the head away from the torso, in the direction up through the knees, feet solidly on the ground and the thought of the back lengthening and widening. If one does this for several 5-minute sessions a few times a day, one notices positive changes quite quickly: more ease in the shoulders and neck, thereby more freedom in the voice, more sense of ease in movement, and more of a sense of ease of height. Often, an added benefit is an improved sense of well-being.

Ways to Deal with Monotone Delivery

An actor speaks in monotone when he or she has not fully comprehended the "geography" of the text; that is, how one phrase and thought builds into the next. The actor needs to allow the voice to reflect the rhythm of the text and the pitch to appropriately reveal the meaning, using the sounds of the words to convey the message. Here are some ways to help the actor discover the connection of the meaning to pitch and rhythm in an intuitive manner. The actor can sing and dance the text and then go back to speaking it. This exercise achieves two things. One, the actor becomes more physically relaxed, allowing the natural breath support to take over and, two, the movement and singing help the actor find the inherent rhythm and musicality of the text, which allows the actor to connect to the language in a deeper and more released way. Often it is useful to ask the actor what kind of music he or she likes. Then one says to the actor, "Here are the lyrics (the actor's text) and you are the composer. You need to find the right music for these lyrics that fit the meaning." With verse speaking, actors have achieved great success with country and western delivery, rap, jazz, and opera singing. This gives the actor the opportunity to experience the words in a new way. In general, when the actor returns to speaking the text after this exercise, the actor speaks it with much more variety and vocal build of ideas.

Another exercise involves the coach at the piano. The coach gives the actor a lower pitch to start with and then gives the actor a new ascending pitch for each new idea, as the thoughts build. Once the thought idea is completed, the coach can then return to a lower pitch and build again. The actor chants the text on the particular pitch, rather than speaking it or fully singing the text. Then the actor goes back to speaking the text without the piano and usually approaches the text with more variety and nuance.

Precision of Language

If the actor is having difficulty finding precision in the language, then have the actor speak the line of text word by word, (ie, to . . . to be . . . to be or . . . to be or not . . . to be or not to . . . to be or not to be . . .) then repeat the whole thought. This is an exercise I learned from Patsy Rodenburg and I have nicknamed it "Lego blocks," because the actor begins to sense the shape of each idea and how each word builds on the word before. Actors tend to run words together, which obscures clarity of meaning. Awareness of each word as a string of thoughts, like a string of pearls, is particularly important in classical text, but any text benefits from this exploration.

Exploring Imagery

Often, vocal tension arises out of a lack of clarity about what the character actually is saying. A simple exercise I have developed has proven quite useful. The actor draws each new image on a blackboard as specifically as possible, even abstract ones. This often helps the actor grapple with each new part of the thought, which the actor may have overlooked. The time taken to really delve into each image specifically helps the actor relax into the language, deepen the support, and hence use less tension in the speaking.

Asking the actor to close one's eyes and visualize each image as the actor says it is a tool I have found particularly effective for dealing with tension. Often, tension stems from the physical manifestation of not giving each image and idea its full importance. Picturing the text helps find the specific image behind each thought.

One can also take a similar approach in a group by using sound. This idea came to me when I led a workshop of Buffalo storytellers in a workshop a number of years ago. One participant was sight impaired and I was quite shocked by the fact that almost my entire repertoire of metaphors involved sight. So when this gentleman performed his story, the group developed appropriate sound effects to support the images in the story. When he spoke the text again, without the group's sound effects, he was able to find many more levels in the ideas and the voice responded accordingly, expressing the ideas with changes in pitch, rhythm, dynamic, and so forth. I have often since asked students to close their eyes and have the group make sound effects and often this has quite a dramatic impact. Working individually with an actor, one might ask the actor to think through the text and just make sounds appropriate to the ideas. Then the next time the actor speaks the text, the actor should have a more kinesthetic response to the language, with more vivid images and textures to the ideas.

SUMMARY

Unless one fully takes into account the specifics of each thought, one cannot really help an actor fully realize his or her vocal potential. It is not enough to free the sound, but the thought must be carved out with commitment and precision and a full kinesthetic relationship to the *language*. Coaches need to approach the actor with a sense of openness as a guide. This works much better than taking a "corrective" attitude, which usually serves to render the actor self-conscious. Finding vocal ease requires commitment to healthy technique, daily vocal preparation, openness, and a genuine desire to communicate. The actor and coach must delve into the text as deeply as possible to allow the thought to propel the sound, the nuances, and delicate dynamics of thought. Both coach and actor must include the overall personality of the actor in addressing vocal tension.

REFERENCES

1. Linklater K. *Freeing the Natural Voice.* New York, NY: Drama Books; 1976. (Basic introduction to the Linklater approach to voice work.)
2. Wade A. *Voice and Text Professional Workshop* through VASTA (Voice and Speech Trainers Association); University of Arizona, Tempe, Ariz; January 1994.

3. Berry C. That secret voice. In: Hampton M, Acker B, eds. *The Vocal Vision.* New York, NY: Applause Books; 1997. (A collection of essays including Catherine Fitzmaurice's article "Breathing Is Meaning" and other articles related to voice pedagogy, controversial issues in teaching, and various techniques.)
4. Gelb MJ. *Body Learning.* New York, NY: Owl Books; 1996. (History and explanation of the Alexander Technique and resources for further study.)

ADDITIONAL RESOURCES

Berry C. *Voice and the Actor.* New York, NY: Applause Books; 1991.

Berry C. *The Actor and the Text.* New York, NY: Applause Books; 2000. (Deals with the visceral connection of voice and text as well as text analysis.)

Linklater K. *Freeing Shakespeare's Voice.* New York, NY: Theatre Communications Group; 1992. (Explorations of voice/text and psychophysical work.)

McCallion M. *The Voice Book.* New York, NY: Theatre Arts Books/Routledge; 1998. (Explores many aspects of voice/speech/text; particularly good in dealing with the Alexander technique and voice.)

Rodenburg P. *The Right to Speak.* New York, NY: Theatre Arts Books; 1992. (Basic vocal approach; deals with the voice as it relates to the "right to express" and self-image in our society.)

Rodenburg P. *The Need for Words.* New York, NY: Theatre Arts Books; 1993. (More voice/text explorations.)

Rodenburg P. *The Actor Speaks.* New York, NY: St. Martin's Press; 2000. (Deals with voice curriculum and vocal demands in various performance situations.)

Sataloff RT. *Professional Voice: The Science and Art of Clinical Care.* San Diego, Calif: Plural Publishing, Inc; 2005. (Basic medical overview, explanation of voice disorders, with color illustrations.)

Sataloff RT. *Vocal Health and Pedagogy.* San Diego, Calif: Plural Publishing, Inc; 2006. (Good overview of interdisciplinary voice care from both medical and artistic perspectives.)

Plural Publishing has many books on voice and voice care. CDs and tapes on voice and voice care are available from the Voice Foundation (1721 Pine Street, Philadelphia, Pa 19104.).

Chapter 18

TREATMENT OF INJURED SINGERS AND PROFESSIONAL SPEAKERS: THE SINGER/ACTOR, SINGER/DANCER, AND SINGER/MUSICIAN

Jeannette L. LoVetri

Actors, dancers, and musicians are often called upon to sing. Each of these groups of professional voice users will encounter unique challenges in singing and will have specific issues to address if they are to remain vocally healthy or to recover from vocal injury. To assist a performer to return to healthy vocal use for singing and speaking, it is necessary to understand as many factors as possible that could contribute to vocal injury.

THE SINGER/ACTOR—THE LARGER CONTEXT

In New York City and other major theatrical centers, there is a difference between someone who sings and can act (singer/actor) and someone who acts and can sing (actor/singer). This may sound odd, but it comes from the fact that actors and singers are trained very differently and think of themselves in ways that are distinct from each other. This is also true of those who are primarily dancers (dancers who sing) and musicians (someone who can play and sing). These are not inconsequential differences, as they are significant factors in

how each of these performers uses his or her voice when singing. In New York professional circles, "actor" is a term that can be used to refer to both men and women. In this chapter, the use of this word will be a reference to both males and females.

The following are quotes from ads for auditions that appear in the weekly New York theatrical trade publication, *Back Stage*:

> "Thoroughly Modern Millie"—Seeking male dancers who sing . . .

> "Evita"—Seeking singers who move, dancers who sing, male and female . . .

> "Disney Cruise Line"—Seeking musical theater performers, trained vocalists and actors who move well, or trained dancers who can sing on key.

> "Floyd & Clea Under The Western Sky"—Seeking Singers: male or female, who are also instrumentalists, must be proficient on the dobro/acoustic guitar/pedal steel guitar, etc. Singers who are not proficient musicians cannot be considered.[1(p8,22)]

THE SPEAKING/SINGING INTERFACE

All singers discover through life experience that the speaking voice has a direct impact on the singing voice. (Perhaps this is why we divide them into two categories even though the voice source is from the same two vocal folds). It is also true in reverse in that singing can have an impact on how an actor speaks. To ascertain the interface between speaking and singing, it is useful to take a look at the training of performers' speaking and singing voices. Training, or lack thereof, has a direct impact on the vocal patterns habitually used by the singer/actor or actor/singer so, before attempting to return a performer to healthy singing, it is important to know what these patterns are and how they were developed. Retraining an injured voice implies bringing it back to a state of normalcy, and deviation from the functional norm can have deep and old roots that must be unearthed before they can be removed.

TRAINING HISTORY—A NECESSITY

Regardless of whether the training is for singing or speaking, as has been stated, singers and actors are trained very differently. Because the level of training available runs the gamut from poor to excellent, and because not all singers and actors have formal training, performers bring a wide range of patterns with them when they begin professional work. Training *should* be helpful, but this is, unfortunately, not always the case. Some types of training can be useless, some can be confusing, others will set up conflicts between how the voice is used for singing and how it is used in speech, and still others may actually be harmful to the voice in general. Remember, too, that some singers, dancers, and musicians have no training at all for speech or singing yet work professionally.

> A *singer/actor* is someone who is trained first to sing and then learns to act. This performer would answer the question "what do you do?" with the answer, "I am a singer."

Singing training involves learning very different skills than those used in acting. Singers focus on learn-

ing to read music and on singing with enough carrying power to be heard over an orchestra without electronic amplification. A singer needs to make a clear tone, using a wide range of pitches, with deliberate control over the use of the breath and with a constant vibrato. "A good vibrato is a pulsation of pitch, usually accompanied with synchronous pulsations of loudness and timbre, of such extent and rate as to give a pleasing flexibility, tenderness, and richness to the tone."[2] Singing training will also involve learning to sing in several foreign languages and learning to use complex musical decorations called ornaments. It may or may not include formal acting training (which is separate from that used in a musical production) or movement/dance training. The goals of training someone to sing are still almost totally classical; that is, training is aimed toward opera, oratorio, art song, chamber, or other classical music. These are primarily musical goals.

Singers who are called on to act in plays without music can be quite challenged by use of the speaking voice, as frequently it will have been largely ignored during singing training. In theatrical productions, women especially are often asked or expected to use a speaking voice that sounds deep, low, and robust but may not have the ability to do so as they have only been trained as singers to sound high, sweet, and warm. Singers who find themselves in a nonmusical play may find speaking for long periods of time fatiguing. Lighter voices, especially, can be worn out by long rehearsals with continuous repetition of scenes.

An *actor/singer* is trained first in "straight" drama (no music is involved) and is asked to investigate his or her own memories, history, and points of view in learning to develop and express a character in a dramatic work. Movement training is frequently involved, and sometimes there is training for the speaking voice. Actors also analyze historic and contemporary plays and playwrights and types of productions and directing. Generally, no musical training is given. The actor may or may not at some point have some lessons in singing and/or learn songs that may or may not be classical.

Actors can be quite confused when asked to sing something that requires very precise pitch control in a range that is far above that of conversational speech, as musical ability can be divorced entirely from speaking well. If the performer is able to use a vocal quality in singing that is very similar to the same vocal quality used in speech, it is likely that things will work out well.

A QUICK LOOK AT THE BASICS

All healthy voice use, including singing, is based upon a few of the same principles. A *professional singer* is someone who gets paid for singing and must deliver musical sound on demand. The following list of prerequisites for good voice use applies to every vocal professional, both singing and speaking:

1. Excellent posture
2. A strong open chest and rib cage
3. Strong but flexible abdominal muscles
4. Relaxed strap muscles in the neck
5. The ability to take a free, full inhalation, well down into the bottom of the lungs
6. Coordination between the ribs and abdominal muscles during exhalation (This is usually called "breath support".)
7. The ability to open the mouth by dropping the jaw freely and easily and with more than the usual amount of space between the teeth
8. The ability to articulate clearly—using the lips and tongue easily and freely
9. Comfortable vocal expression in song and speech— no strain, no forcing, and no discomfort
10. A pitch range of an octave and a half to two octaves, and enough power to be heard without electronic amplification in a moderately sized room with good acoustics.

Interference with the function of any of the above can exacerbate vocal problems for anyone but lack of these skills can be a serious issue for those singer/actors, dancer/singers, and musicians who wish to sing well.

THE BODY/VOICE CONNECTION

Anyone who is in good health and physically fit has an advantage in keeping the voice functionally strong, as these things go together well.[3] Beyond this, however, the vocal performer draws on the body and its ability to move when expressing emotion and becomes acquainted with the body's sensations and feelings in order to create a character in a play or musical.[4] Skilled performers learn to be intimately aware of the body

and what it can do or handle.[5] The enhanced awareness that a performer has of his or her body is also very valuable to vocal health, as performers can often sense when something is wrong, even if they do not have the specific medical terms to describe it.

RANKING THE SINGER'S TASKS

In musical theater, the amount and type of singing varies from show to show, so it is difficult to generalize about vocal function in singer/actors and actor/ singers or dancer/singers. A performer who is in the chorus of an older musical show (something written before 1968) is less likely to encounter vocal problems. The earlier music was written so differently for singers than is the music of today's composers that it is usually easier to sing.

Singer/actors who must add movement or dancing into their work are also more likely to incur vocal problems because the added activity can interfere with correct use of the voice or be fatiguing to the body, or both. Singers who are in leading roles of rock musicals such as *Tommy*, *Jesus Christ Superstar*, or *Rent* are performing music that is extremely demanding emotionally, physically, musically, and vocally and must not only be very skilled but must monitor how the voice is used outside the performance to be able to maintain a full 8-shows-a-week schedule. When there are so many factors affecting the way the voice is used, even the best actor/singer or singer/actor could encounter vocal trouble, particularly if other things such as illness or stress are also present.

Any specialist who works with a singer in this last category must understand that this performer is the vocal equivalent of an Olympic athlete who needs to be treated accordingly.

FACING THE UNKNOWN: WHEN THE ACTOR IS THROWN INTO SINGING

Actors who are inexperienced singers can face a wide range of difficulties that could have a negative impact on the voice when asked to sing in a musical. This situation is not particularly unusual, and when such a performer is expected to sing, she will have little prior experience from which to evaluate her ability or the materials she is being asked to execute. This insecurity can undermine even a very confident actor. If the music is difficult or badly written, she can unwittingly push the voice or alter her breathing pattern while struggling to sing the song, and this may cause vocal fold irritation. Music directors, too, can ask the performer to do things that are musically viable but beyond the capability of the novice singer. The music director is usually a pianist and conductor who has dealings with singers but may have no training in singing or be unable to sing him- or herself. Some music directors are intimidating to young performers and have the effect of making the performer afraid to speak up lest he or she seem unqualified to be in the show.

OTHER FACTORS THAT MATTER

Because all professional shows except opera and other forms of classical music are now electronically amplified, a lot depends on the sound system and the sound engineer of any given show. The "sound man" can make or break the performer if he is unfamiliar with singers and the sound system plays a big role in what the performer hears. Without a good monitor (stage amplifier facing the singer) or good acoustic feedback within the theater or performance space, the performer will hear his voice in a distorted or muffled way. This, too, will cause him to push the voice and can lead to vocal problems.

Typically, actors will attempt to sing using the same sound for music as for speech. This is an excellent way to begin and for most music it is the correct approach. However, some of the most popular shows that have appeared on Broadway over the last 40 years are quite demanding, particularly rock-and-roll based shows. Singing this music demands a strong vocal instrument, lots of power in the breathing mechanism, and a good deal of physical movement. The range of the songs is typically high and can involve powerful emotional expression as well. Those who do not have strong vocal technique may quickly run out of options in terms of vocal resources.

Certain roles demand very loud singing or speaking, sometimes in unusual or difficult positions (lying down, bent over, twisted alignment, etc). In productions that use heavy or restrictive costumes, the performer may have a great deal of weight in the costume itself. It may be made out of restrictive materials that can affect head/neck alignment or place stress on the neck and throat muscles or the rib cage position and interfere with the ability to freely inhale and strongly exhale. For example, the Broadway musical *The Lion King* has a number of roles in which the actors play animals, and must both sing and speak with "animal" voices and wear heavy costumes. Singing or speaking in a very high pitch range or a very rough vocal quality can cause fatigue if done repeatedly over an extended period of time.

THE DANCER'S DILEMMA

Many dancers are professionally mute for their entire careers. Those who belong to a dance company can survive well without ever uttering a sound while flying across the stage on their winged feet.

Dancers who are lucky enough to belong to a professional dance company where no vocal utterances are ever required, however, are the rare exceptions. More often, at some point in his or her career, a dancer will be called on to speak or sing as a part of a performance. The dilemma faced by these dancers is that they may not be prepared, psychologically or vocally.

Dancers who have not had speech or singing training or who have had little experience using the voice professionally are often quite frightened by the prospect of doing so. This fear only makes it more difficult to produce a free healthy sound, as it inhibits both the breath and the voice itself. Additionally, dancers who have had no vocal training may suffer from habitually restricted movement of the muscles that affect vocal production, making it difficult for the dancer to learn new vocal skills quickly even if the dancer is willing and unafraid.

Professional dancers usually begin training at an early age. No matter what style of dance is studied, little anatomy or physiology is included in dance training except at the most elite schools, so the dancer may not have a good grasp of any of the vocal muscle systems, and likely knows very little about the voice and how it works or how it relates to the body as a whole.

All of this means that dancers are ripe for vocal problems if they are also in a situation where the voice must be used similarly to those just described for singer/actors. Even though they are coordinated and strong, dancers can be very specifically focused on using the body for dancing, *and only for dancing*, and be unable to include awareness of the voice and how it is being used. The issues of using the voice well would become doubly difficult, as the dancing would be a diversion of mental and physical energy, away from the voice itself.

Dancers frequently have tension in the genioglossus, hyoglossis, mylohyoid, diagastric muscles,[6] and the muscles of the root of the tongue connecting to the hyoid bone. They can have tight, stiff jaw (masseter and medial pterygoid[6] muscles), making it difficult to get the mouth open enough to be useful in terms of volume and acoustic efficiency or resonance amplification. Because a long "swanlike" neck is considered a mark of beauty in a ballet dancer, dancers often have very stretched sternocleidomastoid (strap)[5] muscles in the neck, which make it difficult for the larynx to float loosely in the throat. The overall tensions, if not released gradually over a period of time, can cause the dancer to push the voice to make it seem louder or more professional, and this in turn actually makes things worse.

Effective treatment of a vocal disorder would warrant looking at the ability of the dancer to easily move and be aware of all the external muscles affecting the sound. Each of these areas would need to be approached individually so that they could be more relaxed, movable, flexible, and eventually stronger. This would include work on stretching the jaw, developing greater flexibility in the tongue, activating the face and mouth muscles, and loosening the neck and shoulder muscles. The stomach muscles (rectus and transversus abdominis, and the obliques)[5] in particular need to be flexible enough to allow for some forward movement during inhalation. Dancers' stomach muscles are very strong and sometimes they are so taut that little movement is possible. This inhibits the ability of the diaphragm to descend during inhalation and consequently restricts the amount of air intake. Ballet dancers are taught to breathe laterally, meaning that the ribs move out to the sides during inhalation so that the rib cage does not rise and fall during dancing. This type of inhalation is less efficient for singing but is better than a locked rib cage which cannot move at all, making inhalation very shallow.

MUSICIANS

A musician has to fall into one of two categories: either she is capable of singing while playing the instrument or she has to stop playing it to sing. The people who play brass or woodwinds are in the second group. The rest of the musicians can sing while they play. The odd group would be the violinists and violists, who could conceivably make vocal sound but would find it difficult to move the mouth to pronounce words, as the jaw has to anchor the instrument to the shoulder in order for it to be stable.

Playing an instrument definitely helps make the performer more musically confident when he or she has to sing, but the postures used in each of the various instruments do affect the way the voice works. Some instruments are less likely to cause vocal problems for the performer than others, but a great deal rests on the way each individual actually plays.

The Alexander Technique is beneficial to instrumentalists both for their own technique in whatever instrument they play and for helping them find a good use of the body for singing as well. If the posture of the musician is relatively good while playing the instrument, learning to breathe correctly and keep good alignment while singing should be an achievable task. If, however, the performer is wrapped around his guitar or saxophone or falling into the piano or cello, things can be more challenging. Also, if the performer is singing early music while gently strumming a lute, it would be much less worrisome than if he is banging a set of drums in a heavy metal band while pumping out background vocals. The second performer would have a more difficult job getting to good vocal production habits unless he or she was quite able to adapt in several areas easily and simultaneously. Also, in the case of someone who has to play with an embouchure, the way in which a player applies the mouth to the mouthpiece of a brass or wind instrument,[7] the function of the lips, jaw, mouth, and the structures inside the mouth itself, including the soft palate, the back of the tongue, and the larynx and the vocal folds all have an impact on the production of the instrument's sound. In a professional musician, these muscles are quite strong and do a different job than they would for someone who is a singer, and only a singer. Horn players who must develop strong air pressure in the mouth and strength in the muscles surrounding the lips will also keep the jaw in a relatively raised position. All these muscle patterns are antithetical to good singing and can cause the musician to sound unpleasant or to experience pitch fluctuations or diminishment of vocal range.

As with dancers, musicians have to be cross-trained to function optimally in both playing and singing. The muscle groups involved in playing need to be massaged (externally, where possible), relaxed, stretched, and moved so that they can allow for greater flexibility and ease of movement. Postural imbalances must be addressed through stretching and strengthening and perhaps also through physical therapy and medical massage. On the positive side, though, brass and wind instrumentalists have good breath control and this facilitates breathing for singing, as it is possible to easily adapt the breathing techniques used for playing to singing.

PITCH-RELATED ISSUES

Actors and dancers and even musicians may also have pitch-matching issues that professional singers do not have. This means that these individuals may not easily "sing on key" or "on the note" or have major issues with pitch control (sharping—singing too high or flatting—singing too low to be accurate). Until these issues are addressed through training (and good singing training can train anyone to sing on pitch accurately), the added insecurity about "being able to stay on pitch" would be yet another stress factor that could inhibit correct and healthy singing.[6]

APPROACHES TO RETRAINING A DISORDERED OR INJURED VOICE

Many of the same principles that apply to working with a disordered or injured speaking voice also apply to working with the voices of those who sing. The primary difference is that the exercises are applied to pitches that are specific (musical scales and arpeggios) and often sustained for longer durations and at louder volumes than necessary for conversational speech. Also, because the work is directed toward vocal fold function rather than articulatory issues, there is an aspect of acoustic acuity necessary, on both the part of the singer and the teacher, that typically would not be called for in speech.

A singing voice specialist (SVS) is a singing teacher who is familiar with healthy vocal function and is able to discuss any vocal health issues with a speech-language pathologist and otolaryngologist. The SVS will understand the diagnosis made by the medical and clinical professionals and be able to work as part of a team in helping the singer return to good healthy singing. Working in this way, the SVS can be assured that others are also able to support and evaluate the progress of the singer and validate the health of the vocal mechanism through objective measures and tools.

BEGIN WITH WHAT CAN BE SEEN AND TOUCHED

All singing training begins on the outside of the body with posture and alignment and with specific exercises for the various parts of the body that affect the way the sound is produced. Training also begins by teaching the singer to have a more deliberate and specific approach to breathing that must be consciously coupled with sound-making for the vocal output to be freely and correctly controlled. It should also teach the singing actor, dancer, or musician how to listen objectively for correct vocal and musical function. Returning to normal singing function means returning to normal function in the following areas.

Posture

The importance of posture cannot be overstated.[6] The larynx works best when situated in the throat without any undue muscle tension from muscles that are not necessary for phonation. The relationship of the head, neck, shoulders, and rib cage to each other is a crucial ingredient in allowing the muscles of the upper torso to function properly. If a singing professional has vocal problems, and if those problems are chronic, it is important to evaluate the relationship between the head and neck, the neck and shoulders, and the upper chest with the lower back. Misalignment or tension in any of these muscles will affect the ability of the larynx to function optimally. It is helpful for the performer to work with a postural alignment system such as the aforementioned Alexander technique, one of the various approaches to yoga, or other bodywork disciplines that facilitate correct alignment. If the head juts forward, protruding out in front of the body, allowing the ribs to sag, the larynx will not be able to move freely and the vocal folds will be affected by this restriction. If the head is dropped back so that the cranium is collapsed into the cervical spine, the neck muscles will shorten and the contraction will restrict the muscles of the neck and throat, ultimately affecting the larynx in a similar fashion. These are just two of the possible problems that can aggravate vocal fold issues and make it more difficult for the singer to function optimally; potentially, there are many more.

Breathing

Singing can demand more than twice the air pressure and as much as five times more range than speech. In order for the singer to be able to generate sufficient air pressure for loud sounds and higher pitches, it is necessary to work on increasing the singer's ability to deeply inhale and to control the air as it goes out during singing. This involves using the intercostal muscles in the ribs and the abdominal muscles in a coordinated and deliberate manner while exhaling during a sung phrase. For this to work properly, the body must stand erect, but without rigidity, and the torso must be balanced so that it is possible to walk and move with grace and ease at all times. The ribs must remain open and stable during both inhalation and exhalation and the singer must inhale by drawing the air down into the bottom of the lungs, simultaneously allowing the abdominal wall to move forward, down, and/or out. When sound is being made, the singer must learn to deliberately contract and tighten the abdominal muscles to keep the air pressure constant while the lungs are emptying. This is a learned behavior that takes time to master. There is some variability from person to person

in how this is accomplished, but breathing patterns that do not generally conform to these principles may not be sufficient to keep vocal production healthy.

The Face and Head

The muscles of the singer's face and head greatly affect the sound that is being sung. The mandible (jawbone) must be able to drop significantly more in singing than it does in speech and remain in a dropped position for long periods of time. The tongue must be relaxed even when the mouth may be wide open, and this is a learned behavior for most people. The jaw can also be dropped too far down and interfere with the muscles of the throat or with the tongue, so the amount of the opening must be evaluated in relationship to other structures. The muscles of the face and the lips change the shape of the mouth, which affects the quality of the sound; and the tongue, both in front and in back, plays a crucial role in shaping the vowel sounds both for accuracy and for purposes of expressiveness. Although most novice singers can make simple movements of the face and lip muscles and the jaw, the exaggerated movements necessary for singing are sometimes beyond the ability of an inexperienced singer to initially control and can require time and patience to develop to optimum responsiveness and efficiency. Singing high notes and loud sounds requires that the jaw be dropped quite a bit. At the same time, the face and lips must also be shaped and the tongue positioned so that there is no interference with the muscles inside the mouth and throat, and there must be good solid help from the breathing mechanism. This, too, requires a high degree of coordination and also takes time to learn.

Internal Structures

The musculature in the velopharyngeal port (the back of the mouth and throat) has a profound affect on the singer's voice. The shapes made inside the mouth and throat, and the modifications of those shapes by the tongue, determine not only what vowel we hear but how that vowel sound comes across as acoustic output. Singer's call this "resonance" and it is the crucial ingredient in most singing, as it is a part of what makes the singer's voice unique. Because none of these structures are deliberately movable, except perhaps in a very skilled and experienced singer, creating change in them is often an elusive and confusing process unless the SVS understands how to stimulate vocal function through specific exercises. If internal change does not occur, the sound remains the same and the faulty habits that produced that sound also continue.

The larynx has a very important role to play, as the vocal folds determine both the pitch and the basic tonal quality of the sound.[8] They also regulate the airflow, depending on the quality of the sound the singer is producing. Much has been written and discussed regarding vocal production but it is generally conceded by the scientific and academic voice communities that the main body of the folds, the thyroarytenoid muscle, is responsible for producing the vocal quality that is called *modal* or speaking voice quality. The muscle that stretches and thins the folds, the cricothyroid, helps produce the quality that is called *loft*.[8]

There are many other terms or names for these vocal qualities. The most common term is *vocal register*.[8] A register is essentially a group of tones that have the same texture or quality. This definition, which is an aural one, says that one group of tones sounds like speech and the other does not. Typically, vocal sounds are divided into two basic qualities: chest register and head register, named by the sensations felt in the body while the sounds are being made. *Modal* would be chest register and *loft* would be head register or "falsetto." The easiest way to understand this difference is to think of a man speaking in his normal voice and in a falsetto or childlike quality. The simultaneous combination of these two qualities would give a balance of both.

The use of registers is a key ingredient in style and a primary element in singing voice training. Classical singers are taught to "blend" the registers so that there is a smooth sound from the lowest to highest pitches. Theater singers, and others who sing the various styles of commercial and pop music, do not necessarily blend the vocal registers. In fact, some styles specifically require that the singer stay in the chest or modal quality throughout the entire sung range (see "belting" below). If the performer does not understand how to sing in the correct register quality, he or she might be unable to produce the appropriate sounds for the music being performed.

Proper use and development of registers is a key ingredient in helping a singer/actor, dancer, or musician understand healthy vocal production. Development and strengthening of both chest and head registers assist the entire vocal mechanism to work freely and efficiently. Lower voiced males typically need to develop the head or falsetto register to strengthen it and help expand their range upward and lighten the amount or pressure on the larynx and vocal folds in higher pitches. They can then also integrate the head register quality into their lower pitch range, making it warmer and more appealing. Women sometimes need to do the same, as not all women's voices are head register dominant, as was the case a generation ago. Lighter higher voices (including classically trained tenors and sopranos, lyric mezzos, and baritones—particularly those who have been trained in an older more conservative approach) also usually benefit from developing the chest register on the lower pitches to give the voice more strength and richness.

Contemporary commercial music, the new term for all nonclassical styles, places a strong emphasis on the use of chest register. Learning to sing with this quality in a free and healthy way is of paramount importance to all contemporary performers.[9] It is possible to produce high tones in a speech-based chest register quality, but this is more likely to cause vocal dysfunction issues as, to be done safely, it requires greater and more efficient output of all the systems involved in producing vocal sound. Singers of any kind of commercial music who have been injured must be guided toward correct register function in order to sing well and remain healthy.

Emotional Issues

All artists are emotional. It comes with the territory. Performing often magnifies emotional response and asks for its powerful expression, repeated on demand, over and over. No one's throat was meant to do this, day in and day out. In music that is particularly demanding, adding emotional factors into the mix is often enough to overload the vocal system and cause the vocal folds to become fatigued or injured. Singers must learn to deal with these demands, as it is part of what they are expected to deliver as professionals, but it can require enormous stamina, skill, and care to do that successfully. Tension brought on by chronic or acute stress tightens the muscles, inhibits breathing, and takes a toll on the voice and body, so adding personal emotion to professional emotion can complicate things still further. Any singer who has had vocal problems is stressed, and this must be addressed as the voice is guided back to healthy function, so that the worry does not also cause vocal function issues.

CONSTRICTION—THE BIGGEST ISSUE

The biggest vocal difficulty of singers who perform in shows that have vigorous, demanding music, as is found in many of today's musicals, is constriction. The three groups of constrictor muscles (superior, middle, and inferior) often become engaged when the singer has to hit high pitches in a loud chest register or "belt" quality and does not have sufficient strength in the muscles of the body and throat to manage this task.

> The nature of the belt: it is an attempt to extend the normally "short" female chest register upward.) When secure, the belt produces an edgy, driving sound. Because of the tension involved in holding the position, vocal qualities associated with relaxation as well as all those associated with the integrated head register, are not possible. Sweetness of tone, ductility in phrasing, flexibility of movement are closed out. There is no such thing as a quiet belt, or a beautiful one. (Osbourne, as cited in Potter[10])

Men belt, too. Carrying the chest register quality above approximately E/F/G$_4$ without modifying or darkening the vowels, at a loud volume, would constitute belting.

The constriction narrows the sidewalls of the pharynx, raises the base of the tongue, pulls the larynx up, and tightly compresses the vocal folds. Sometimes, but not always, the external throat and neck muscles bulge or protrude. In all but the most unusual singers, this constriction is not deliberate, nor desired, and often becomes a chronic pattern affecting all vocal production. The performer may be unaware that anything is wrong until and unless the vocal folds them-

selves develop problems or until professional musical standards can no longer be met.

The side effects of this type of constriction are numerous and varied. Aside from pathology, they can include loss of high range or certain pitches, loss of pitch control, difficulty with sustained notes, breathiness in middle pitches, easy fatigue of the voice, extreme nasality, and difficulty with articulation, as words can become swallowed or garbled.

This problem is the most difficult one to address, as it cannot be handled directly. In general, the tension must be taken off layer by layer, starting on the outside of the body with the head position and with the jaw. The head must remain level and positioned directly over the shoulders and torso, and the upper chest must be lifted but only from below by the abdominal and back muscles and not by the pectoralis muscles or shoulders. The tongue must be loosened, but in the back, and this is only possible indirectly through exaggerated movements initiated in the front. Furthermore, the pressure must be taken off the larynx so that the folds can release, and this must be done through a combination of lowered volume and pitch range. All of this, hopefully, will have an effect on the inner musculature where the constrictive patterns reside and, secondarily, on breathing patterns as well. Constriction in the throat will inhibit a free and easy inhalation/exhalation cycle, and release of constriction will allow the larynx to rest in a lower, more comfortable position in the throat, facilitating easier and fuller breathing.

If the problem is long-standing, the patterns can be resistant to change and the retraining can take too long to be of practical value, in which case the SVS and the performer may have to accept less constriction overall, rather than the elimination of constriction, as the final outcome of their work together. If the vocal folds are diagnosed as being healthy, this is sufficient.

SUMMARY

Many factors that have an impact on the vocal health of singing actors, dancers, and musicians can be generalized but, in the final analysis, each individual performer must be evaluated uniquely. Each person will have a current vocal health status or diagnosis; a history of training; habits of speech, singing, breathing, and movement; and specific performance needs and demands. All these factors must be incorporated into any retraining or treatment program. The SVS must work as a member of the voice care team of otolaryngologist, speech-language pathologist, and perhaps other professionals, to serve the performer's need to return to healthy singing in a timely and efficient manner.

REFERENCES

1. *Back Stage*, September 29–October 5, 2005, New York, NY: 8, 22.
2. Seashore CE. *Psychology of Music*. New York, NY: McGraw-Hill; 1938.
3. Emmons S, Thomas A. *Power Performance for Singers*. New York, NY: Oxford University Press; 1999:67.
4. Bunch M. *Dynamics of the Singing Voice*. 4th ed. Wien: Springer-Verlag; 1997:14.
5. Perkins WH, Kent RD. *Functional Anatomy of Speech, Language, and Hearing, A Primer*. Boston, Mass: College-Hill Press; 1986:28–32,132–140.
6. Sataloff RT, Carroll L. The singing voice. In Sataloff RT, ed. *Professional Voice: The Science and Art of Clinical Care*. New York, NY: Raven Press; 1991:381.
7. *Oxford Essential Dictionary of Difficult Words*. American ed. New York, NY: Berkley Book, Oxford University Press; 2001:151.
8. Sundberg J. *The Science of the Singing Voice*, Dekalb, Ill: Northern Illinois University Press; 1987.
9. LoVetri J. Contemporary commercial music: more than one way to use the vocal tract. *J Singing*. 2002;58(3):249–252.
10. Banfield S. (1979). Stage and screen entertainers in the twentieth century. In: Potter J, ed. *The Cambridge Companion to Singing*. Cambridge, UK: Cambridge University Press; 1979:65.

Chapter 19

PERFORMANCE ANXIETY: IDENTIFICATION, ASSESSMENT, AND TREATMENT

Philip J. Lanzisera

Performance anxiety is one of the most common experiences involving negative emotions. Indeed, it is ubiquitous in human experience. Most individuals will acknowledge such anxiety, and the most commonly reported "social" fear is public speaking, a form of performance anxiety. Virtually all musicians, instrumental and vocal, experience some degree of performance anxiety.[1,2] For experienced musicians, stressful performance situations may actually enhance musical performance.[3] Performance anxiety, however, can seriously impair the musician. Powell[4] estimates that 2% of the population is susceptible to "debilitating" performance anxiety. In this chapter we describe the nature of performance anxiety including its place in human experience, its physiologic and cognitive components, its phenomenology, the differentiation between normal and clinical varieties, self-management, and formal treatment.

PERFORMANCE ANXIETY AS A HUMAN PROCESS

Anxiety is a process whereby danger is recognized, information is obtained relevant to the perceived danger, and the organism is mobilized to solve the prob-
lems posed by the danger. It is an innate mechanism and can be observed in infants. The brain mechanisms that perceive danger are primitive parts of the brain residing in the brainstem and limbic system. Those brain centers communicate with "higher" cortical areas and produce the more overt cognitive components of the experience. For the most part this system is cue-based, meaning that it is responsive to discrete sensory configurations some of which are innate (eg, fear of snakes) and some of which are acquired by cue-based conditioning. This system can be responsive to linguistic processes when language serves to "transform the function of a stimulus."[5] These conditioning processes do not require conscious awareness to operate. Indeed, most of the processing that occurs in anxiety occurs outside of awareness and, actually, prior to full conscious appraisal of the situation.[6] The extent to which these "outside of awareness" processes influence the conscious appraisal of the situation varies.

As one can imagine, because anxiety serves a realistic protective function, evolution perfected the capacity to detect danger and experience and respond to anxiety. As with most functional capacities, the capacity (or propensity) to experience anxiety is not simply present or absent. Some individuals will experience anxiety much more easily or intensely, and others will experience it much less so.

Part of the evolutionary process is the ability of the brain to be "perfected" after birth. Thus, as with most propensities, early experience will shape it so that it is more responsive to some stimuli than to others, more or less easily soothed, more or less easily generalized, and attached to some symbolic representations and not to others. It is important to realize that this early shaping causes modifications in neuroanatomy both at the synapse and intraneuronally.[7] Different neurobehavioral functions have different "critical periods"[8] during which neurodevelopment is most easily modified by environmental shaping and after which such shaping occurs with great difficulty and only to a lesser extent.

Finally, as is implied by the above, one will experience anxiety only if relevant triggering stimuli are detected in the environment. Thus, the likelihood that a given individual will develop clinically significant performance anxiety is a function of many genetic influences, key early shaping experiences, and how all those things tend to bring the individual into contact with situations in which performance anxiety is relevant.

Although one might wonder whether it would be better to have very low anxiety susceptibility, we should note that without the capacity for anxiety, humans die at younger ages because they take risks that "wiser" individuals avoid, as a result of which they are not available for reproduction. Simply put, we need anxiety to survive. But, we should ask, does performance anxiety fit into this scheme, do we need it for survival?

Indeed we do. Humans, like primates and many other animals, are social creatures. Simply put, without others of our own kind, we have a difficult time surviving. First, we have a very prolonged period of helplessness during which we are fully dependent on our mother's (or mother surrogate's) care for sustenance and protection. Second, we need the group to which we belong to supply secondary protection (from outsiders and other predators) and to provide food (via hunting). We need to remain a member of our group. Virtually all social creatures form hierarchies and individuals have to fit into that hierarchy in some way to keep their places in the group.

Modern humans live in very complex social spaces so that we can rightly say that each of us is a member of several different communities and that those communities may be complementary or competitive with one another. I am, for example, a member of my family of birth together with my parents and siblings, and I have a place in that community. I am also a member of my own nuclear family together with my spouse and our children; I have a place in that community as well. In addition, I am a member of my work community, my professional community, and various other communities. There may be conflicting loyalties and demands, and my place in one community might be far more secure than my place in another community. As long as I perceive my place to be secure, I am not likely to feel much anxiety. As I perceive that place to be less secure, I am likely to feel more anxiety. What will "tell" me that I am or am not secure will vary depending on how my anxiety sensitivity was shaped by my early experience.

Performance anxiety occurs when we feel that our place in the community of musicians, for example, is threatened by the judgment of those for whom we are performing. Performance anxiety requires that we detect that our performance in a specific situation will have a bearing on our place in a community of value and that we determine that there is some chance that we might not perform well enough to keep our place in that community. We do not have to be consciously aware of either of these components. Indeed, we can feel anxious when we consciously believe that we are quite capable of performing well and will do so. Our conscious beliefs are often not our only beliefs and often not the beliefs most fully activated in a situation.

Performance anxiety tends to occur in individuals who have high expectations and demands for themselves[4] and occurs when the individual believes he or she will not live up to those expectations or those of the audience and will be negatively evaluated by self and others.[9,10] If the individual believes he or she "must" perform well but cannot and will suffer some terrible social loss because of failure, the situation will be very threatening. Anxiety is the natural response in such a situation and alerts the individual to take appropriate action. That one is likely to gain confidence in one's ability to meet expectations with experience is the most likely explanation for the fact that more experienced musicians tend to feel less anxiety than less experienced musicians.[2]

Performance anxiety has cognitive, somatic, and behavioral components. These components feed back on one another in such a way as to create a positive feedback system helping to create more and more anxiety. It may lead to "split attention," which has been demonstrated to lead to impaired performance, particularly in individuals who are just learning complex skills.[11] This may be because the novice needs to be able to direct attention to the mechanics of performance. If the more experienced performer attempts to cope with anxiety by focusing on the mechanics of musical performance, the problem could be seriously compounded. The experienced performer relies on having automated certain musical skills. "Choking" in experienced individuals appears to be related to excessive self-monitoring and self-coaching during performance.[11,12] This is particularly true for highly practiced sensorimotor skills such as musical performance.

THE PHENOMENOLOGY OF PERFORMANCE ANXIETY

Most commonly, individuals begin to experience anxiety prior to beginning a performance. For some the first recognized experience is somatic but for others it may be a thought. There is almost always some kind of thought that helps to trigger the anxiety. This is because as soon as the performer gets ready to perform, he or she begins to think about what the performance is going to be about, how prepared he or she is, and how the performance is likely to go. In addition, the performer thinks about the audience and about what the audience is likely to think of the performer. To the extent that the performer thinks the audience will be critical, anxiety is more likely to occur. If there is a formal critic in the audience, the performer is more likely to feel anxious,[13] and as the size of the audience increases the likelihood of anxiety increases. The performer may flitter back and forth between thoughts about the audience and thoughts about his or her own capacity to perform up to perceived expectations. If there is a discrepancy, and often performers have a more negative view of their capacity to perform than does the audience,[14] that discrepancy gives rise to the perception of danger and risk, which initiates the somatic responses. Some thoughts may be "hot thoughts," thoughts that have a powerful emotional significance to the person and which are not easily questioned. It is as if the danger the thought points to is so important that it has to be taken seriously.

Remember, the anxiety system is designed to overpredict danger not "miss" it.

The somatic components are those of which the performer is usually most aware. These include increased heart rate, altered breathing, nervousness, sweating, jitteriness, muscle tension or spasm, and gastrointestinal sensations including nausea. Not everyone will experience each of these symptoms, but most will experiences several of them. These experiences may be mild in some cases but may be overwhelming and incapacitating in others, and individuals tend to experience their anxiety symptoms in a sequence that is characteristic for them.

There are a number of behavioral consequences of this process. For the vocal artist of great concern are the effects on tone and on the smoothness in the respiratory and vocal apparatus. As the performer becomes aware of the sense of tightness in these areas, the sense of danger can be intensified by negative thoughts such as "I must sound terrible." In addition, increased arousal can interfere with working memory,[15] which can result in forgetting a line or losing place in the score. Such a lapse will further increase anxiety.

Wilson[16] in his discussion of performance anxiety compares the commonly held belief that performance increases as arousal increases from zero to some specific point after which performance deteriorates gradually (the well-known inverted-U function) with a competing notion that at some point the combination of physical arousal and worry becomes catastrophic after which performance precipitously decreases. Anxiety is, at its heart, an arousal mechanism. Although it can facilitate appropriate arousal, communicate importance to the performer, and energize the performance, combined with worry it can be disastrous.

As anxiety (or physical arousal) increases one becomes more aware of one's surroundings and of one's own internal physical experiences. This can help to make our behavior more accurate and in tune with the demands of the external world. Individuals prone to social anxiety tend to shift their attention toward internal cues as sources of information about threat far more than to the demands of the external environment.[17] This results in an excessive focus on internal cues. This can lead to impairment of attention and concentration leading to errors. Motor functions can become impaired by tremor or spasm. Working memory can become impaired[15] leading to difficulty unless the material is learned to the point of automatic functioning. Together these result in decreased performance. As anxiety increases further, the anxiety itself becomes traumatic. The anxiety takes over more and more of the individual's focus of attention and becomes all the individual sees. Even if the performance is "adequate," the level of anxiety might be so high that the individual cannot recognize the information value of the "adequate" performance but only experience the trauma of the anxiety.

A lapse or excessive focus on anticipated negative evaluation can lead to a catastrophic response during which the individual feels that the world is caving in and the somatic symptoms increase in intensity. The performance may quickly deteriorate at this point. The deterioration of the performance confirms all the negative thoughts that the performer had about his or her capacity and sets up expectations for what will happen in future performance situations. Such a situation can be traumatic to the performer and lead to avoidance of performing. The performer dwells on the experience of failure, and the recollections may become even more dramatic and devastating than the original experience. Furthermore, avoidance tends to intensify anxiety rather than decrease it. Thus, the problem can worsen even though the individual successfully avoids having even a second failure experience.

NORMAL VERSUS CLINICALLY SIGNIFICANT PERFORMANCE ANXIETY

The above is a description of the worst kind of outcome, terror and fright during a performance that leads to severe withdrawal from performance. This is not, of course, the most common outcome. Almost everyone experiences performance anxiety, usually much more mildly than the terror described above. It is important to review, then, the difference between "normal" and "clinically significant" performance anxiety.

As with most psychological problems, the boundary line is not always clear. The single most important point of distinction is the degree of functional impairment. "Normal" range anxiety tends to be self-correcting or mild in terms of its impact on a person's functioning. Typical social support or "self-help" is sufficient to

correct the problem. We should go just a bit further, however, and assert that some degree of "normal" performance anxiety is critical to good performance.

The mere presence of anxiety in performance situations, however, does not warrant a formal diagnosis. Performance anxiety should be considered normal and even helpful when it is at lower levels. It helps to heighten awareness and motivate behavior. It might even help the individual "feel" the audience and enliven the performance. When, however, it either impairs the actual performance or causes so much distress that performing hardly becomes enjoyable, we should consider the problem to be a diagnosable disorder. The formal diagnosis is that of social anxiety and requires that physical symptoms of anxiety occur when the individual is exposed to a feared social situation (the performance), the individual recognizes that the anxiety is unrealistic, the situation is either avoided or endured with intense anxiety, and the anxiety interferes significantly with functioning or leads to preoccupation with having the anxiety.[18] (The anxiety must not be due to drug use or other medical conditions.) So, if the individual avoids performance situations, "freezes" at times, or becomes so distressed before or after a performance that other aspects of life are interfered with, a formal diagnosis is warranted.

SELF-MANAGEMENT OF PERFORMANCE ANXIETY

There is a wealth of self-help material for anxiety problems, and the interested individual should look through them in a local bookstore to find one that is appealing. It is probably more important that the book seem to fit the individual's style of thinking and solving problems than describe any specific techniques to a psychologist's satisfaction. That having been said, we can look at some general principles and specific techniques of self-help applied to social anxiety. The professional interventions are built upon the same basic approaches. Figure 19–1 depicts the key processes and decisions involved in both self-management and professional management of performance anxiety.

Prior to discussing the more "psychological" approaches to self-management, it is critical that we

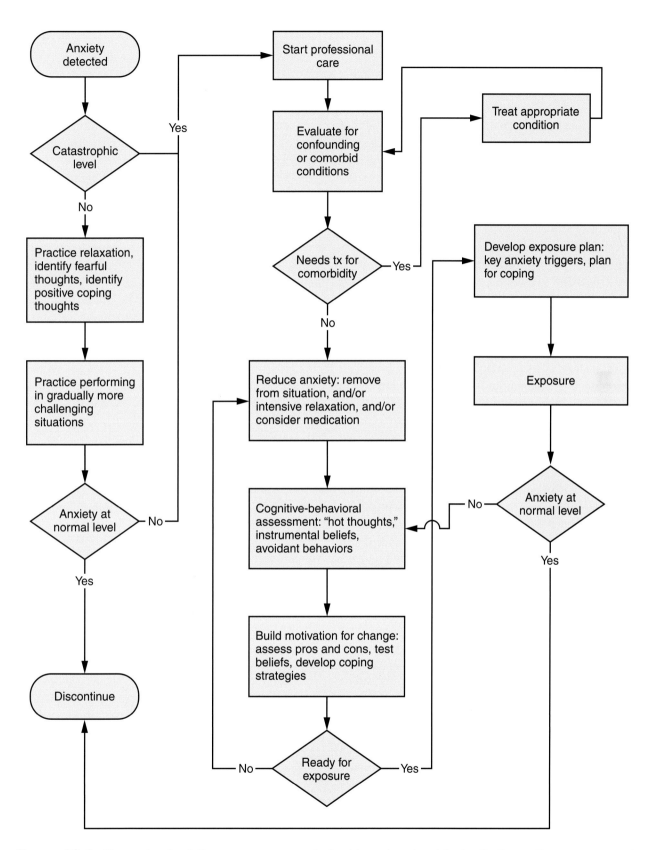

Figure 19-1. Flow chart of the processes and decisions involved in both the self-management (*left-hand side*) and professional treatment (*middle and right-hand side*) of performance anxiety.

discuss the role of preparation. It is unrealistic to think that one will perform adequately if one is not prepared. Not only is the performer's level of experience (and, hence, overall preparation) relevant to the degree of anxiety experienced, but also performers report that worry about their level of preparation is a typical anxiety thought.[2] When possible, practice a piece to the point that its performance is automatic. This reduces the likelihood that divided attention will impair the performance. If one is in a situation in which a performance is required for which one is not adequately prepared (hopefully, for reasons beyond one's control), one has to be realistic about evaluating one's own performance. At the very least the performer should set his or her sights on a level of performance that is realistic for the situation.

Most self-help and formal treatment approaches for performance anxiety are based on a cognitive behavioral approach to treatment, and the foregoing discussion was based on a cognitive-behavioral understanding of anxiety. Relaxation training, stress inoculation training, mindfulness and acceptance, and exposure and rehearsal are the primary components.

Relaxation training involves learning how to relax in the face of stress and how to control or moderate anxiety symptoms or the intensity of those symptoms. We use these methods not to end the anxiety symptoms but to help an individual manage the symptoms. They are not designed to eliminate anxiety but to make working with it easier. There are several approaches to relaxation training. The two basic components are breathing control and muscle relaxation.

Anxiety often leads to a shortening and quickening of the breath. This is, obviously, not good for a singer. The experience of such breathing changes can trigger a precipitous increase in anxiety as the singer has thoughts such as "I won't get through that passage." It is of great advantage for the signer to learn to slow the breath and deepen it. (As with everything else discussed in this section, it is very important that the individual practice this frequently when not under stress so that this practice can make this something the individual can do even under stress.) Count from one to five over a period of 5 seconds all the while breathing in. Be sure that the lungs are completely full at the end of the count. Then begin to breathe out over the same length of time, counting to five, and be sure that the lungs are empty at the end of the count. As you are breathing out, be aware of how letting the breath out is relaxing. You can picture all the tension in your body going with that breath. Repeat that in-and-out sequence 12 times (or for 2 minutes). By the end of that sequence, most individuals report feeling far more relaxed and calm physically. Deen[19] found that a similar exercise designed to integrate relaxed breathing and awareness of relaxation during that breathing had a significant effect on performance anxiety among vocal performers.

Muscle tension may develop anywhere in the body, but tension in the vocal apparatus, neck, and shoulders may be of particular concern to the vocal performer. For many individuals, using the above breathing exercise is enough to facilitate relaxation of these muscles, particularly if some focus is placed on them and allowing them to relax passively during the breathing exercise. If, however, the muscles are very tense, progressive muscle relaxation[20] may be more effective at helping individuals reverse this tension and produce deep states of relaxation. Often we begin with a few minutes of relaxed breathing as above, and then proceed through the muscles of the body in a systematic way. Start with one arm and hand, then the other, then the legs, trunk, shoulders, neck, tongue, jaw, and face. In each case tense those muscles briefly, hold the tension long enough to be aware of it, and then release those muscles suddenly, fully and completely. Let each of those muscles relax further for a minimum of 30 seconds and for up to 2 minutes being aware of the relaxation that is deepening in the muscles. Repeat the same muscle group a second time before moving on to the next group. Note that we save those muscles of greatest concern to the musician for last. These muscles are often those that tense earliest in anxiety and that are hardest to relax. Relaxing other, easier muscles makes relaxing these less difficult. After going through all the sets of muscles, return to relaxed breathing for a while longer. Be sure to do this slowly, taking sufficient time with each muscle group to allow it to relax deeply.

Once one has learned these breathing and muscle relaxation techniques well, one can usually find ways of abbreviating them. Sometimes one or two quiet, deep breaths together with picturing all the muscles relaxing is sufficient to reduce tension and bring about a greater sense of relaxation. Incorporating some image such as picturing the muscles to be rubber bands that are unwinding may be helpful, or thinking of how a dog lies in the sun breathing quietly may be very helpful in inducing relaxed feelings. Doing this before a rehearsal, practice, or performance can help make it a regular part of one's routine, making it more likely that one will be at least physically relaxed prior to performance.

Self-administered stress inoculation involves identifying thoughts that are involved in the anxiety response, learning to test those thoughts, and developing alternative thoughts. The first step is for the individual to observe him- or herself in the performance situation to identify the thoughts that tend to occur. Write them down as quickly as possible after the performance situations. After a few occasions, one can then find which ones occur most frequently and which ones seem to be the most powerful triggers. One can use a "Thought Record" to help in this process. Once you have identified some key thoughts, ask yourself what there is about that thought or idea that is so threatening or what really could go wrong. Ask what the worst possible outcome could be.

Then ask yourself how likely it is that each of these things could really happen or how realistic the thought is. Suppose the thought is, "the audience will think I'm terrible." Maybe the worst possible outcome is that the critics will say such terrible things about you that you will be banished from the stage forever and become penniless and homeless. Then ask yourself two key questions: is there any evidence that the audience would really have such thoughts, and how likely is it that the worst-case outcome would come true. In addition, one should ask how useful that thought is to promoting a good performance. Usually this helps foster more realistic thinking. Then, develop realistic but helpful coping thoughts. For example, in response to the thought "the audience will think I'm terrible," a more appropriate thought might be, "I'm likely to do well and the audience will likely see that, but even an error or two won't make them think I'm terrible." You might have the idea that you will "choke" and make a fool of yourself. It would be more realistic to think, "I might make an error or two but am not likely to "choke," and I have had many good performances." You might add that a good enough performance is much more likely than a horrible one. Review all the times you have coped well with the pressures of performance.

Finally, if possible reframe the situation from one of danger and threat to one of possible opportunity and challenge. Skinner and Brewer[9] found that individuals who focus on a situation as a challenge rather than a threat experience much less anxiety in a performance situation. For example, work on thinking of the performance situation as an opportunity to feel more and more comfortable with an audience and one's own capacities. Again, be realistic.

Write down a very brief summary of what you have learned. Include the thoughts you developed to reframe the situation or counter the "hot" thoughts that you tend to have. That summary should fit on a small index card you can keep with you or put in your musical score. Just before a performance, go through your relaxation routine and, while relaxed, review your "coping card" to set your mind on helpful and adaptive thoughts.

Note that the thoughts developed to counter the anxiety thoughts are not "pie in the sky" hopefulness. You are not counting on winning the lottery. You are being realistic. You are anticipating some errors (as that is very common in musical performance). You are also recognizing that the consequences will not be dire and that they are of such a sort that you can live with them. It does no good to tell yourself things you cannot really believe.

You can help the process of cognitive restructuring along if you remember that identical situations can be viewed differently by different people or by the same person at different times. Individuals who see performance situations as challenges or opportunities rather than threats feel more comfortable in the situation.[2,9] One can reframe a threat into a challenge or opportunity by the way one phrases the situation to oneself.

Mindfulness or acceptance[21] is a key component in anxiety management. We often develop true fears of our emotions and attempt to avoid experiencing them,[22] and we sometimes think of the anxiety as the danger rather than merely serving to suggest there could be a danger present. As much as one might want to order anxiety away, one cannot do that; we have to accept the fact that it will be there. Mindfulness involves letting oneself experience a feeling in detail while not getting "caught up" in that emotion. It is a skill that has to be developed over time by practice. Start by observing mild emotions and "seeing yourself" having them. Notice how they affect you and how you can still act and function despite them. As you build this ability, you will develop a greater ability to accept the anxiety. This is important because were you to insist that you not feel anxiety before or during a performance, you would almost never perform, and you would likely feel even more distress when the anxiety refused to submit fully to your efforts at control. One has to be willing to feel anxiety. The more willing you are to feel the anxiety, the less distressing the anxiety becomes. The less willing you are to feel the anxiety, the more distressing it becomes (you become anxious about being anxious). Remember you can feel anxiety and still perform. Recall how many great musicians have had very intense performance anxiety. They have had to be willing to experience the anxiety and perform anyway.

The above strategies are all preparatory for the "real" component of self-management, exposure. The functioning of the brain structures that produce anxiety can only be changed by experience. That experience occurs during exposure when you discover that you can be successful and that disaster does not occur. It is very important that the level of anxiety that one feels not be so great that it becomes traumatic. Except when under professional care, it is best to engage in exposure gradually. Fortunately, music teachers often help students do this naturally. Children first perform in front of their loving parents, then in front of peers, and then perform small recitals before performing larger ones. In this way they move from a supportive and encouraging environment in which performing is an opportunity to receive praise to situations in which performing could be met with higher expectations and some degree of critical appraisal. Thus, when the individual has little experience and could justifiably worry about being adequate, the situation will evoke, instead, thoughts of reassurance and support from the audience. As training goes along and the individual has reason to anticipate more and more "adequate" performances, that individual will find it easier to deal with an audience that is more critical.

One can engage in a partial form of exposure without any risk at all. One can imagine the scene of the performance in great detail and even imaging making an error. One can picture oneself recovering from the error. One can picture the audience's response and even a less than ideal response. One can practice quieting oneself during the performance. It is very important to make what one imagines as real as possible. Rather than making it "just a daydream" in which one is performing wonderfully to the audience's intense rapture with your music-making, imagine being anxious. Over time intensify the image. Feel the butterflies in the stomach; feel the tightness in the chest; think of the heart rate going up; think of the audience having paid for a great performance Then, use all the techniques discussed above to deal with those images and experiences. This becomes practice in managing anxiety in a real situation.

All this work in imagination is a preparation for "real" exposure. Perform first in situations that are relatively low in threat or challenge and build to those that are more threatening or challenging. You should feel "comfortable enough" and able to perform adequately at a lower level of threat before going on to a higher level of threat. Performance anxiety has been found to increase as size of the audience increases and when the audience contains critics.[23] One should build the "threat or challenge" into one's exposure with this in mind.

PROFESSIONAL TREATMENT OF PERFORMANCE ANXIETY

One should seek professional treatment if the above self-management approaches are not successful in reducing performance anxiety or if the level of anxiety is "catastrophic" and one's ability to perform is seriously threatened. Even though most common professional treatment approaches will be quite similar to the above, the professional will be able to catch some parts in the anxiety response that the one experiencing the anxiety will not catch and will have tools available to help identify hidden thoughts and fears. Most clinicians will use a cognitive-behavioral approach such as that outlined by Rodebaugh and Chambless.[24]

Evaluation

First, the clinician will perform a thorough evaluation of the individual with performance anxiety with a view toward the presence of confounding and comorbid conditions. Powell,[4] summarizing the literature in the area, concludes that about one-third of individuals with performance anxiety will have some other psychiatric disorder. It is not uncommon for someone with performance anxiety to have generalized anxiety disorder (GAD),[19] which is a debilitating, chronic, and intrusive worry about all sorts of common problems. Social anxiety disorder is also frequent. Depression may be less frequent, but it must be recalled that persistent difficulty doing one's job (making music) can generate a strong feeling of failure and serve to precipitate a depressive episode. Still, Powell reminds us that two-thirds of those with performance anxiety do not have other psychological conditions.

The clinician must also look for substance use problems. Not only are substance use problems fairly common among the general population, but also it is fairly common for individuals to treat their own anxiety with a variety of substances both pharmacological and recreational. Unfortunately such self-medication seldom works and can often lead to other problems because individuals, erroneously thinking that it is merely that they are not using enough medication, tend to increase their use of self-medications when they don't work.

The clinician should also recall that there is a significant difference between performance anxiety and many other forms of social anxiety disorder. In performance anxiety, there is often a much greater emphasis on negative self-appraisal. In most forms of social anxiety, the emphasis is almost totally on a negative appraisal coming from others. The clinician should carefully explore the performer's self-expectations and the presence of perfectionistic demands. Finally the role of the demands placed on the performer by family and teachers must be considered. How the performer views these demands and what the performer sees as the consequences of failing to live up to those expectations may be of great importance in the creation or maintenance of the anxiety. It is even possible, although not common, that the anxiety serves to solve some interpersonal conflict for the individual. The anxiety, then, would be reinforced by the reduction in anxiety the individual feels by virtue of avoiding the conflict. This form of reinforcement is called "negative reinforcement" and is the strongest type of reinforcement, and the resultant learning is hardest to extinguish.

Cognitive-Behavioral Therapy

Very commonly, the clinician will use some form of "stress inoculation" training as a part of the treatment. Stress inoculation training consists of identifying likely stressful situations, what the individual sees as "the problem" in the situation, and then developing specific ways of coping with those problems. The clinician will help the individual to identify specific actions or self-statements that can be used at various points in the situation that the person finds stressful. For example, the clinician will help the individual develop a strategy for self-soothing or refocusing on one's abilities and past successes. Through this, the individual gains confidence that he or she will be able to manage the stressful situation. Of course, it is the real-life management of the stressful situation that "stamps in" the newfound confidence. In a meta-analysis of 37 studies, Saunders[25] found stress inoculation training to be quite effective at reducing anxiety and enhancing performance under stress. Even though just one session of stress inoculation training can be helpful, one should expect treatment to last a minimum of six to seven sessions. It is probably realistic to think that individuals who have tried the self-management techniques above and have not been able to manage their own anxiety will require even more sessions as there are likely to be many hidden obstacles or cognitions that will take time to find and confront.

Confronting one's anxiety is difficult. Often the clinician has to work with the performer to help the latter develop the will and desire to confront the anxiety. The clinician will assess the performer's readiness to start each stage of the treatment and will reassess that readiness and the individual's response to the interventions attempted. It may be necessary to "cycle back" to an earlier stage in the treatment when an obstacle is met or a new "hot thought" discovered during the process of exposure.

The individual will be asked to engage in "homework" between sessions. Because in all psychological treatments it is the "patient" not the "therapist" who does the changing,[26] this homework becomes critical to the change process. Much of what constitutes professional treatment is helping the individual identify the internal obstacles to change and organizing him or herself toward changing those obstacles. The individual has to work on those changes between sessions for the treatment to be efficient and effective.

Because the individuals who present to a professional, as distinguished from those who manage their own anxiety successfully, will present a number of challenges to the clinician, it is important that the approach be flexible and incorporate strategies most likely to affect that individual's particular combination of difficulties.[27] The clinician should draw from cognitive, behavioral, interpersonal, and psychodynamic approaches.

Exposure is the basic tool in treating almost any anxiety disorder. Most commonly one starts with identifying situations that tend to be anxiety provoking and then ordering them in ascending order of intensity of anxiety. Then the key features of those situations are determined and the list refined further taking those key features into consideration. Once the list is complete, the clinician leads the individual up the list starting with situations that provoke very little anxiety. Once such "easy" situations no longer trigger any appreciable anxiety, the clinician invites the individual to move up the list. This is done progressively so that the individual never has to experience more anxiety than can be managed. Very commonly this is combined with careful relaxation training so that the experience of relaxation can be "paired" with the cues that have triggered anxiety in the past. This sets up a new conditioned (learned) experience that is incompatible with the previous anxiety.

This process has to be highly flexible and the clinician will most commonly go back and forth between exposure and a cognitive-behavioral analysis of the problem. At each point in exposure, the clinician will test the effectiveness of the exposure and, implicitly at least, the prior cognitive-behavioral analysis. The clinician will not assume that a reduction in anxiety is due to having challenged the cognition previously identified as relevant but will be open to the possibility that a different cognition was operative in this instance. Failure of a particular intervention is as much data for the assessment as is the earlier assessment, and such failures are a routine part of the treatment of even moderately complex cases.

At times psychodynamic approaches might be useful in managing performance anxiety, particularly when the individual has strong tendencies toward feeling shame and inadequacy or when the anxiety "solves" an interpersonal conflict. Psychodynamic approaches examine how various thoughts and behaviors serve to protect one from anxiety or other emotions about which one has felt conflicted. There is always a personal story behind these types of fears and conflicts. For example, if one has been shamed in the past for proud or boastful behaviors, one can develop a fear of performance because it is (sometimes literally) blowing one's own horn. The clinician helps the individual to recognize those fears and confront them mentally before encouraging behavioral exposure. McCullough[28] describes the use of a behaviorally enlightened psychodynamic therapy for performance anxiety. This will involve careful identification of the nature of the guilt or shame together with an exploration of the "narrative" behind that experience. This facilitates a more appropriate appraisal of the situation and greater tolerance of the affect.

Pharmacotherapy

A number of medications have been used to manage anxiety disorders. In general, and with some exceptions, the research data do not demonstrate any superiority for medications over psychological treatments in the management of anxiety and no real advantage to combining them except in the most severe cases. Furthermore, individuals who are treated with medications are very likely to need to use them for a very long time and may not be able to discontinue them without difficulty. There is an old saw in medicine, "what gets you well keeps you well." Long-term maintenance on medications for anxiety is more and more common. Because they have no major advantage over behavioral therapy as monotherapy, their use should likely be limited to more severe situations in which the individual is on the verge of making damaging choices to quit performing or needs some initial help in starting the process of behavioral treatment.

Most commonly today, SSRIs (selective serotonin reuptake inhibitors) are used to manage anxiety disorders in general clinical practice. These drugs, which include such household words as Prozac (fluoxetine) and Zoloft (sertraline), are used to treat anxiety and depression and can be quite effective in doing so.

They must be used consistently and are useless on an "as-needed" basis. Because they can not be used on an as-needed basis and have some significant side effects, they should probably be reserved for use when the individual with performance anxiety has other comorbid conditions for which they would be appropriate.

There is one class of drugs that should clearly be avoided for performance anxiety, the benzodiazepines. These include Xanax (alprazolam), Valium (diazepam), Klonopin (clonazepam), and a number of other compounds. These drugs are central nervous system depressants and can impair cognitive and motor functioning.[29] In addition, these drugs interfere with exposure.[30] This may result from one or more of several processes including the tendency of these drugs to interfere with short-term memory and their function as cues which signal safety in the exposure situation preventing the individual from learning that the situation is not dangerous. Finally, benzodiazepines may lead to a bias toward perceiving internal cues of anxiety.[31] This, as noted above, can lead to an increase in anxiety experience and interfere with performance.

Many performers rely on beta-blockers on an as-needed basis. These drugs are commonly used for hypertension and cardiac arrhythmias. One of their effects is to slow cardiac acceleration. The individual does not feel as much of a rise in heart rate and is, supposedly, less likely to respond to that experience as a signal of impending anxiety. Turner and colleagues[32] found that there was no difference between atenolol (a beta-blocker) and placebo in reducing social anxiety in a performance situation. There is little doubt that knowing they are "in the system" might give the performer some confidence, but it is most likely more a placebo effect than a pharmacologic effect. If the individual comes to believe that having such a drug on board is critical to controlling anxiety, the lack of it, for whatever reason, may actually intensify anxiety.

In all, then, unless there are significant comorbid conditions that would justify the use of one of these medications or the anxiety has gotten so highly disruptive and traumatic that some immediate, short-term pharmacological reduction in anxiety is needed to enable the individual to start the process of behavioral treatment, behavioral treatments should be the sole treatment modality for performance anxiety.

SUMMARY

Performance anxiety is a near-universal problem for vocal musicians. For most it does not cause disability but it can interfere with one's functioning and make music-making far less enjoyable than it should be. One's own demands for excellence and an intolerance for imperfection can predispose an individual to develop more problematic performance anxiety. Performance anxiety can most often be managed on one's own with the use of cognitive and behavioral techniques. If one cannot manage it on one's own, clinicians will most commonly use similar cognitive-behavioral techniques and will add strategies for identifying covert thoughts and beliefs that block change and will build motivation and tolerance for exposure. While medication is not usually indicated and often contraindicated, it is occasionally useful for the most acutely impaired. Above all, it is important to know that the pressure a performer experiences that can lead to performance anxiety is also a motivator to move toward excellence and can energize the performer and the performance. In this way, what might otherwise be experienced as anxiety could be experienced as the thrill of performance.

REFERENCES

1. Kaspersen M, Gotestam K. A survey of music performance anxiety among Norwegian music students. *Eur J Psychiatry.* 2002;16:69–98.

2. Tamborrino R. *An examination of performance anxiety associated with solo performance of college-level music majors* [dissertation]. Bloomington, Ind: Indiana University; 2001.

3. Hamman DL. An assessment of anxiety in instrumental and vocal performances. *J Res Music Ed.* 1982;30:77–91.

4. Powell DH. Treating individuals with debilitating performance anxiety: an introduction. *J Consult Clin Psychol.* 2004;60: 801–808.

5. Hayes SC, Barnes-Holmes D, Roche B. *Relational Frame Theory: A Post-Skinnerian Account of Human Language and Cognition.* New York, NY: Kluwer Academic/Plenum Publishers; 2001.

6. Yiend J, ed. *Cognition, Emotion, and Psychopathology: Theoretical, Empirical, and Clinical*

Directions. Cambridge: Cambridge University Press; 2004.

7. LeDoux J. *The Emotional Brain: The Mysterious Underpinnings of Emotional Life.* New York, NY: Touchstone; 1996.

8. LeDoux J. *Synaptic Self: How Our Brains Become Who We Are.* Harmondsworth, UK: Penguin Books; 2003.

9. Skinner N, Brewer N. The dynamics of threat and challenge appraisals prior to stressful achievement events. *J Pers Soc Psychol.* 2002;83:678-692.

10. Tobacyk JJ, Downs A. personal construct threat and irrational beliefs as cognitive predictors of increases in musical performance anxiety. *J Pers Soc Psychol.* 1998;51:779-782.

11. Beilock SL, Carr TH. On the fragility of skilled performance: what governs choking under pressure? *J Exp Psychol:Gen.* 2001l;130:701-725.

12. Beilock SL, Kulp CA, Holt LE, Carr TH. More on the fragility of performance: choking under pressure in mathematical problem solving. *J Exp Psychol: Gen.* 2004;133:584-600.

13. Maroon MT. *Potential Contributors to Performance Anxiety Among Middle School Students Performing at Solo and Ensemble Contest* [dissertation].

14. Rapee RM, Lim L. Discrepancy between self- and observer ratings of performance in social phobics. *J Abn Psychol.* 1992;101:728-731.

15. Ashcraft MH, Kirk EP. The relationships among working memory, math anxiety, and performance. *J Exp Psychol:Gen.* 2001;130:224-237.

16. Wilson GD. *Psychology for Performing Artists.* London: Whurr Publishers; 2002.

17. Pineles SL, Mineka S. Attentional biases to internal and external sources of potential threat in social anxiety. *J Abn Psychol.* 2005;114:314-318.

18. American Psychiatric Association. *Diagnostic and Statistical Manual.* 4th ed. Washington, DC: Author; 1994.

19. Deen DR. *Awareness and Breathing: Keys to the Moderation of Musical Performance Anxiety* [dissertation]. Lexington, Ky: University of Kentucky; 1999.

20. Bourne EJ. *The Anxiety and Phobia Workbook.* 3rd ed. Oakland, Calif: New Harbinger Publications; 2000.

21. Hayes SC, Strosahl KD, Wilson KG. *Acceptance and Commitment Therapy: An Experiential Approach to Behavior Change.* New York, NY: Guilford; 1999.

22. McCullough L. *Changing Character: Short-Term Anxiety Regulating Psychotherapy for Restructuring Defenses.* New York, NY: Basic Books; 1997.

23. LeBlanc A, Jin YC, Obert M, Siivola C. Effect of audience on music performance anxiety. *J Res Music Ed.* 1997;45:480-496.

24. Rodebaugh TL, Chambless DL. Cognitive therapy for performance anxiety. *J Consult Clin Psychol.* 2004;60:809-820.

25. Saunders T, Driskell JE, Johnston JH, Salas E. The effect of stress inoculation training on anxiety and performance. *J Occup Health Psychol.* 1996;1: 170-186.

26. Tallman K, Bohart AC. The client as a common factor: clients as self-healers. In Hubble MA, Duncan BL, Miller SD, eds. *The Heart and Sole of Change: What Works in Therapy.* Washington, DC: American Psychological Association; 1999.

27. Lazarus AA, Abramovitz A. A multimodal behavioral approach to performance anxiety. *J Consult Clin Psychol.* 2004;60:831-840.

28. McCullough L, Osborn KAR. Short term dynamic psychotherapy goes to Hollywood: the treatment of performance anxiety in cinema. *J Consult Clin Psychol.* 2004;60:841-852.

29. Streufert S, Satish U, Pogash R, et al.. Effects of alprazolam on complex human functioning. *J Applied Soc Psychol.* 1996;26:1912-1920.

30. Birk L. Pharmacotherapy for performance anxiety disorders: occasionally useful but typically contraindicated. *J Consult Clin Psychol.* 2004;60:867-879.

31. Steward SH, Westra HA, Thompson CE, Conrad BE. Effects of naturalistic benzodiazepine use on selective attention to threat cues among anxiety disorder patients. *Cog Therapy Res.* 2000;24:67-85.

32. Turner SM, Beidel DC, Jacob RG. Social phobia: a comparison of behavioral therapy and atenolol. *J Consult Clin Psychol.* 1994;62:350-358.

Part V

When Is Surgical Treatment Necessary?

Chapter 20

SURGICAL ANATOMY, PLANNING, AND CONSENT

Michael S. Benninger

SURGERY IN THE SINGER

It is not by chance that the section on surgical therapy in the singer is the last treatment section in this book. Fortunately, surgery is only rarely needed to manage a voice problem in a singer. Most voice disorders in singers can be improved or completely resolved through appropriate assessment, diagnosis, and non-surgical treatments. These may include lifestyle changes, modification of voice use, speech therapy from a voice pathologist, or ongoing voice instruction from a singing voice teacher.[1]

There are times, however, when surgery is the preferred treatment option. This chapter discusses decision-making processes to identify those singers who should consider surgery, the preoperative evaluation, surgical planning, the critical surgical anatomy, and the informed-consent process and documentation.

IDENTIFYING THE PATIENT WHO IS A SURGICAL CANDIDATE

There are numerous singers who present with findings that theoretically could be amenable to surgery. In principle, most mass lesions can be removed with sur-

gery, yet few truly require it. So, how do you determine which patient should be considered for surgical treatment? This question is not easily answered. There are as many variables that need to be considered as there are voice-disordered patients. Those variables include the singer, the environment, the time needed for recovery, and the comfort levels of the singer and the surgeon. Needless to say, the determination of surgical candidacy requires a caring, thoughtful, and empathetic approach. Singers must understand that surgical treatment is only one step in the rehabilitation of a vocal injury. Once determined, candidacy does not mean that surgery will result, as candidacy is only the initial step in the ultimate decision to perform surgery.

The evaluation techniques that have been discussed in the preceding chapters are particularly important in an individual who is being considered for surgery. A thorough history and physical examination should be bolstered by appropriate objective tests and subjective observations to make the diagnosis and to confirm the degree of voice dysfunction. Videostroboscopy is particularly useful in assessing the impact on vocal fold vibratory characteristics, as well as giving an impression of firmness and chronicity.[2] The VHI, as described in chapter 7, is very useful in helping to determine the impact of the lesion on overall life quality. A person who has notable dysphonia but is still able to perform within defined expectations and scores well on the VHI may not be a good surgical candidate even if he or she has a chronic lesion that is poorly responsive to conservative treatments.

All pertinent evaluations should be performed at the initial visit and then again following behavior modifications, voice therapy, and singing instruction. It is imperative to assess whether or not further nonsurgical therapy may be of value. It is also important to understand the degree of the singer's compliance with these treatments, as poor compliance prior to surgery will usually mean poor compliance after, with the potential for less than optimal results. It is my opinion that it is better to err on too long a period of time for conservative treatment before surgery than too short. I have been surprised more than once that a patient who had gone through a long period of conservative treatment with suboptimal results eventually had positive results later.

A failure of conservative treatment does not alone determine which singers are surgical candidates. A singer with nodules and chronic dysphonia secondary to vocal nodules who is still able to perform (even if suboptimally), and who is not able to change performance schedules, may not have significant improvement until the schedule can be changed. A singer with reflux and persistent hoarseness will not benefit from laryngeal surgery for Reinke's edema, but after failing aggressive reflux treatment might benefit from surgical fundoplication. By maintaining open communication among voice team members and the patient, a clear and conservative treatment plan is shared by all and open to change when appropriate.

The primary indications for laryngeal surgery in singers are mass lesions on the vocal folds. Although there has been considerable debate and a lack of consensus regarding nomenclature for vocal fold mass lesions, some constant descriptive terms are helpful in describing the lesions and allowing for a general understanding of what the pathology is among health care providers. These descriptive terms may vary somewhat between centers so it is important for the members of each vocal care team to have consistency within their group. It should also be noted that the tentative diagnosis used to describe the preoperative lesion may be altered at the time of surgery when the surgeon has been able to carefully palpate, assess, and examine the lesion directly. I try not to give my definitive impression to the patients preoperatively, as there

have been a number of times where my diagnosis changed in the operating room.

That all being said, I prefer to classify lesions based on the location on the vocal fold, the likely histopathology, the effect on vibration seen during videostroboscopy, whether or not the lesion is unilateral or bilateral, and a general impression of firmness or chronicity. Although this is a clear simplification, bilateral and nearly symmetric lesions in the mid to anterior one-third of the vocal folds are often vocal nodules in women.[3] Similar appearing lesions in men are typically not nodules. Most otolaryngologists and voice pathologists have seen lesions that have been defined as "nodules" but did not respond appropriately to voice therapy; and the results after surgery revealed a cyst with a contact nodule on the opposite vocal fold (Figures 20-1A and 1B). "Vocal nodules" that have responded little or not at all to voice therapy and vocal hygiene are of particular concern. Not only is it possible that one or both masses is a cyst but there also may be a sulcus vocalis. Videostroboscopy has been found to be useful in clarifying the nature of some of these lesions.[2]

On occasion, it is difficult to identify whether or not a unilateral lesion should be classified as a cyst or a polyp. In some cases this distinction may be relatively simple (Figure 20-2), while in others it may be quite difficult. It is also often difficult to determine the difference between chronic nodules and more insidious lesions such as sulcus vocalis (Figure 20-3). It is critically important to inform patients that a suspected diagnosis made preoperatively may be changed once the lesion is better evaluated in the operating room. It is also important to inform patients that the magnitude of the procedure may need to be changed in the operating room, or, on rare occasions, may need to be aborted based on the intraoperative assessment and diagnosis.

Granulomas are typically found on the posterior aspect of the vocal fold, usually on the vocal process of the arytenoids, and although usually unilateral, they may also be bilateral (Figure 20-4A). Granulation tissue can also form on other areas of the vocal folds, and some refer to them as granulomatous polyps (Figure 20-4B). Typical granulomas rarely require treatment, as aggressive reflux treatment and appropriate behavior modification and voice therapy will usually allow them to resolve spontaneously, whereas granulomatous polyps more often require surgery.

A.

B.

Figure 20–1. Poorly responsive "vocal nodules." **A.** Low magnification suggesting asymmetric nodules. **B.** Higher magnification revealing cyst on the right vocal fold with contact nodule on the opposite vocal fold.

A.

B.

Figure 20–2. A. Unilateral laryngeal polyp. **B.** Unilateral laryngeal cyst.

A.

B.

Figure 20–3. Chronic, recalcitrant "nodules" failing conservative treatment. **A.** Chronic appearing bilateral swelling. **B.** Intraoperative palpation reveals deep bilateral sulci.

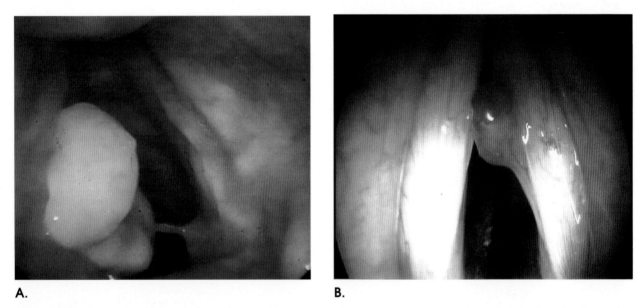

A.

B.

Figure 20–4. A. Classic vocal fold granuloma on the vocal process of the arytenoids. **B.** Granulomatous polyp on the free margin of the vocal fold.

Even if obvious mass lesions are noted on the vocal folds, it does not necessarily imply that surgery is necessary. When a singer is evaluated in the clinic, it is sometimes difficult to determine if the lesion is new or has been there for some time. I have been impressed with the number of singers who have had an acute change in voice where a mass is noted, and where there were older photographs or videos of the larynx that show that the mass had been there for some time, even when there was an intervening period of normal voice quality. Making decisions regarding surgery in these situations may be difficult. If possible, and if the singer has been seen in the past, it is always helpful in obtaining any older medical records or images. In some cases, a chronic mass lesion may have been present for a long time and some other factor resulted in the recent voice change. In such cases, surgery may not be of great value.

Another critical and important issue is the singer's expectations from the evaluation and recommendations. Some singers are not concerned about the impact of the mass (which could potentially be surgically removed). In some cases they just want reassurance that the problem will not progress or permanently affect their voice. In other cases, they are concerned about the possibility of a cancer, particularly in those singers who smoke. There are singers where the raspy or breathy voice afforded by the mass lesion is actually part of their voice signature and is, therefore, desirable. This is true for some cabaret singers where removing the lesion could be catastrophic. The bottom line is that every singer is different, with different voice demands, and different expectations. It is important for the voice surgeon to establish a strong relationship with the singer, know his or her singing style and demands, then be honest about the problem and explain the treatment options and their ramifications. Then, the surgeon should take the time to hear the singer's concerns and allow him or her to participate in the discussion and ultimately make the decision. When the surgeon is specifically asked what he or she feels is the best option for the singer, taking a balanced approach and being honest about the expectations is the best approach.

During the preoperative evaluation it is very important to identify any other significant medical problems that need to be considered. In some cases other physicians may need to be brought into the care team. A thorough history of medications is mandatory to be certain that they will not adversely affect the surgical outcome (see chapter 14). With the number of alternative and homeopathic medications available, it is also important to identify these as some of them may be contraindicated in the surgical patient. For a full description of the potential side effects of these products please refer to chapter 15.

INFORMED CONSENT

This is the basis of the informed-consent process. The singer should be aware of each available and reasonable option, their advantages and disadvantages, and a consistent plan for each. If the singer has not already achieved appropriate resolution of the voice problem from nonsurgical therapy, and if a significant impact on the singing voice remains that is potentially amenable to surgery, then surgery should be discussed with the singer. The first question that a surgeon should ask is, "Am I comfortable with my own skills in surgically managing this problem?" If the answer is "No," then there should be follow-up questions: "Are there others that are more competent to surgically manage this patient?" or "Is the problem complex enough that others would also be uncomfortable in managing this?" These questions allow the surgeon to re-evaluate his or her role in the rehabilitation of the singer. The surgeon may then perform the surgery, refer the singer to another surgical laryngologist, or consider that the risks could potentially outweigh the benefits at this time and pursue other avenues.

Once the surgeon has determined that surgery is the best option, and that he or she is competent to perform the surgery, then the benefits and risks of the surgery should be discussed with the patient in detail. These should not only include the risks related to the effect on the larynx and voice, but also other potential issues such as anesthetic complications, injury to the teeth, postintubation laryngospasm with pulmonary edema, or other risks specific to the patient's health. These discussions should be thoroughly documented in the medical record and a consent form should be signed and witnessed with a copy for the patient. The patient should never be coaxed into surgery. In addition, it is important to discuss with the singer that it is impossible to determine how one will heal and that there is a risk that the voice may not improve or could theoretically worsen due to the aforementioned risks, and that the results could be permanent. These discussions will vary based on the severity of the surgical problem. In most cases they should be part of an open discussion, emphasizing the positive aspects, suggesting that improvement is expected, and allaying the singer's fears while increasing the singer's confidence in the surgeon. Reviewing photographs and videos and drawing templates on paper are very helpful in describing the surgery and in gaining the patients understanding of the surgery. It is also helpful to describe the entire process from preoperative steps to leaving the recovery room. The more informed the patient, the greater their psychological comfort and the stronger the relationship with the surgeon. This will also help to buffer any potential litigation issues if there is a suboptimal outcome (see chapter 25).

Other objective tests may also be helpful to clarify the need for surgery and may be useful in assessing the effectiveness of surgery when comparing preoperative to postoperative results. These tests may be more relevant based on the specific test and the nature of the problem. For example, airflow analysis may be useful in vocal fold paresis or paralysis or very large masses, but may be less valuable in Reinke's edema. Objective tests are useful for monitoring nonsurgical treatments but do not take the place of laryngeal videostroboscopy (LVS). In addition to LVS, outcomes instruments like the Voice Handicap Index (VHI) are important. They help not only to assess the severity of disease and the response from the patient's perspective to treatment but may also help clarify whether or not the patient is a surgical candidate.

SURGICAL PLANNING

Once the determination has been made to proceed with surgery, and the informed-consent process has been completed, a number of important issues need to be considered as part of the surgical planning. The first is the timing of the surgery. How does it fit into audition, recital, or performance schedules? How does it fit into family, social, or other occupational schedules? When does the patient want to proceed? It is important to be flexible, understanding, and supportive of the singer's schedule and timing needs. As there will be some recovery time before singers can resume their voice use after surgery, this also needs to be built into the schedule. In general, for superficial vocal fold masses such as nodules or superficial polyps, it is not unreasonable that the singer may begin some gentle singing within 4 to 6 weeks following surgery. They can gradually advance their voice use so that they can perform by 2 to 3 months after surgery. If the problem

appears more significant, then it may take longer. It is reasonable and preferable to overestimate the time to recovery. It is often easier for the performer to add in an engagement than to cancel one because recovery was underestimated. It also helps to emphasize that the healing process may be slow and that postoperative voice use should be tempered.

I typically tell patients that they should have little voice use for at least 2 weeks following surgery. I see them around that time and obtain LVS assessment. If there is a return of vocal fold vibration, and if the mucosa is healing well, I will begin advancing their voice use. I see them again 2 weeks later, and if they continue to do well, I will ask them to begin some gentle singing vocalizations. I generally do not allow them to begin dramatically advancing their volume or range until 6 weeks and only then if everything is going perfectly. The value of a singing voice specialist at this time is important as the singer will often discuss details of singing with that person rather than anyone else. The typical patient can begin performing between 8 to 12 weeks. It is important to note that this time frame may vary significantly. Close observation and examination of patients is critical to optimize their return while still avoiding any potential setbacks. It is generally best to err on being conservative. If recovery is planned prior to surgery and then adjusted, if necessary, once the magnitude of the surgery is known, all involved will be comfortable with the recovery time.

Another consideration that should be made preoperatively about the perioperative treatment is the importance of integrating the voice pathologist and singing teacher into the treatment plans. It is important to coordinate these visits, determine the appropriate roles for each practitioner, and elucidate to the patient the specific roles. Treating a singer is a multidisciplinary endeavor and this is particularly true for the surgical patient. It may be important to begin singing instruction before the surgery to maximize the effectiveness of these treatments postoperatively.

SURGICAL PLANNING: MICROANATOMIC CONSIDERATIONS

The other part of surgical planning is conceptualizing the surgery and what may be expected to be encountered based on the evaluation of the lesion and the relevant surgical anatomy. Although the anatomy of the larynx is well described in chapter 3, a review of the microanatomic principles of the larynx and how they relate to surgery is valuable. The layered structure has been well defined by Hirano[4,5] (Figure 20–5). There is mucosa, three layers of the lamina propria, with the most superficial being Reinke's space and the deepest layer being the vocal ligament. Deep to the ligament is the thyroarytenoid (vocalis) muscle.[4] These layers tend to vibrate independently at lower frequencies and more as a unit at higher frequencies. These layers are relatively independent and with differing composition of collagen and cellular matrix with the predominant collagen fibers of the vocalis ligament running parallel to those of the mucosa. Injury to both the mucosa and the ligament will cause disruption of this orientation so that there are adhesions between these deep layers and mucosa.[5] This can lead to stiffness and limitations in the vibratory characteristics of the vocal fold.

Fortunately, most lesions of the vocal folds such as nodules, polyps, and superficial cysts such as mucus-retention cysts, are limited to the mucosa and superficial layer. Surgery, therefore, confined to the mucosa and Reinke's space as is usually possible in such lesions, will lead to maintenance of the orientation of the layers with normal or near-normal vibratory characteristics.[5] Deeper lesions, such as epidermoid cysts and sulci, may not result in completely normal vibration.

The surgeon needs to plan the type of anesthesia, perhaps even having a discussion with the anesthesiologist prior to surgery. Although venture-jet ventilation is an appropriate consideration, with this technique the surgeon and anesthesiologist need to work closely together to make sure that the ventilation does not move the vocal folds while the laryngeal surgeon is manipulating the vocal folds.

Specialized equipment for laryngeal surgery should be available. There have been great advances in laryngeal microsurgical instruments that recognize the microanatomic principles of vocal fold surgery. Smaller instruments that allow for atraumatic manipulation of the vocal folds have been developed. Although most surgeons have moved away from laser surgery for many benign lesions, in skilled hands the outcomes would be expected to be similar to those obtained with microinstruments.[6] Another significant innovation in surgical instruments has been the orientation of the handle of the instruments. In these instruments, thumb activation does not result in any perceptual movement of the distal, active part of the instrument (Figure 20–6). This results in better stability and may potentially reduce the risk of movement error.[7]

Figure 20–5. The microanatomy of the vocal fold showing the mucosa, three layers of the lamina propria, and vocalis muscle.

A.

B.

Figure 20–6. Laryngeal microinstrument with thumb-activated handle that allows for minimal distal movement with closure. Notice the difference between the lower (traditional handle) and upper (thumb-activated handle) instruments in relationship to distal tip motion. **A.** Instrument open. **B.** Instrument closed.

SUMMARY

Planning for surgery in a singer requires the establishment of a strong relationship between the surgeon and the singer. In essence, they need to develop a partnership of care. In most cases, the diagnosis should be confirmed with appropriate objective tests, LVS, and a trial of voice therapy prior to determining the need for surgery. The decision to proceed with surgery should lead to a thorough discussion of the risks, benefits, and alternatives (informed consent) and this should be properly documented. The surgery should be planned where possible around the schedule of the performer and a contract should be developed regarding the approximate timing of the postoperative voice use and performance schedule. The surgeon should plan the surgical technique but be flexible to modify the technique based on the intraoperative findings. He or she should make sure that suitable instruments are available to treat the problem. The surgeon also is responsible for coordinating the surgery with other health care providers including the anesthesiologist. Finally, the surgeon should be involved in the postoperative care along with the speech pathologist, the voice teacher, and the singer's agents or managers.

REFERENCES

1. Benninger MS, Johnson A, Jacobson B, eds. *Vocal Arts Medicine. The Care and Prevention of Professional Voice Disorders.* New York, NY: Thieme Medical Publishers; 1993.
2. Sataloff RT, Spiegel JR, Hawkshaw MJ. Strobovideolaryngoscopy: results and clinical value. *Ann Otol Rhinol Laryngol.* 1991;100:725-727.
3. Benninger MS, Jacobson B. Vocal nodules, microwebs and surgery. *J Voice.* 1995;9:326-331.
4. Hirano M. Phonosurgery. Basic and clinical investigations. *Otologia (Fukuoka).* 1975;21:239-262.
5. Benninger MS, Alessi D, Archer S. et al. Vocal fold scarring: current concepts and management. *Otolaryngol Head Neck Surg.* 1996;115:474-482.
6. Benninger MS. Microdissection or microspot CO_2 laser for limited vocal fold benign pathology: a prospective randomized trial. *Laryngoscope.* 2001;110 (Suppl 92):1-17.
7. Benninger MS. Laryngeal microinstrumentation: a novel design to reduce movement. *Otolaryngol Head Neck Surg.* 2003;129:280-283.

Chapter 21

MICROLARYNGOSCOPIC PROCEDURES AND OPERATIONS

Seth H. Dailey
Charles N. Ford

INDICATIONS

Microlaryngoscopic surgery must be performed with utmost technical skill in singers and professional voice users. Keys to success are often related to factors other than the technical skills of the surgeon. Making the proper diagnosis, knowing when to operate, and managing the whole patient are essential. Although some lesions are obvious, there are some that require study over time and others that require microlaryngoscopic examination to secure a diagnosis. In the singer, suspicion of a surgical lesion should be high with complaints of progressive dysphonia. However, many singers are able to overcome the mechanical challenge of a pathologic larynx through technical finesse. That is why painful phonation or vocal fatigue is such a red flag in singers.

Certain physical findings are highly suggestive of underlying vocal fold pathology. Lesions on the surface are usually obvious in the case of leukoplakia, vascular ectasias, granulomas, polyps, and papillomas. Deeper lesions like cysts, sulci, and scars are often more subtle and require stroboscopic or microsopic examination to confirm. There are clues to underlying pathology that warrant further study, for example endoscopic evidence of dilated or misaligned vessels on the superior vocal fold surface, or tenacious mucus stranding at points of contact on the medial vocal fold edge. Stroboscopic evidence of aperiodicity, focal areas of stiffness, or recalcitrant supraglottic hyperfunction often indicate surgical pathology.

Singers tend to be very compliant with voice therapy, so failure to respond to an adequate course of voice therapy is often another indicator of vocal fold pathology. Surgical intervention is seldom indicated in the professional singer without a trial of voice therapy and perioperative work with a speech pathologist, phoniatrician, or vocologist. With the help of these voice specialists, it is important to choose the correct time for operative intervention. Surgery should not be planned within a 4-week period of a performance; the interval might be longer depending on the nature of the surgery and demands for healing. Optimal healing may be compromised if surgery is undertaken within 5 days of menses. Other considerations include adequate control of laryngopharyngeal reflux, allergies, and situational stresses.

The actual phonosurgical approach, techniques, and intrumentarium are not unique for singers. As with all phonomicrosurgery, the operative technique must focus on careful microlaryngoscopic assessment of pathology, delicate handling of tissue, and sparing of normal tissues. Structurally, there is not a great difference between the larynx of a professional singer and that of a nontrained voice user. The geometric contours, delicate layered architecture, cellular and extracellular matrix of the vocal fold lamina propria, and the supporting exoskeleton are essentially the same.

INFORMED CONSENT

The informed consent process is an exploration in various steps to understand if elective surgery is right for a given patient. Essential factors in this process include first the development of a trusting relationship where open dialogue is encouraged. A healthy and trusting relationship is essential so that information can be freely shared and questions asked on both sides. For professional and performing voice users an understanding of their personal and vocal demands is essential in building this bond as is an appreciation that a vocal deficit can be devastating to their professional confidence and progression.

The physician is obliged to provide the patient with a full exposition of the risks, benefits, and alternatives to the proposed procedure, allowing ample time and opportunity to answer questions. A descriptive phase often helps familiarize the patient. Anxiety-relieving details include that no skin will be cut, that the procedure is under general anesthesia so that no recollection of the surgery is likely, and that it is performed in an ambulatory setting. After the description of microlaryngoscopy for benign lesions it is essential to understand if the likely outcome of the procedure is aligned with the patient's expectations. For example, if a professional voice user is seen to have scarring or more involvement of the vocal fold than anticipated then full disclosure up front is mandatory to help attenuate the anticipation of a "perfect voice" postoperatively. One might explain, perhaps, that resection of a vocal fold polyp should improve symptoms of vocal fatigue, effort, and projection, but that contralateral pre-existing scarring may impede return of the upper register. Furthermore, the vocal folds need time to heal fully, making voice improvement a gradual process that should be anticipated. Education through the use of video playback from digitally recorded stroboscopic examinations greatly enhances the patient's ability to grasp some of these concepts. Many vocalists have been taught to think of their voice with imagery to enhance resonance (eg, think of your voice as a bird),

a construct which can be confusing. Conceptual reduction of the impaired glottis to something as simple as a "leaky valve" can help to relate how this inefficient system yields symptoms of vocal fatigue, increased effort, and reduced projection accompanied often by a breathy or thready vocal quality. Given that the glottis is hidden from plain sight and that many vocal professionals have never seen their vocal folds prior to evaluation for surgery, this rapid and effective education is critical. Some prior studies dealing with informed consent have demonstrated that educational materials in written formats with or without illustrations can enhance the retention of facts discussed during the consent process.[1-5] Furthermore, younger and more educated patients may recall risks better.[6]

Following the educational segment of the discussion, it is imperative to assess whether the patient can follow through on perioperative adjustments to maximize the eventual outcome. Management of excess life stressors, and reduction of laryngeal irritants such as alcohol and primary or second-hand smoke are required. Medical conditions such as laryngopharyngeal reflux and allergies should be accounted for. Timing of the surgery must be optimized so that there is minimal loss of professional revenue. For women, the surgery should not be performed in the 5-day period before menses as there may be an increased risk of bleeding from the vocal folds.[7] Pre- and postoperative voice therapy are often part of the management. A common cause of hesitation is lost revenues from the need to take time off work. In professional singers there is also a fear of being perceived as injured by one's peers and, therefore, of lesser professional standing. If the patient appears reluctant to adhere to these standard recommendations, the physician is required to address that hesitancy immediately. Further education and counseling will frequently assuage any concerns, but if the patient's reluctance persists, then postponing or aborting the procedure may be necessary.

Discussion of the specific risks of suspension microlaryngoscopy will recapitulate prior discussions, but also takes on a medicolegal component. A written checklist that details bleeding, infection, temporary or permanent hoarseness, mucosal injury to the oral cavity or oropharynx, throat pain, dysesthesia of tongue, taste impairment, need for further surgery, cervical spine injury, and chipped teeth may prove useful. Reference to prior studies reporting particular risks frames the dialogue, and helps to alleviate anxiety and anticipate short-term concerns postoperatively. For example, Klussman et al found that 75% of their patients undergoing suspension microlaryngoscopy had minor mucosal lesions within the pharynx or oral cavity.[8] Furthermore, dental injury was found in 6.5% of cases and temporary injury to the lingual or hypoglossal nerve in 3.8% of cases. In a prospective study, Rosen et al recently found a dental injury rate of 0%, but found that 18% had taste alterations and 12.5% had partial tongue hypesesthesia.[9] Reassurance that the mean duration of these side effects of surgery is 11 days is helpful. Fortunately, major risk of cardiovascular compromise appears to be low and risk of reintubation after laryngoscopy for otolaryngologic disease is about 1%.[10,11] Specific information related to a worsened voice quality is somewhat scarce. However, Johns et al found that the Vocal Handicap Index values improved significantly following phonomicrosurgical resection of vocal fold cysts and polyps.[12] Patients with Reinke's edema and vocal fold scar did not experience statistically significant improvement after surgery. Also, men tended to experience less improvement than women. Zeitels et al found improvement of aerodynamic and acoustic measures following phonomicorsurgery for benign lesions in vocal professionals.[13] Finally, there is emerging evidence that between 9 and 36% of patients who undergo microlaryngoscopy for a benign lesion identified by office endoscopy will have an altered diagnosis at the time of surgery.[14,15] Sulcus vocalis, mucosal bridges, and intracordal lesions are the most commonly unidentified entities prior to surgery. This evidence suggests that a detailed discussion must take place so that the surgeon has enough freedom to act appropriately when new information is gleaned intraoperatively.

SURGICAL PRINCIPLES: INCISIONS, MICROFLAPS, AND PLANES OF DISSECTION

Many fundamentals of surgery apply to phonomicrosurgery for benign disease. Adequate exposure, careful tissue handling, hemostasis, preservation of normal tissues, and primary healing are necessary to preserve vocal fold function. As we have learned more about

vocal fold structure and function, efforts to preserve the cellular and amorphous components of the vocal fold lamina propria have influenced phonosurgical refinements. Surface lesions usually arise from the superior, medial, or infraglottic surface of the vocal fold. It is important to recognize the site of origin and to avoid sacrificing any uninvolved surface in order to reduce the demand for re-epithelialization. For benign lesions deeper within the vocal fold (eg, cysts/sulcus), the lateral microflap cordotomy approach (Figure 21–1) involves making an incision on the superior-lateral surface of the vocal fold, and often extending this incision with microscissors or a spreading technique. This relatively long incision facilitates blunt dissection in the superficial lamina propria plane and allows easy identification of the vocal ligament. Although initially described as the basic microsurgical approach to benign lesions located deep to the superficial layer of

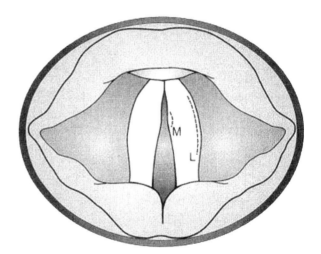

Figure 21-1. Diagram showing the fundamental difference between the lateral (*L*) and medial (*M*) microflap. The medial incision is limited by the approximate dimensions of the lesion. (After Ford CN, Advances and refinements in phonosurgery. *Laryngoscope.* 1999;109:1891–1900.) The diagram is used to illustrate the difference between the lateral microflap incision, placed superolaterally, and the medial microflap, placed medially. (Mention of microscissors and spreading in the text may lead the reader to believe that an operative photo will be shown; when they see the diagram, however, it should be clear that the point to be emphasized is how different incisions are planned.)

the lamina propria, it is now preferred mainly in cases where the lesion is large or diffuse, or where identification of the vocal ligament might be problematic. For example, in the scarred vocal fold with a poorly defined lesion, it is easier to first identify the vocal ligament laterally and then proceed to dissect around the lesion.

Sataloff was one who proposed a "mini-microflap" approach to minimize damage to the complex basement membrane attachments to the superficial lamina propria.[16] The essential difference with this approach is in the placement of the incision near the free edge of the vocal fold (Figure 21–1). Unlike the lateral incision, it is relatively short with anterior-to-posterior extension only as long as necessary to expose the lesion. Such an approach minimizes tissue damage and the risk of postoperative scarring. Courey[17] distinguished the medial microflap approach from the lateral microflap approach. The medial microflap is ideally suited for situations where: (1) the lesion involves only the medial surface of the vocal fold, (2) the overlying cover is very thin, (3) there is redundant cover, or (4) it appears easy to separate the lesion from the vocal ligament.[17] With the medial microflap approach, it is possible to use a more focal incision, separate the pathologic tissue, and spare normal tissue. The key concept here is to spare not only the vocal ligament, but also avoid damaging uninvolved superficial lamina propria. The superficial lamina propria regenerates poorly, and stiffness will result from re-epithelialization over deficient tissue.

Concern about the integrity of the superficial lamina propria (SLP) is particularly relevant to current methods for microsurgical management of Reinke's edema. It is uncommon for the overlying epithelium to exhibit substantial changes worrisome for premalignancy (ie, leukoplakia or "white plaque"), so surgery for Reinke's edema has focused on removal of the pathologic tissue with suction while sparing nonredundant epithelial covering tissues. Zeitels stressed the importance of preserving as much lamina propria as possible to prevent the epithelial basement membrane from adhering to the vocal ligament.[18] Such adherence decreases oscillation and results in a stiffer vocal fold due to iatrogenic scarring. This phenomenon may be responsible for some prolonged postoperative dysphonias in patients with Reinke's edema. He also demonstrated that cold instrumentation is better suited than CO_2 lasers for resection of small superficial vocal fold lesions.[19] In earlier work, Lumpkin also noted that, when compared to laser surgery, cold lateral microflap surgery led to quicker healing and rehabilitation in patients with Reinke's edema.[20] In contrast, Benninger demonstrated no differences in vocal outcome in a randomized trial comparing the use of cold instruments versus microspot CO_2 laser for benign glottic lesions.[21] With increased understanding of the cellular and acellular components of the superficial lamina propria, it appears the explanation for this lies in the extent of lamina propria destruction. Gray stressed the importance of the superficial lamina propria in preserving optimal viscoelasticity for vocal fold oscillation.[22] Surgical damage to the lamina propria causes the normal beneficial proteins, elastins, and hyaluronic acids to be replaced with collagen fibers and fibronectin. This increases tissue viscosity, which means that greater energy is required to overcome frictional forces to permit oscillation. In phonosurgery, it is therefore obviously expedient to preserve the superficial lamina propria. When lamina propria is lost, correction should consider replacement with substances that restore freedom of motion and decrease tissue viscosity.

HISTORICAL NOTE

Phonomicrosurgery is the application of the microscope and micro-instrumentation in endoscopic laryngeal surgery. Magnification and tissue sparing are the keys to success, and this is especially important in operations on singers. Recent advances might be considered refinements of the important, visionary contributions of microlaryngoscopy pioneers. The concept of phonosurgery was introduced by Albrecht, whose use of a gynecologic colposcope for microlaryngoscopy was met with skepticism by the otolaryngologic community. von Leden recalled this event and his personal interactions with Lewy, Kleinsasser, Jako, Lynch, and others who catalyzed the evolution of laryngoscopes and optics.[23] These seminal advances, which allowed the surgeon magnified vision while performing bimanual surgery through a laryngoscope, have facilitated the continued development of phonomicrosurgical tools and techniques. Hirano emphasized the parallel advances in basic anatomy and physiology of phonation, pathophysiology of vocal fold diseases, and vocal function evaluation.[24] Continued refinement of techniques is dependent on accurate, objective voice assessment to precisely diagnose disorders and measure the results of surgical intervention.

Many of the technical advances in phonomicrosurgery involve improved visualization of the pathology and operative field. The keys to any direct laryngoscopic examination have not changed over the years. These principles were nicely summarized by Zeitels and Vaughan: (1) position the patient supine with the neck flexed on the chest and extended at the occipitoatloid joint, (2) apply external counterpressure (usually with tape) to direct the laryngeal framework posteriorly, (3) conform the laryngoscope to the triangular shape of the glottis, (4) provide independent laryngeal suspension so the surgeon has both hands free, and (5) induce internal laryngeal distension to move the supraglottal tissues away from the true vocal folds.[25]

EQUIPMENT

Microinstrumentation

A full set of microlaryngeal instruments is enormously helpful for manipulation of the epithelium and lesion alike. For example, gentle grasping of the epithelial flap along a broad base with a heart-shaped forceps will present a reduced risk of tearing the flap when compared to the use of an alligator forceps; the pressure on the tissue is reduced as the surface area employed is larger pressure = force/area. Also, when the lesion is densely adherent to the undersurface of the epithelium, only sharp dissection will be effective in establishing a tissue plane between the two; if the scissors are too dull or if blunt dissection is selected due to a lack of instruments, undue epithelial loss is likely to occur. Furthermore, given the small size of benign vocal fold lesions (often 2–3 mm in size), instruments with working ends that are twice the size of the lesion are awkward and usually ineffective; having instruments with small distal tips allows greater precision. For example, in the excision of ectasias and

varices, without proper instruments such as fine picks, a surgeon might resort to the use of CO_2 laser which has been reported to induce more scarring than cold instrument dissection.[26] Subepithelial infusion of saline or epinephrine solution helps to delineate the interface of normal and abnormal tissue during surgical exploration and will also reduce bleeding.[27]

Surgical instruments are only as stable as the surgeon using them, however. Stability in turn is enhanced by physical comfort. Mayo stands, rolling chairs with adjustable arms supports or other devices will help to ensure rest of major arm and back muscles groups so that fine muscle groups of the forearms and hands are not unduly fatigued. In Otolaryngology–Head and Neck Surgery we are often too willing to sacrifice physical comfort for speed. For microlaryngoscopy this is a liability, as physical discomfort will lead to excessive muscle tension, hand tremor, and possibly suboptimal results.[28] Therefore, attention to the neck, back, arms, and hand position relative to the patient is valuable, especially as the length of the case increases. Removing the instruments and relaxing for a moment now and then is helpful. Use of one instrument as a stabilizing fulcrum for the other has been advocated by Woo (personal communication). Hockstein et al have demonstrated the use of robotics for microlaryngeal surgery in animal and cadaveric models for elimination of hand tremor.[29,30] High cost and further development of the robotic system limit its immediate application.

Magnification and Endoscopes

With improved techniques, the reliance on magnification has become essential in both intraoperative diagnosis and precision techniques. As with all surgery, it is important to see what you are cutting. Magnification and adequate lighting provide the surgeon with the best opportunity for assessment of color, tissue pliability, vasculature of the cover, and assurance of proper tissue contouring. The differentiation of normal from abnormal tissue can be quite difficult and loss of this opportunity can lead to poor tissue plane definition and the sacrifice of normal SLP.[31] The advent of xenon light sources and higher-resolution microscopes is helpful in this regard. Angled telescopes are also of use in the examination of the inferior vocal fold edge and the ventricle. Hemostasis enhances visualization. When bleeding from small vessels in the cover is encountered, reduction of bleeding can be controlled with different modalities each having relative benefits. Tiny cotton balls soaked in epinephrine (1:10,000 dilution) can be gently applied to the area. Care must be taken not to wipe away normal SLP and not to tear the epithelial flap. Microbipolar forceps (Microfrance SKU#-MCL34) have been produced for control of vessels and are effective when used conservatively. Thermal injury, especially to the cover, can induce an exuberant inflammatory reaction and lead to scar. Larger unipolar devices are to be avoided for this reason.

Various laryngoscopes of different size and shape have been designed to achieve improved exposure. The very versatile Holinger laryngoscope proved useless for binocular microsurgery; however, the basic design features of this scope formed the basis for several useful laryngoscopes that are widely used. Dedo modified this design by opening the proximal end to accommodate binocular microscopic vision while flattening and recessing the barrel where the scope meets the maxillary incisors. The Ossoff-Pilling is one modification that allows increased anterior commissure exposure. Bouchayer designed a useful laryngoscope that affords a large working field. Kantor and Berci introduced a novel approach to avoid the optical disadvantage imposed by looking through the laryngoscope.[32] In their system, a rigid telescope with an attached camera is passed through a separate channel within the laryngoscope. The surgeon operates while viewing a magnified, high-resolution image that fills the entire field. Yanagisawa et al compared this approach to conventional microlaryngoscopy, noting its many advantages but also demonstrating the slight distortions introduced by the earliest version of this instrument.[33] Zeitels has introduced a triangular laryngoscope (modular glottiscope) that affords excellent visualization of the true vocal folds, although its design requires an modified approach whereby the scope is passed lateral to the tongue and advanced toward the midline to avoid compression injury to the lingual nerve.[34] An alternative use of rigid endoscopy allows the surgeon to use 0-, 30-, and 70-degree telescopes through any laryngoscope to enhance visualization in difficult exposure cases, but this requires an assistant if the surgeon is not to be limited to a single-handed approach.[35]

Photodocumentation

Photodocumentation of microlaryngoscopic procedures benefits education of patients, students, trainees, and colleagues. Since the first reported attempts to photodocument the larynx in 1892 and 1893 by French, capturing still images has undergone a huge transformation.[36,37] From capturing images in the office with a camera attached to an endoscope to applying a camera directly to the eyepiece of an operative microscope, documentation of laryngeal pathology has helped to shed light on an area hidden from the naked eye.[38-40] Since the advent of digital recording apparatuses within the last decade, immediate playback, selection of still images, improved color and resolution, and videoediting have taken the experience to a new level. It is now possible to review a stroboscopic examination that was just performed with a patient or even to allow *simultaneous* visualization through the use of a video monitor. Additional benefits relate to medicolegal aspects. Postoperative stroboscopy can also help assure patients that a lesion has actually been removed and can help to corroborate any sensations they might be having with altered voice (eg, glottic swelling). This office-based technology can be used in conjunction with office-based interventions that are becoming commonplace.

Office-Based Procedures

Office based procedures fell into disfavor when the availability of general anesthesia and endotracheal tube intubation became possible in the latter half of the 20th century. Because of advancing age and the associated cardiovascular risks thereof, laryngeal procedures accomplished using only topical anesthesia have become more popular. Transoral, transnasal, and transcervical approaches with needles to deliver injectables have been described. Injectable substances have included Teflon, Gelfoam, collagen, micronized dermis, hydroxyapatite, and many others. Medically active drugs such as steroids and cidofovir for papilloma are also deliverable through these routes. Office-based lasers such as the 585-nm pulsed dye laser and CO_2 equivalents with flexible fibers are now used routinely without the need for general anesthesia or sedation.[41] Distal-chip camera technology also permits not only transnasal esophagoscopy but also tracheoscopy and bronchoscopy.[42] In the office setting, diagnostic and therapeutic accuracy may be sacrificed for convenience and reduced morbidity in some instances. For the professional singer, however, accuracy of diagnosis and meticulous preservation of native tissue are of such importance that direct microlaryngoscopic surgery is often the most conservative approach. For example, one would most likely not choose an office-based polyp resection in a professional singer when a brief procedure under general anesthesia is likely to yield better diagnostic and technical precision. In some instances office procedures are advantageous. Vocal fold augmentation, for example, might be just as well managed in the office using a glottic injectable such as micronized dermis as it would allow for immediate voice assessment and incremental adjustment. Better outcomes in the office are afforded by a cooperative, well-informed patient who can tolerate a transient period of discomfort without excess motion.

CASE STUDIES

Case A

This 28-year-old jazz vocalist had intermittent hoarseness for over one year. She was referred for management of vocal nodules but on examination exhibited asymmetric vocal fold fullness and inflammation. With substantial vocal behavior modification, treatment of laryngopharyngeal reflux, and voice therapy her speaking voice improved but she was still unable to achieve the high end of her range and experienced breaks at low intensity. Examination revealed a right cystic-appearing lesion in the midmembranous vocal fold with only slight impairment of mucosal wave. Microlaryngoscopy was performed for excision (see Figures 21–2A through 21–2E).

This patient had an uneventful recovery, maintained good vocal hygiene, and resumed normal vocal activity with no restrictions after 4 weeks. At one year there was no evidence of recurrence and she was enjoying a successful singing career in New York. This is a case where the diagnosis of pseudocyst was made at surgery and superficial excision was facilitated by miniflap elevation and undermining.

Case B

A 37-year-old woman presented for evaluation for progressive hoarseness of one-year duration. She affirmed vocal fatigue and increased vocal effort along with reduced projection. She affirmed loss of her upper register during avocational singing. She is a nonsmoker and denied prior voice difficulty as well as swallowing

Figure 21–2A. Microscopic examination revealed a well-circumscribed cystic lesion of the right vocal fold.

Figure 21–2B. A microflap was elevated and no cystic lesion was present in the superficial lamina propria.

Figure 21–2C. Having elevated the flap preserving lamina propria tissues, the superficial pseudocyst was removed.

Figure 21–2D. Gentle eversion displays the intact superficial lamina propria tissues and delicate vasculature.

Figure 21–2E. Postoperative appearance.

problems. Her vocal load was heavy including a job as a waitress, singing, and managing three children including a teenager. On physical examination she was found to have a breathy, effortful, irregular voice quality that never improved with register changes. Passagio into the upper register yielded no high notes. Stroboscopic examination revealed an hourglass-shaped glottic closure pattern and midmusculomembranous vocal fold lesions consistent with phonotrauma. She underwent 3 months of resonant voice therapy and did well with significant reduction in her vocalizing pressures. However, her symptoms persisted as did her vocal fold lesions at the time of follow-up. After informed con-

sent was obtained she was taken to the operating room for microlaryngoscopy with subepithelial excision of both vocal fold lesions. The more polypoid right-sided lesion and the sessile left-sided lesion were reduced in size to allow for smooth straight contours to the vocal folds with epithelial preservation (see Figures 21–3A to 21–3D).

One month postoperatively she reported marked reduction of her vocal effort and fatigue and noted return of her high range. The passagio into her high range still was unsteady. She underwent postoperative voice therapy to maintain the benefits of her surgery and to help smooth the passagio.

Figure 21-3A. Digital image of the glottis with the patient under suspension microlaryngoscopy. The right vocal fold lesion is noted to be polypoid and the left sessile.

Figure 21-3B. Exposure of the right vocal fold supepithelial pathology after subepithelial infusion with epinephrine, epithelial cordotomy, and retraction of the overlying epithelium medially with microforceps.

Figure 21-3C. Removal of a portion of the subepithelial pathology on the right vocal fold using microcup forceps.

Figure 21-3D. Digital image of the glottis after excision of bilateral subepithelial pathology.

REFERENCES

1. Makdessian AS, Ellis DA, Irish JC. Informed consent in facial plastic surgery: effectiveness of a simple educational intervention. *Arch Facial Plast Surg.* 2004;6:26-30.
2. Layton S, Korsen J. Informed consent in oral and maxillofacial surgery: a study of the value of written warnings. *Br J Oral Maxillofac Surg.* 1994;32:34-36.
3. Langdon IJ, Hardin R, Learmonth ID. Informed consent for total hip arthroplasty: does a written information sheet improve recall by patients? *Ann R Coll Surg Engl.* 2002;84:404-408.
4. Dawes PJ, O'Keefe L, Adcock S. Informed consent: the assessment of two structured interview approaches compared to the current approach. *J Laryngol Otol.* 1992;106:420-424.
5. Chan Y, Irish JC, Wood SJ et al. Patient education and informed consent in head and neck surgery.

Arch Otolaryngol Head Neck Surg. 2002;128: 1269-1274.

6. Hekkenberg RJ, Irish JC, Rotstein LE, Brown DH, Gullane PJ. Informed consent in head and neck surgery: how much do patients actually remember? *J Otolaryngol.* 1997;26:155-159.

7. Abitbol J, Abitbol P, Abitbol B. Sex hormones and the female voice. *J Voice.* 1999;13:424-446.

8. Klussmann JP, Knoedgen R, Wittekindt C, Damm M, Eckel HE. Complications of suspension laryngoscopy. *Ann Otol Rhinol Laryngol.* 2002;111: 972-976.

9. Rosen CA, Andrade Filho PA, Scheffel L, Buckmire R. Oropharyngeal complications of suspension laryngoscopy: a prospective study. *Laryngoscope.* 2005;115:1681-1684.

10. Wenig BL, Raphael N, Stern JR, Shikowitz MJ, Abramson AL. Cardiac complications of suspension laryngoscopy. Fact or fiction? *Arch Otolaryngol Head Neck Surg.* 1986;112:860-862.

11. Hill RS, Koltai PJ, Parnes SM. Airway complications from laryngoscopy and panendoscopy. *Ann Otol Rhinol Laryngol.* 1987;96:691-694.

12. Johns MM, Garrett CG, Hwang J, Ossoff RH, Courey MS. Quality-of-life outcomes following laryngeal endoscopic surgery for non-neoplastic vocal fold lesions. *Ann Otol Rhinol Laryngol.* 2004;113:597-601.

13. Zeitels SM, Hillman RE, Desloge R, Mauri M, Doyle PB. Phonomicrosurgery in singers and performing artists: treatment outcomes, management theories, and future directions. *Ann Otol Rhinol Laryngol Suppl.* 2002;190:21-40.

14. Poels PJ, de Jong FI, Schutte HK. Consistency of the preoperative and intraoperative diagnosis of benign vocal fold lesions. *J Voice.* 2003;17:425-433.

15. Dailey SH, Spanou K, Zeitels S. The evaluation of benign glottic lesions: rigid telescopic stroboscopy vs. suspension microlaryngoscopy. (submitted).

16. Sataloff RT, Spiegel JR, Heuer RJ et al. Laryngeal mini-microflap: a new technique and reassessment of the microflap saga. *J Voice.* 1995;9:198-204.

17. Courey MS, Garrett CG, Ossoff RH. Medial microflap for excision of benign vocal fold lesions. *Laryngoscope.* 1997;107:340-344.

18. Zeitels SM, Hillman RE, Bunting GW, Vaughn T. Reinke's edema: phonatory mechanisms and management strategies. *Ann Otol Rhinol Laryngol.* 1997;106:533-543.

19. Zeitels SM. Laser versus cold instruments for microlaryngoscopic surgery. *Laryngoscope.* 1996; 106:545-552.

20. Lumpkin SM, Bennett S, Bishop SG. Postsurgical follow-up study of patients with severe polypoid degeneration. *Laryngoscope.* 1990;100: 399-402.

21. Benninger MS. Microdissection or microspot CO_2 laser for limited vocal fold benign lesions: a prospective randomized trial. *Laryngoscope.* 2000;110:1-17.

22. Gray SD, Bielamowicz SA, Titze IR, Dove H, Ludlow C. Experimental approaches to vocal fold alteration: introduction to the minithyrotomy. *Ann Otol Rhinol Laryngol.* 1999;108:1-9.

23. von Leden H. Microlaryngoscopy: a historical vignette. *J Voice.* 1988;1:341-346.

24. Hirano M. Phonosurgery: past, present, and future. *Transactions ABEA.* 1995:25-30.

25. Zeitels SM, Vaughan CW. "External counterpressure" and "internal distention" for optimal laryngoscopic exposure of the anterior glottal commissure. *Ann Otol Rhinol Laryngol.* 1994; 103:669-675.

26. Hochman I, Sataloff RT, Hillman RE, Zeitels SM. Ectasias and varices of the vocal fold: clearing the striking zone. *Ann Otol Rhinol Laryngol.* 1999; 108:10-16.

27. Zeitels SM, Vaughan CW. A submucosal true vocal fold infusion needle. *Otolaryngol Head Neck Surg.* 1991;105:478-479.

28. Hemal AK, Srinivas M, Charles AR. Ergonomic problems associated with laparoscopy. *J Endourol.* 2001;15:499-503.

29. Hockstein NG, Nolan JP, O'Malley BW, Jr., Woo YJ. Robot-assisted pharyngeal and laryngeal microsurgery: results of robotic cadaver dissections. *Laryngoscope.* 2005;115:1003-1008.

30. Hockstein NG, Nolan JP, O'Malley B W, Jr., Woo YJ. Robotic microlaryngeal surgery: a technical feasibility study using the daVinci surgical robot and an airway mannequin. *Laryngoscope.* 2005;115: 780-785.

31. Zeitels S. *Atlas of Phonomicrosurgery and Other Endolaryngeal Procedures for Benign and Malignant Disease.* San Diego, Calif: Singular Publishing Group; 2001.

32. Kantor E, Berci G, Partlow E, Paz-Partlow M. A completely new approach to microlaryngeal surgery. *Laryngoscope.* 1991;101:676-679.

33. Yanagisawa E, Horowitz JB, Yanagisawa K, Mambrino LJ. Comparison of new telescopic video microlaryngoscopic and standard microlaryngoscopic techniques. *Ann Otol Rhinol Laryngol.* 1992;101:51-60.

34. Zeitels SM. Universal modular glottiscope system: the evolution of a century of design and technique for direct laryngoscopy. *Ann Otol Rhinol Laryngol Suppl.* 1999;179:2-24.
35. Yeh AR, Huang HM, Chen YL. Telescopic video microlaryngeal surgery. *Ann Otol Rhinol Laryngol.* 1999;108:165-168.
36. French T. On photographing the larynx. *Trans Am Laryngol Assoc.* 1883:59-68.
37. French T. *Trans Am Laryngol Assoc* 1882:32-35.
38. Yanagisawa E, Yanagisawa R. Laryngeal photography. *Otolaryngol Clin North Am.* 1991;24:999-1022.
39. Bass RM, Kilbourne CS. Intraoperative laryngeal photographic techniques. *Otolaryngol Head Neck Surg.* 1982;90:408-412.
40. Benjamin B. Indirect laryngeal photography using rigid telescopes. *Laryngoscope.* 1998;108:158-161.
41. Zeitels SM, Franco RA, Jr., Dailey SH, Burns JA, Hillman RE, Anderson RR. Office-based treatment of glottal dysplasia and papillomatosis with the 585-nm pulsed dye laser and local anesthesia. *Ann Otol Rhinol Laryngol.* 2004;113:265-276.
42. Postma GN, Cohen JT, Belafsky PC, et al. Transnasal esophagoscopy: revisited (over 700 consecutive cases). *Laryngoscope.* 2005;115:321-323.

Chapter 22

NONLARYNGEAL PROCEDURES IN THE PEFORMER

Glendon M. Gardner

In this chapter, we focus on surgery that does not directly involve the larynx. The surgery discussed here can be divided into that which involves the vocal tract, the other regions of the head, neck and upper chest, and the remainder of the body.

Anesthesia issues and postoperative vocal considerations are addressed.

ANESTHESIA CONCERNS/AIRWAY MANAGEMENT

For any surgery done under general anesthesia, injury to the vocal folds during endotracheal (ET) intubation is a risk. Although most complications related to intubation occur with long-term intubation (days to weeks), problems can arise after an "easy" intubation that lasts only the duration of the surgery (hours). Acute injuries, which include vocal fold edema, mucosal tears, vocal fold hemorrhage, arytenoid cartilage dislocation, and vocal fold paralysis, have been reported in 6 to 73% of patients undergoing short-term intubation with the more severe injuries occurring very rarely.[1-4] Prior to surgery, the patient should always advise the surgeon and the anesthesiologist that he or she is a vocalist. The anesthesiologist will then take even more care to avoid a traumatic intubation. A smaller tube (6.0 for women, 7.0 for men) is preferred unless the patient is very large or has poor pulmonary reserve and requires maximum ventilation.[5,6] Even after a completely normal atraumatic intubation, development of a vocal process granuloma is possible. This manifests itself with globus sensation, the urge to clear the throat, and sometimes voice changes weeks after the intubation. Gastroesophageal reflux is thought to be the factor that causes granulomas to form in a small number of patients. Preoperative antireflux/antacid prophylaxis with proton pump inhibitors or H2-antagonists might be considered, whether the patient has a history of gastroesophageal reflux disease or not.[5] Preoperative corticosteroids may also help reduce vocal fold edema.[6]

Loucks et al propose a protocol for "vocal athletes" who will be undergoing endotracheal intubation. This includes preoperative counseling by a speech-language pathologist (SLP) regarding the importance of vocal hygiene both before and after intubation. Next is a thorough discussion with the anesthesiologist concerning alternatives for intubation (regional anesthesia, laryngeal mask airway), use of a small tube, attention to humidification and cuff pressures, tube positioning, and exceptional care during the actual intubation. A complete voice assessment is carried out preoperatively by both SLP and otolaryngologist and any medical conditions (allergies, reflux) and maladaptive vocal behaviors are identified and treated prior to the intubation. After extubation, maintaining vocal hygiene is stressed. Important factors include voice rest for 24 hours, maintaining adequate hydration either intravenously or orally, humidification of inspired air, treatment of reflux, and avoidance of nausea and vomiting with appropriate medications. Assessment of the larynx immediately after extubation and again within one month of extubation allows for early identification and treatment of any injuries that may have occurred and any maladaptive vocal behaviors that may have developed.[1]

Another option is the laryngeal mask airway (LMA). This device has a cuff that seals off the airway at the level of the supraglottis rather than passing a tube between the vocal folds. The airway is not quite as secure as with an ET tube.[7] Short-term voice changes were noted to be less common in patients ventilated with the LMA rather than standard ET intubation.[8] There have, however, been cases of injury to the larynx reported with the LMA, although it is rare.[9]

Chipped teeth are an unlikely, but known, complication of endotracheal intubation. This is a concern for all patients, but especially for performers whose appearance is a factor in obtaining employment. Making the anesthesiologist aware of any cosmetic dental work (caps, bridges, crowns) and wearing a protective tooth guard is helpful in avoiding dental injury.

RESUMPTION OF SINGING AFTER ENDOTRACHEAL INTUBATION

Although significant injury to the larynx is unlikely after a general anesthetic, the entire experience is likely to affect normal function at least minimally. These minor effects include mild sore throat, dry throat, decreased level of alertness (sedation), mild vocal fold edema, decreased sensation, susceptibility to nausea, decreased muscle strength, poor respiration, and overall fatigue. Additionally, many patients will be treated with narcotic analgesics that sedate, decrease motor function, and cause nausea. Any combination of these factors may adversely affect singing technique. It is, therefore, advisable that the singer abstain from singing of any sort until these various symptoms have completely resolved. If the speaking voice is affected in any way, the singer should seek an otolaryngologic evaluation immediately. If the speaking voice is normal, the singer can resume singing with

typical warm-up exercises. Should there be any abnormalities with the singing voice, again, otolaryngologic evaluation is indicated immediately. Assuming that all is well with both speaking and singing voice, the singer can carefully resume full activity. Any problems discovered in the postoperative period will alter this plan, of course. Most singers will be able to resume singing without medical or SLP intervention after a routine endotracheal intubation. The most conservative approach is that described by Loucks discussed above.[1] Also, the various surgeries discussed in the remainder of this chapter add other factors that influence when a vocalist can resume full activity and these issues are described below.

SURGERY OF THE HEAD, NECK, AND UPPER CHEST

Paralysis of one or both vocal folds can result from a variety of surgical procedures in the neck and chest. The most common of these are thyroid and parathyroid surgeries, anterior approach to the cervical vertebrae, and carotid endarterectomy. The likelihood of a permanent paralysis after thyroid surgery is less than 5%.[10] For carotid endarterectomy, this number is less than 0.5%.[11] Anterior approach to the cervical vertebrae has been reported by Jung to have an incidence of vocal fold paralysis as high as 24% immediately after surgery and 11.3% at 3 months, whereas others have reported only a 1.4% rate.[12,13] Additionally, dysphagia after this surgery is reportedly as high as 50% at 1 month and still 12.5% at 1 year.[14] Apfelbaum has suggested that decreasing the ET tube cuff pressure after the retractors have been placed will reduce the likelihood of a recurrent laryngeal nerve (RLN) injury.[15] For each of these procedures, the surgeon must counsel the patient about this potential, and likely career-ending, complication. A frank discussion of the likelihood of this problem and the surgeon's own experience may frighten the patient, or reassure her or him that it is unlikely to occur. Use of an ET tube with electromyography (EMG) capabilities may be helpful in avoiding injury to the vagus or RLNs.[10] Injury to the superior laryngeal nerve will impair high pitch vocalization.[16] This is more likely to occur with surgeries that put the vagus nerve at risk (carotid endarterectomy or skull base surgery) or with thyroid surgery. During thyroid or parathyroid surgery, the strap muscles, which control the position of the larynx in the neck during phonation and swallowing are retracted and sometimes cut. Care should be taken to avoid cutting or denervating these muscles as this may adversely affect pitch control.[6,17]

Surgery in the mediastinum (mediastinoscopy with biopsy, thymectomy) can also result in injury to the RLN as can any surgery of the upper chest.[18] The left RLN is at greater risk than the right due to its longer course. Surgery of the aortic arch, which is usually emergent, will often result in injury to the left RLN. Surgery for lung cancer has become a more common cause of surgically caused unilateral vocal fold paralysis in several series.[19,20] Unfortunately, in these cases, preservation of life often supercedes preservation of the normal voice.

Skull base surgery puts at risk a number of cranial nerves (CN) including nerves V, VII, VIII, IX, X, XI, and XII. The other cranial nerves can also be damaged, depending on the exact area where the surgery takes place, but those listed are most prone to injury that could adversely affect voice and articulation. Skull base surgery is usually performed for removal of tumors, both benign and malignant, as well as vascular anomalies. The need to preserve life in these cases often takes precedence over maintaining function, but the professional voice user must be made aware of the potential injuries and sequelae before surgery is undertaken. As discussed above, injury of the vagus nerve (CN X) will result in a paralyzed vocal fold with resultant breathy, weak voice and possible aspiration. A high vagal injury will also cause paralysis of one side of the soft palate with velopharyngeal incompetence, (hypernasal voice and nasal regurgitation of liquids). The pharynx and tongue base receive sensory and motor innervation from the glossopharyngeal nerve (CN IX). Injury to this nerve affects swallowing and articulation. Likewise, injury to the hypoglossal nerve (CN XII) causes paralysis of the ipsilateral anterior two-thirds of the tongue and a resultant problem with articulation, although people compensate surprisingly well from this injury even without recovery of nerve function, at least with regard to speaking and swallowing. Whether an isolated CN XII paralysis would make it impossible to sing well is not known. Unfortunately, large skull base resections often result in injury to sev-

eral of these nerves at once which results in patients with severe dysphagia and dysarthria.

Rhytidectomy (face-lift) and salivary gland surgery puts the facial nerve (CN VII) at risk. Permanent injury with rhytidectomy is rare (0.1%) and temporary injuries are only 3%.[21] An injury to that nerve causes paralysis of different parts of the face and may include the orbicularis oris muscle which controls the lips. This would impair articulation. Injury to other branches of the facial nerve causes a cosmetic deformity and may lead to ocular problems. The amount of tightness of the facial structures after rhytidectomy may adversely influence a singer's technique and should be taken into account by the surgeon and the patient when he or she resumes singing.[4,6]

Injury to acoustic and vestibular nerves (CN VIII) will cause unilateral sensorineural hearing loss and imbalance and/or vertigo, respectively. These injuries are most likely during surgery of the temporal bone for chronic ear disease or tumors that arise from CN VIII itself, most commonly the acoustic neuroma. Hearing loss is obviously a problem for a vocalist, although the other ear is usually fully functional and adequate. The dysfunction of the vestibular system, however, can be disabling for an extended period of time, interfering with balance.

Surgery for chronic ear disease (mastoidectomy) also puts the entire facial nerve at risk. Injury results in paralysis of the entire side of the face with possible damage to the eye and an obvious cosmetic problem as discussed above.

SURGERY OF THE VOCAL TRACT

The vocal tract includes all the spaces above the vocal folds including all of the pharynx, the oral cavity and lips, nasal cavities, and paranasal sinuses. The vocal tract is the resonating chamber for the voice and is as important as the vocal folds and may account more for the individual quality of one's voice than the vocal folds. Commonly performed surgeries that can affect the vocal tract include tonsillectomy, adenoidectomy, septoplasty, rhinoplasty, inferior turbinate surgery, sinus surgery, and a variety of procedures for snoring and sleep apnea that involve the palate, oropharynx, and tongue base.

The adenoids are usually removed due to large size and obstruction of the nasopharynx, which causes the voice to be hyponasal. Removal almost always results in a better voice with better balance between oral and nasal resonance with the person able to control this with the soft palate. Problems arise when the soft palate is not normal, either weak or too short, and unable to effectively close off the nasopharynx when needed. This leads to velopharyngeal insufficiency with a hypernasal voice and nasal regurgitation of liquids similar to when the palate is paralyzed. If the adenoids are not significantly enlarged and are being removed due to chronic adenotonsillitis, usually no change in voice occurs. Adenoid surgery is uncommon in adults and is usually performed in children.

Tonsillectomy is performed because of chronic infections or as part of treatment for obstructive sleep apnea. If the tonsils are quite large, they can cause muffling of the voice or a "hot potato" voice. Removal clears up the voice. Changes have been noted in the speech spectrum following tonsillectomy by some authors and no changes noted by others.[22,23] In general these have been very mild, often beneficial, and frequently return to preoperative status.[24,25] The risk of removing tonsils as it relates to the singer is that scarring may occur as the tonsillar fossae heal that could affect the vocal tract. Fortunately this rarely occurs. The surgeon must take care to avoid damaging the fascia surrounding the tonsillar capsule and the pharyngeal constrictor muscles deep to that fascia. A careful dissection in the appropriate plane should avoid that complication.[6] Scarring could affect the singer's ability to easily change the shape of the vocal tract and may affect the resultant sound or increase the effort required to achieve a certain sound. The decision to undergo tonsillectomy at all must be based on the reason it is being done. If a person is experiencing frequent and/or prolonged bouts of tonsillitis, he or she is likely to be feeling poorly often and is likely to miss much work. This will affect both the patient's singing and ability to progress with his or her career. Singers who are always sick do not succeed. After surgery, the singer should not resume singing until the pharynx is completely healed, which often takes a month. While the pharynx is healing, pain with swallowing and phonation is common. This negative feedback may cause the singer to alter what is otherwise excellent singing technique to avoid the pain. This could lead to an undesirable change in technique. The singer should wait until he or she is comfortable with the changes in sensation and resonance before arranging an important engagement. The time that it takes to return to performing may vary and it is important to inform the singer of this.[26]

Sleep apnea is a condition in which the airway collapses while one is asleep blocking the flow of air through the throat. The person must wake up slightly, restore muscle tone in the throat, which opens the throat, breathing resumes, the person falls back asleep, snores, obstructs, and the cycle repeats. This results in a less than restful sleep and fatigue during the day. The problem is often due to large tonsils, a long soft palate, or a posteriorly positioned or short mandible which puts the tongue farther posteriorly. These people are often obese.

Surgery for sleep apnea aims to increase the diameter of the airway through the throat. To achieve this, surgery must involve the soft palate, pharyngeal walls, tonsils, tongue base, and often the nasal cavities, in other words, the entire vocal tract. As discussed above for adenoidectomy, soft palate paralysis, and tonsillectomy, alteration of these structures may have an effect on the voice or the effort required to produce a particular sound.[6]

Sleep apnea is a serious condition that can lead to hypertension, heart disease, stroke, and auto accidents (from falling asleep while driving). It is a condition that warrants treatment either with continuous positive airway pressure through the nose (nasal CPAP) or surgery. If a patient chooses CPAP, she or he should arrange to have a humidifying device attached so that it will not dry the vocal tract. Weight loss is usually an important component of treatment as well. The risks of the treatment must be weighed against the potential complications of untreated sleep apnea when deciding on how to proceed.[26]

In most cases, there are no complications following such surgery and no excessive scarring. As above for tonsillectomy, the patient should be counseled not to resume singing for at least 1 month after the surgery.

Surgery of the nose is done either for obstruction or cosmetics or both. When the indication is the former, improving the patency of the nasal cavities can only have a positive effect on the voice. This surgery is usually a septoplasty as well as a procedure to decrease the size of the inferior nasal turbinates.[24] A cosmetic rhinoplasty is done to improve the appearance of the nose. Often this involves making it smaller. This can result in a narrower internal nasal airway and nasal obstruction. A hyponasal (less than normal nasal resonance) voice may be the outcome. This can be very difficult to repair. The singer must make it clear that no compromise of nasal airflow can occur as a result of the rhinoplasty. Augmentation of the nose to change its shape, rather than aggressive reduction, is less likely to cause a smaller nasal airway. A complication of septal surgery, perforation, can cause crusting and whistling, especially during deep inspiration. This would be particularly troublesome for a vocalist.[4] Fortunately, these complications are rare, particularly if the surgery is performed by an otolaryngologist. In general, cosmetic surgery can safely be performed on singers with little to no risk. Like all surgeries, the potential benefits of cosmetic surgery should be weighed against the risks.[6]

Surgery to remove nasal polyps or remove chronically inflamed sinus tissue will also usually help nasal resonance. This surgery has become much less invasive and painful since the advent of telescopes/endoscopes that allow an excellent magnified view of the inside of the nose and sinuses. The postoperative period is still an uncomfortable time, however, with the need for frequent nasal irrigation and debridement. It is wise not to make any significant performance commitments for the first month after surgery, but it is safe to continue singing.

SURGERY OF THE CHEST WALL AND ABDOMEN

The chest wall, diaphragm, and abdominal muscles are all structures that generate the power that drives the voice. Although surgery is rarely aimed directly at these structures, they are frequently traversed en route to other organs that are the target of the surgeon. In the past, large incisions were always necessary to access the intrathoracic or intra-abdominal cavities. These approaches involved many layers of muscle and sometimes cutting or separation of ribs and resulted in very painful, often slow-healing wounds that made every breath or cough an unpleasant experience. Needless to say, providing proper breath support to the voice is difficult, if not impossible, in this situation. After healing, that function should be restored, likely

in full. Overexertion or too early resumption of physical activities could also lead to development of incisional hernias that, themselves, can continue to impair proper breathing and support and may require further surgery to repair.[6]

Currently, many abdominal surgeries are accomplished with a laparoscopic approach in which several small incisions are made through the abdominal wall to allow the passage of a telescope and several instruments. The resultant wounds are much less painful and heal much faster. This allows the singer to be able to resume singing with proper technique much earlier. The operations frequently performed with this approach include cholecystectomy, appendectomy, gastric fundoplication, and many gynecologic procedures. Within the chest, thoracoscopy allows biopsies without causing severe damage to the chest wall. The smaller wounds that result will still cause significant pain with respiration, but should heal much faster than traditional thoracotomy incisions.

Unfortunately, many medical conditions, most notably cancer, still require the more traditional open approach to both the chest and abdomen. The surgeon is expected to use the approach that will provide adequate exposure while causing minimal morbidity afterward, but the patient should always discuss the approach that will be used as well as the activity limitations after the surgery, keeping in mind that the severity of his or her medical condition may supercede concerns about singing. Because abdominal support is very important in the production of voice, the singer should make sure that abdominal strength has returned prior to a performance or aggressive rehearsing or practice. With large chest and abdominal incisions, this may take months.

SURGERY OF THE MUSCULOSKELETAL SYSTEM

Proper posture and stance contribute to efficient vocalization. Injuries to the extremities or back may affect this aspect of a singer's technique. Likewise, surgery to repair such an injury can have the same effect as the original injury on technique.

If a singer is experiencing musculoskeletal pain, he must be cognizant of how he might change his stance and how he might tense muscles that would ordinarily be relaxed while singing. Excess tension anywhere above the waist can lead to strain in the cervical musculature, the strap muscles, and finally lead to vocal fatigue and pain when singing.

Should surgery for a musculoskeletal problem be considered, it is wise for the surgeon and patient to understand thoroughly how the resultant wound will affect the simplest of activities, such as standing. The patient should have a clear understanding of how long the recuperative period is likely to be, to plan for upcoming performances.[6] This will vary dramatically, depending on the type of surgery (eg, back versus hip versus foot surgery).

Much surgery of the extremities can be done with regional anesthesia blocks or a spinal anesthetic. This avoids the need for endotracheal intubation and potential injury to the vocal folds. This should be discussed with the surgeon and anesthesiologist prior to surgery as discussed at the beginning of this chapter.

REFERENCES

1. Loucks TMJ, Duff D, Wong JH, Finley-Detweiler R. The vocal athlete and endotracheal intubation: A management protocol. *J Voice*. 1998;12:349-359.

2. Peppard S, Dickens J. Laryngeal injury following short-term intubation. *Ann Otol Rhinol Laryngol*. 1983;92:327-330.

3. Proschel U, Eysholdt U. Kurzzeit-Veranderungen an Kehlkopf und Stimme nach Intubation. *Laryngo Rhinol Otol*. 1993;72:93-97.

4. Spiegel JR, Sataloff RT, Hawkshaw M. Plastic surgery in professional voice users: special considerations. *J Voice*. 1990;4:86-90.

5. Powner DJ. Airway considerations for professional singers—a survey of expert opinion. *J Voice*. 2002; 16:488-494.

6. Benninger MS. Medical disorders in the vocal artist. In: Benninger M, Jacobson B, Johnson A, eds. *Vocal Arts Medicine: The Care and Prevention of Professional Voice Disorders*. New York, NY: Thieme Medical Publishers, Inc; 1994.

7. Harris TM, Johnston DF, Collins SRC, Heath ML. A new general anaesthetic technique for use in singers: the brain laryngeal mask airway versus endotracheal intubation. *J Voice*. 1990;4:81-85.

8. Lee S, Hong K, Choe H, Song H. Comparison of the effects of the laryngeal mask airway and endotracheal intubation on vocal function. *Br J Anaesth*. 1993;71:648-650.

9. Inomata S, Nishikawa T, Suga A, et al: Transient bilateral vocal cord paralysis after insertion of a laryngeal mask airway. *Anesthesiology*. 1995;82: 787-788.

10. Hermann M, Hellebart C, Freissmuth M. Neuromonitoring in thyroid surgery: prospective evaluation of intraoperative electrophysiological responses for the prediction of recurrent laryngeal nerve injury [see comment]. *Ann Surg*. 2004;240: 9-17.

11. Sannella NA, Tober RL, Cipro RP, et al. Vocal cord paralysis following carotid endarterectomy: the paradox of return to function. *Ann Vasc Surg*. 1990;4:42-45.

12. Jung A, Schramm J, Lehnerdt K, Herberhold C. Recurrent laryngeal nerve palsy during anterior cervical spine surgery: a prospective study. *J Neurosurg Spine*. 2005;2:123-127.

13. Baron EM, Soliman AM, Gaughan JP, Simpson L, Young WF. Dysphagia, hoarseness, and unilateral true vocal fold motion impairment following anterior cervical diskectomy and fusion. *Ann Otol Rhinol Laryngol*. 2003;112:921-926.

14. Bazaz R, Lee MJ, Yoo JU. Incidence of dysphagia after anterior cervical spine surgery: a prospective study. *Spine*. 2002;27:2453-2458.

15. Apfelbaum RI, Kriskovich MD, Haller JR. On the incidence, cause and prevention of recurrent laryngeal nerve palsies during anterior cervical spine surgery. *Spine*. 2000;25:2906-2912.

16. Dursun G, Sataloff RT, Spiegel JR, Mandel S, Heuer RJ, Rosen DC. Superior laryngeal nerve paresis and paralysis. *J Voice*. 1996;10:206-211.

17. Rubin JS, Korovin GS, Epstein R. Special considerations for the professional voice user. In: Rubin JS, Sataloff RT, Korovin GS, eds. *Diagnosis and Treatment of Voice Disorders*. 2nd ed. Clifton Park, NY: Thomson Delmar Learning; 2003.

18. Widstrom A. Palsy of the recurrent nerve following mediastinoscopy. *Chest*. 1975;67:365-366.

19. Gardner GM, Shaari CM, Parnes SM. Long-term morbidity and mortality in patients undergoing surgery for unilateral vocal cord paralysis. *Laryngoscope*. 1992;102:501-508.

20. Benninger MS, Gillen JB, Altman JS. Changing etiology of vocal fold immobility. *Laryngoscope*. 1998; 108:1346-1350.

21. Sullivan CS, Masin J, Maniglia AJ, Stepnick DW. Complications of rhytidectomy in an otolaryngology training program. *Laryngoscope.* 1999;109: 198-203.

22. Saida H, Hirose H. Acoustic changes in voice after tonsillectomy. *Acta Otolaryngol Suppl.* 1996;523: 239-241.

23. Chuma AV, Cacace AT, Rosen R, Feustel P, Koltai PJ. Effects of tonsillectomy and/or adenoidectomy on vocal function: laryngeal supralaryngeal and perceptual characteristics. *Int J Ped Otorhinolaryngol.* 1999;47:1-9.

24. Behrman A. Shikowitz MJ. Dailey S. The effect of upper airway surgery on voice. *Otolaryngol Head Neck Surg.* 2002;127:36-42.

25. Ilk GH, Erogul O, Satar B, Ozkaptan Y. Effects of tonsillectomy on speech spectrum. *J Voice.* 2002; 16:580-586.

26. Gardner GM, Benninger MS. Sleep disorders and the vocalist . *J Singing.* 1997:53:45-48.

Chapter 23

POSTOPERATIVE VOICE CARE OF THE SINGER

Robert H. Ossoff
Thomas F. Cleveland

Postoperative care of singers is important to the long-term success of surgery. Although the approach may vary with the practitioner, a multidisciplinary approach including the surgeon, speech-language pathologist (SLP), and singing voice specialist (SVS), provides the thorough care necessary for postsurgery treatment. Whatever the postsurgery strategy, the goal must be to rehabilitate and equip the singer with the tools necessary to return to optimal voice use as soon as possible. This chapter presents concepts and strategies for the rehabilitation of singers postsurgery. The chapter includes postsurgery and medical protocols, as well as strategies and techniques necessary for equipping the patient with skills that will help the singer minimize the opportunity for reinjury.

TREATMENT STRATEGIES

Postsurgery outcome depends on excellent presurgery advice, screening, and treatment. The screening and treatment received by the patient presurgery can, in some cases, obviate the need for surgery, but in all cases, it can jump-start the postsurgery intervention by making singers familiar with the treatment protocols. Once the patient has completed surgery, and aside

from those noted in the section on exceptions, the postoperative protocol is the same for all benign vocal fold lesions, including vascular lesions that have been addressed via laser.

THE POSTOPERATIVE PROTOCOL

The following protocol is followed by the authors of this chapter. It is one that we have found to be successful over many years of caring for such patients. However, it is a guide and there are other approaches that have been used in successful practices. Because it is delivered in a 4-stage process over a 3-month period, measured postoperative care can accomplish several important goals. First, it can prevent the misuse/abuse of the voice that caused the problem initially, and thereby give the patient down-time for healing. Second, it can give the voice care team time to effect changes in voice production that will help the singer minimize the chances for recurrence. Third, programmed visits for ongoing evaluation can help detect problems early and solve them before they really get started. In the following protocol, postsurgery visits occur at 2 weeks, 4 weeks, 8 weeks, and 12 weeks and coincide with the treatment stages given below.

Stage 1

During the first stage, the patient is placed on voice rest for a period of 2 weeks immediately after surgery. The 2 weeks are the standard that we have used, although the amount of voice rest needed has been debated and excellent surgeons and voice teams have had success with shorter periods of postoperative voice rest. This stage can be a welcome event for a busy patient who needs rest and recuperation, but it can severely test the resolve of a performer to be completely quiet for 2 weeks. To assist the patient with those who would interrupt the singer's silence, the patient receives a button informing an observer that the patient is on voice rest and unable to communicate orally. The phrasing on the button is important because nonverbal behavior typically evokes a similar behavior from the person with whom the patient is seeking to communicate. The button should read as follows: "I am on voice rest and therefore cannot speak, but I can hear so please speak to me in a normal fashion." The interested reader can find in Appendix 23-1 a page of reactions one patient received to her voiceless behavior. It is important for the physician to realize the responses patients receive on voice rest to help them be prepared for any eventuality. Nonetheless, this time of no voice use is crucial to the healing process, if for no other reason than keeping the patient from employing the abusive behaviors that may have caused the initial problem.

Stage 2

At the end of week 2, the patient returns to the clinic for a stroboscopic evaluation and physician examination. At this time, provided the patient has healed sufficiently, the patient is taken off voice rest by a speech-language pathologist, and given instructions as to how the voice is to be used over the coming 2 weeks. The written directions that accompany any verbal instructions by the SLP are given in Appendix 23-2. Essentially, when the patient is taken off voice rest, the protocol needs to be simple and easy for the patient to follow. Although this is also somewhat subjective to differences in practice type, we recommend that the first day should have only 10 minutes of voice use, 5 in the morning and 5 in the afternoon. The next day, the voice use is doubled, and the use continues to double each day thereafter until the patient reaches normal voice use, which occurs by the end of the first week. The patient is precluded from telephone use until the end of the third week and is cautioned not to use the singing voice until the end of the fourth week. Further directives encourage the patient's avoidance of voice use at the extremes, yelling, screaming, and throat clearing. Between weeks 2 and 4, the patient has at least one visit with the speech-language pathologist who further evaluates the singer's voice and makes necessary corrections in the speaking voice.

Stage 3

The third stage is the reintroduction and rehabilitation of the speech and singing voice which takes place between weeks 4 and 12. During this time, the speech-language pathologist and the singing voice specialist assist the patient in the use of the voice in a less costly fashion. The protocol includes education and treatment in the care of the voice or vocal hygiene and modification of the physiology of voice production. The psychological approach taken by the SLP and the SVS during this stage is crucial to the success of the intervention. For instance, a patient who has had a successful singing career does not want to be told that everything he did prior to the surgery was wrong. As the patient made a lot of money singing that way, he will not want to jeopardize his career by changing the way he sounds, as this could end his career. The patient should be informed that he will not be asked to make any changes in his voice production, but will be given some more choices as to how to produce his sound. Imagine how this approach will register with the singer. If told he must change, he will be resistant, but if told he will be given more choices, the singer will be motivated to listen further and explore the possibilities. A patient who depends on his voice for primary livelihood can be very anxious during this stage and want to return to voice use sooner than the protocol allows. However, the patient needs to agree in advance of the surgery to the duration of the postsurgery rehabilitation period and not violate that time commitment.

Stage 4

The fourth stage occurs after week 12 and encompasses the reintroduction of the singer to his or her career. Although some practices have introduced this stage earlier in carefully selected patients, we have followed these protocols after years of successful experience. We estimate that the singer's vocal health is typically far better at this point than it has been for several months, and may be approximately 80% of capacity. Additional percentage points will be gained over the next 18 to 24 months, according to the singers themselves. The singers will be given directives including the incorporation of voice rest times during the show, for example, to add variety to the show by not singing every song but by including a guitar solo, a drum solo, and so forth after every three or four songs. During this time, the singer is able to rest the voice, rehydrate, and get ready for the next group of songs. "Meet and greet" times before or after the show can be dangerous for the singer. Exposure to illness can he heightened, and the noisy environment in which the events occur can compromise the singing voice before the show gets started. Washing the hands after the "meet and greet" can help the patient avoid infections, and managing the surroundings of the "meet and greet" can reduce the chance for injury. By this time, 3 months postsurgery, the patient is allowed to take up professional engagements in a normal fashion. It is hoped that at this time the patient has incorporated the concepts and techniques presented in sessions with the SLP and the SVS.

SECONDARY POSTOPERATIVE CARE

Secondary postop care begins at the end of the third month and singers are re-examined every 6 months for the next 2 years. This re-examination includes stroboscopy each visit, as needed, with intermittent visits to the SLP and the singing voice specialist, as required.

EXCEPTIONS TO THE PRIMARY CARE PLAN

Delayed healing or complications can lengthen any stage of the postoperative care protocol. Complications are usually caused by acute laryngitis due to upper respiratory infection or patient noncompliance to postsurgery protocol. In some rare cases a microhemorrhage can occur requiring the reintroduction of voice rest or limited voice use. The interested reader will find a case study in Appendix 23–3 of a patient who developed complications during his rehabilitation. This case study reveals how complications can postpone the introduction of voice use and singing for an undetermined time, a change that is usually agreed upon by the surgeon, the SLP and the SVS, and the patient.

MEDICATIONS

Patients who are not already on reflux medications prior to surgery are usually given proton pump inhibitors postsurgery. In addition, guaifenesin, 1200 mg twice a day, is standard. Antibiotics are typically not needed and Loratab is given for tongue pain. For patients who develop edema due to postsurgery complications, steroids may be necessary. Depending on the etiology, degree, and frequency, vascular changes are usually addressed with voice rest.

SURGICAL SIDE EFFECTS

Although rare, neuropraxia of the tongue can occur and can manifest as parathesia, ageusia, or gustatory metalica.[1] The neuropraxia subsides in a few days to weeks, but in extremely rare cares, can last for up to 6 months. Singers are told of the possibility of this side effect prior to surgery.

STROBOSCOPY IN THE HEALING PROCESS

Stroboscopy postsurgery provides two important functions. First, reviewing the vibratory patterns of the vocal folds is essential to understanding the healing of the folds. The color, edema, mucosal wave, and vertical phase difference signal certain plateaus of healing. Individuals will respond differently, depending on the degree of surgery, and the patient's own personal healing factors. Stroboscopy is useful in helping to determine timing of onset of vocalization, progression of voice use, or later timing of returning to performance.

Second, the stroboscopic exam provides patients with a yardstick to show improvement in their vocal folds. During the healing process, and even thereafter, any and every twinge of discomfort in the throat can strike fear in the mind of singers making them wonder if they have suffered reinjury. The stroboscopy can help restore a singer's confidence by showing that the folds continue to heal well.

THE ROLE OF THE SLP AND THE SVS

Once the surgery is performed, the SLP and SVS must take the repaired vocal folds, and, over time, correct the technical issues that likely caused the problem initially. Those service providers who do it best are able to sell the concepts and techniques to the singer in a productive, nonthreatening manner, always having the best interest of the singer at heart. Most SLP and SVS have an arsenal of techniques to assist with technical issues.

SPECIAL CONSIDERATIONS FOR SINGERS

Singer surgery affects not only the life of the singer, but a wide array of ancillary people as well. Band members, church congregations, opera companies, management, record companies, and a vast population of fans waiting for the singer to return to professional life as soon as possible, can create undue pressure on the singer. Consequently, singers may want to skip some of the phases of the postoperative protocol and return to work. Regardless, the singer must stay within the time lines of the protocol and not rush the rehabilitation process.

One of the greatest concerns of the singer postsurgery is, "Will I ever sing again?" and if so, "What can I do to keep from injuring myself again?" As a result, singers may use the voice incorrectly, trying to protect it, not realizing that they are actually doing more harm than good. They may have a tendency to speak or sing too softly, thinking that this will protect the voice. Often this creates an underclosure of the folds, preventing efficiency, while promoting voice fatigue and possibly reinjury. The SLP and the SVS need to help the patient learn to monitor voice use efficiency and help prevent this faulty production.

The singer may already have a lack of confidence due to the difficulties experienced prior to surgery. The SLP and the SVS work to assist the singer in regaining lost confidence.

SUMMARY

The postsurgery regimen is extremely important to the success of the surgery and the voice restoration of the singer. A multidisciplinary team, composed of at least a laryngologist, speech-language pathologist, and a singing voice specialist, each with his or her own area of responsibility, should provide the expertise needed for postoperative care. Singers who receive this care have the greatest opportunity to re-enter their career and sustain that career with fewer problems. Nevertheless, just as professional athletes have the need for ongoing monitored care received from coaches, trainers, and physicians, singers should continue to avail themselves of the highest level of care from teams that are trained and experienced in the appropriate disciplines for singers.

REFERENCE

1. Rosen CA, Andrade PA, Scheffel L BA, Buckmire R. Oropharyngeal complications of suspension laryngoscopy: a prospective study. *Laryngoscope*. 2005; 115:1681–1684.

APPENDIX 23-1

Twelve Things I Learned While Being Mute

The following list was composed by a singer after being on voice rest for 2 weeks.

1. Sales clerks yell at you, thinking you are deaf.
2. Even the cat doesn't "meow" to you anymore.
3. Cashiers don't ever count out your change to you.
4. It takes two sandwich creme cookies to rid your voice of the medicine you take. (The patient is probably referring to the oral steroids she was taking at the time.)
5. Friends think they are supposed to write notes back to you instead of answering audibly.
6. A ringing phone can exasperate you or teach you patience.
7. Store employees think you are "dumb" (in more ways than one) and doubt you.
8. You become a more accomplished planner and writer.
9. People think you know sign language, when all you know is motions.
10. The reason deaf people use such exaggerated facial and hand gestures is to express feeling.
11. You are still the same person on the inside—most people just treat you differently.
12. How fortunate I have been for 43 years to have had the blessing of good health.

APPENDIX 23-2

Postoperative Guidelines for Voice Use

First post-op visit—speech-language pathologist takes you off voice rest.

Guidelines for Gradual Return to Voice Use

	AM	PM
Post-op visit	5 minutes	5 minutes
2nd day	10 minutes	10 minutes
3rd day	20 minutes	20 minutes
4th day	45 minutes	45 minutes
5th day	1 hour	1 hour
6th day	2 to 4 hours spread over the day	
7th day	4 to 6 hours spread over the day	

8th day onward: add ½ hour a day to the total talking time.

These are the maximum amounts of cumulative voice use each day.

This is a progression. If you have any trouble, stop and do not progress until you are ready. Everyone heals at different rates.

Remember:

Use an easy, natural voice.

No phone use until the end of the third week after surgery.

Always avoid extremes—yelling, singing, throat clearing, talking for a long period of time without a break, heavy lifting, and strenuous exercise.

If any pain, fatigue, hoarseness call the speech-language pathologist or physician.

Drink lots of water, no caffeine, no alcohol.

Take vocal breaks—for 20 minutes of use, take a 10-minute break.

Specific instructions and exercises will be given to you by your speech-language pathologist.

APPENDIX 23-3

Case Study

Patient presented 07/14 with Right TVF vascular polyp.
Reported loss of upper and lower range, voice fatigue, and hoarseness.

Pt had been placed on 20 mg of Nexium and Humibid by the referring physician. 07/29. DML microflap excision. Acoustic and airflow measures taken presurgery. VHI and SF-36 taken. See Figures 23-1 and 23-2.

Figure 23-1. Preoperative photo of vocal folds.

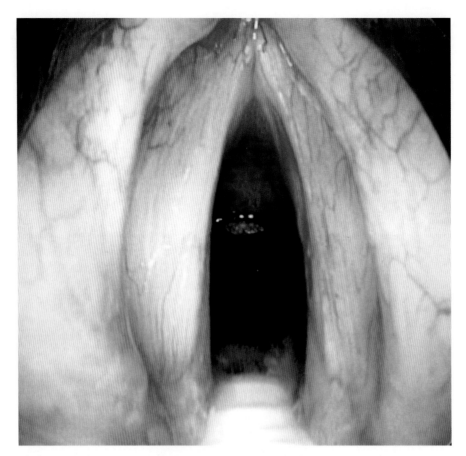

Figure 23–2. Postoperative photo of the vocal folds.

08/14/ pt was healing well. Placed on normal rehab program with SLP.

08/26/ there was reduced mucosal wave on the R, VPD was beginning to return. Perceptually the voice was slightly hoarse and slightly breathy. Pt work leave was continued until 09/13/.

POSTOPERATIVE VOICE CARE OF THE SINGER

09/29/ the voice was hoarse and the pt reported fatigue by the end of the day. Still had stiffness with divot on the right TVF. A-P squeeze at the upper F_0. R reduction in wave. See Figure 23-3.

Figure 23-3. Vocal fold appearance showing divot on right vocal fold (9/29).

11/03/ recurrent polyp R. Stay on meds, modified voiceuse. See exam (Figure 23–4) below.

12/01/ pt improving, lesion R improved, wave improving, microphone approved so pt to use microphone in work.

03/29/ R TVF continues to improve, edema R, stay on meds and continue therapy.

09/09/ slight erythema medial edge R. Obvious wave B, obvious VPD B, good closure, stay on meds, and therapy.

Figure 23–4. Recurrent polyp (11/03).

10/03/ TVF healing well. See Figure 23-5.

10/27/ re-examined. Polyp lower leading edge R returned, pitch lower than normal and voice was slightly rough, erythema R. Pt had URI with cough, yellow-green production. Placed on voice rest 1 week, augmentin 875 mg × 10 days, prednisone 40 mg for 4 days, taper for 4 days. Return in 7 to 10 days.

11/17/ no evidence of recurrent polyp. Patient has no complaints.

Figure 23-5. Vocal fold healing well (10/03).

Part VI

Building a Professional Voice Practice

Chapter 24

THE PROFESSIONAL VOICE PRACTICE

Robert T. Sataloff

*E*ven for a well-trained laryngologist, the task of building a practice specializing in the care of voice professionals may seem daunting. However, with forethought, passion, and diligence, it should be possible to build an excellent and gratifying professional voice practice in most communities. In remote, rural areas, such a practice is unlikely to attract high volumes of metropolitan opera stars; but there are many other voice professionals who make up the majority of patients in the practices of most laryngologists who specialize in voice. Such patients may include teachers, politicians, clergy, sales personnel, shop foremen, football quarterbacks, secretaries, choral conductors, avocational singers, actors in community theater, attorneys, physicians, and practitioners of many other disciplines who depend on vocal quality and endurance to succeed in their careers.

The "three As" of building a successful medical practice are known to virtually all interns and residents, and they should not be forgotten when establishing a voice practice. They are Availability, Affability, and Ability (in that order). Although this guidance has been given in somewhat "tongue in cheek" to medical trainees for decades, there is certainly some wisdom in it. A physician's availability to see voice patients in the office, perform in-hospital consultation, perhaps make the occasional house call or a theater call, and talk to referring professionals (not just physicians, but also nurses, speech-language pathologists, singing teachers, and others) is critical to establishing and maintaining a successful practice. Affability is important not only between physician and patient, but also between the physician and other physicians, other health care providers, secretaries, and everyone else with whom we interact. Every physician should be (and sound) enthusiastic every time he or she is called on to consult in the care of a patient. Although it has been said (only somewhat facetiously) that "ability" is less important than availability and affability in establishing a successful practice, ability is certainly central to caring for the challenging, fragile, and highly self-analytic population of professional voice users. In considering the establishment of a professional voice practice, this author takes the "three As" as given and thinks in terms of "three Cs": competence, communication, and compassion. Although all three Cs must be addressed, each practitioner has to decide the scope of his or her planned practice initially, and over time. If it is not possible to put all desired components of a voice practice in place initially, a 5-year strategic and business plan should be developed to codify strategies through which an optimal voice care environment will be established.

COMPETENCE

The Voice Care Team

Optimal voice care is delivered by an interdisciplinary team consisting of physicians and nonphysicians. The physician may be an otolaryngologist (a specialist who practices all aspects of ear, nose, and throat medicine) or a laryngologist, who specializes in voice disorders. The physician commonly collaborates with other professionals, such as a speech-language pathologist, singing voice specialist, acting-voice specialist, voice scientist, and others who constitute the voice care team.[1] Under the best of circumstances, all the members of the team (including the otolaryngologist) have received special training in not just the general aspects of their disciplines but also additional training in care of the voice. Although even the best training does not guarantee clinical excellence, it does improve the probability that a practitioner will provide superior, state-of-the-art voice care.

A voice care team is ordinarily under the direction of a physician who is usually a laryngologist. In addition to the physician who diagnoses and provides medical treatment for voice disorders, the team includes the speech-language pathologist, who provides voice therapy and attends to problems that affect the speaking voice; a phoniatrist in countries without speech-language pathologists; a singing voice specialist; an acting-voice specialist; a nurse and/or a physician's assistant; and consultant physicians in other specialties. It is helpful for patients to understand the background and role of each member of the voice team, as reviewed in a chapter by Sataloff et al,[1] from which part of this discussion has been modified. The core voice team may practice in one location or be located in different offices. Either model can serve patients well, as discussed below.

Otolaryngologist/Laryngologist

The leader of the voice care team is ordinarily an otolaryngologist. Laryngologists are otolaryngologists who specialize in care of disorders of the larynx and, in some cases, related problems such as swallowing. Most otolaryngologists' clinical practices include many or all components of the specialty, such as otology (disorders of the ear and related structures), laryngology, head and neck cancer, head and neck neoplasms (including benign or malignant lesions), facial plastic and reconstructive surgery, allergy and immunology, bronchoesophagology (lower airway and swallowing disorders), rhinology (nose, sinus, taste, and smell disorders), and pediatric otolaryngology (ear, nose, and throat disorders of children). Most otolaryngologists and laryngologists care for patients of all ages from early childhood through advanced years. Some otolaryngologists subspecialize, caring for disorders in just one or two areas of otolaryngology. This subspecialization can either be a keen interest in a specific area while still providing a broad range of ear, nose, and throat care, or the focused practice of only one or two of the subcomponents of otolaryngology. Laryngology is one such subspecialty.

Most of the physicians specializing in laryngology today did not receive laryngology fellowship training. That is always the case as a new field develops. Modern laryngology evolved out of an interest in caring for professional voice users, especially singers. The first comprehensive article guiding otolaryngologists on care of professional singers was published in 1981[2]; the first major modern American otolaryngology textbook with a chapter on care of the professional voice was published in 1986[3]; and the first comprehensive book care of the professional voice was published in 1991.[4] So, most of the senior laryngologists practicing at the turn of the 21st century were involved in the evolution of the field before fellowships were developed. Most fellowship training programs started in the 1990s, although a few informal fellowship programs existed in the 1980s and earlier. It is reasonable to expect most voice specialists who finished residency training the 1990s or later to have completed a fellowship in laryngology. There are approximately a dozen laryngology fellowship-training programs in the United States, and they are highly competitive. At present, completion of a fellowship is a reasonably good indicator of superior knowledge and clinical training in laryngology. Most laryngology fellowships include training in the diagnosis and treatment of voice disorders in adults and children, neurolaryngology, swallowing disorders, airway reconstruction, and laryngeal cancer. The training includes both medical diagnosis and treatment and sophisticated laryngeal surgery. Typically, laryngologists care for both routine and complex problems that affect the voice. Such problems include voice dysfunction associated with something as simple as a common cold, especially when it affects the voice of a professional singer or actor. However, laryngologists also are called on to diagnose and treat structural lesions such as nodules or polyps, prolonged infections of the vocal folds, cancer, traumatic injury from fracture or internal trauma (intubation injuries from anesthesia, vocal fold injuries from previous surgery), neurologic disorders, and other voice problems. The laryngologist is responsible for establishing a medical diagnosis and implementing or coordinating treatment for the patient. The laryngologist may prescribe medication, inject botulinum toxin, perform delicate microsurgery on the vocal folds, or operate through the neck on the laryngeal skeleton. He or she is also usually responsible for initiating evaluation by other members of the voice team and for generating referrals to other specialists as needed.

Laryngologists may practice in university medical centers or private offices; and in major cities in the United States, they are usually affiliated with a voice team including at least a speech-language pathologist, a singing voice specialist, and sometimes an acting-voice specialist or voice scientist. Laryngologists should also have, or have access to, a clinical voice laboratory with equipment to analyze the voice objectively and a stroboscope to visualize the vocal folds in slow motion. They should be familiar with physicians in other specialties who have an understanding of and interest in arts medicine. Even for patients with a voice disorder who are not singers and actors, such knowledge and sensitivity is important. Just as nonathletes benefit from the orthopedic expertise of a sports-medicine specialist, voice patients receive more expert care from physicians trained to treat singers, the "Olympic athletes" of the voice world.

Currently, there is no official additional certification for those who have completed a laryngology fellowship. However, there are organizations with which many of the leading laryngologists are affiliated. Essentially all laryngologists in the United States are fellows of the American Academy of Otolaryngology-Head and Neck Surgery (http://www.entnet.org), and laryngologists in other countries are members of their nation's analogous organizations. A few are also members of the American Laryngological Association (ALA), the most senior otolaryngology society in the United States

(http://www.alahns.org). The ALA also accepts "associate members" from other countries. Some laryngologists belong to the American Bronchoesophagological Association (http://www.abea.net), and the Voice Foundation (http://www.voicefoundation.org). The Voice Foundation was founded in 1969 and is the oldest organization dedicated entirely to voice education and research. It provides seed grants for research, sponsors an annual symposium on care of the professional voice since 1972, and fosters voice education through conferences, educational videotapes, books, and publications such as the *Journal of Voice* and the *Voice Foundation Newsletter*. In recent years, several countries have developed organizations similar to the Voice Foundation, such as the British, Canadian, and Australian Voice Foundations. Laryngologists in such countries are usually members of their national organization, and many are also members of the Voice Foundation (Philadelphia, Pa). Although membership in these organizations is not a guarantee of excellence in practice, it suggests interest and knowledge in laryngology, particularly voice disorders.

Speech-Language Pathologist

The speech-language pathologist is a certified, licensed health care professional, ordinarily with either a master's degree (MA or MS) or doctorate (PhD). Like otolaryngology, speech-language pathology is a broad field that includes care of patients who have had strokes or other neurologic problems affecting speech and swallowing, have undergone laryngectomy, have swallowing disorders, have articulation or stuttering problems, have craniofacial disorders, or have other related fluency disorders of speech. Some speech-language pathologists subspecialize in voice, which includes the care of voice disorders and swallowing disorders. The speech-language pathologist affiliated with a voice team is usually such a subspecialist and may call himself or herself a "voice pathologist" rather than a speech-language pathologist, although "voice pathologist" is not a term recognized officially by the American Speech-Language-Hearing Association (ASHA, the organization that certifies speech-language pathologists in the United States), yet. Relatively few speech-language pathology training programs provide extensive education in voice, and there are virtually no voice fellowships for speech-language pathologists. Many speech-language pathology training programs do not include even a single comprehensive course on voice disorders. Thus, it cannot be assumed that all speech-language pathologists are trained in or comfortable with caring for individuals with voice problems. Most acquire the subspecialty training they need through apprenticeships, extra courses, and symposia or by obtaining doctoral degrees that include voice-related research.

Speech-language pathologists are responsible for voice therapy and rehabilitation, which is analogous to physical therapy. The speech-language pathologist analyzes voice use and teaches proper voice support, relaxation, and voice placement to optimize use of the voice during speaking. A variety of techniques are utilized to accomplish this goal. Speech-language pathologists do not ordinarily work with the singing voice, although they are involved in the treatment of speaking voices of singers.

Speech-language pathologists may be found in universities, private offices, or freestanding speech and hearing centers. In the United States, most are members of ASHA and its voice-related special interest division (SID-3), which can be accessed on the Internet. Many speech-language pathologists with special interest in voice in the United States and elsewhere are also members of the Voice Foundation. Like otolaryngologists, speech-language pathologists who subspecialize in voice provide more incisive, state-of-the-art treatment for voice disorders than most general speech-language pathologists who care for patients with various problems encompassing the entire field. So, it is worthwhile for patients with voice disorders to seek out a subspecialist to improve the likelihood of a rapid, excellent treatment result. Referrals to speech-language pathologists specializing in voice are usually obtained through a laryngologist or otolaryngologist.

Phoniatrists

Phoniatrists do not exist in the United States, but they provide voice care in many European countries. The phoniatrist is a physician who is in some ways a hybrid of the laryngologist and speech-language pathologist. Phoniatrists receive medical training in diagnosis and treatment of voice, swallowing, and language disorders, including voice therapy; but they do not perform surgery. In countries with phoniatrists, surgery is performed by otolaryngologists. In many cases, the phoniatrist and otolaryngologist collaborate as a team, just as otolaryngologists and speech-language pathologists do in the United States and elsewhere. A physician who has completed training in phoniatry is generally well qualified to diagnose voice disorders and provide nonsurgical medical care, as well as voice therapy.

Singing Voice Specialist

The singing voice specialist is a singing teacher with special training equipping him or her to practice in a medical environment with patients who have sustained vocal injury. Most singing voice specialists have a degree in voice performance or pedagogy, although some have only extensive performing and teaching experience without a formal academic degree. Nearly all have professional performance experience, as well as extra training in laryngeal anatomy and physiology of phonation, training in the rehabilitation of injured voices, and other special education. The singing voice specialist must acquire knowledge of anatomy and physiology of the normal and disordered voice, a basic understanding of the principles of laryngology, familiarity with medications, training in the rehabilitation of injured voices, a fundamental knowledge of the principles and practices of speech-language pathology, and other special education. This information is not part of the traditional training of singing teachers. Moreover, so far there are no formal training or fellowship programs that assist singing teachers in becoming a singing voice specialist. Their training is acquired by apprenticeship and observation. Many take courses in speech-language pathology programs, but usually not as part of a formal degree or certification program,[5] because there is no certification of singing voice specialists. A few of the best singing voice specialists are also certified, licensed speech-language pathologists. This combination is optimal, provided the speech-language pathologist has sufficient experience and training not only as a performing artist but also as a teacher of singing. In patients with vocal injuries or problems, the fundamental approach to training the singing voice is different in important ways from that used by many teachers for healthy students. Hence, even an excellent and experienced voice teacher may harm an injured voice if he or she is not familiar with the special considerations for this population. In addition, most voice teachers do not feel comfortable working with a singer who has had a vocal injury or surgery.

Virtually all singing voice specialists are affiliated with voice care teams. Most are members of the National Association of Teachers of Singing (NATS), or the equivalent organization in another country, and of the Voice Foundation. In many cases, their practices are limited to work with injured voices. They work not only with singers, but also with other patients with voice disorders. As a member of the voice treatment team working with nonsingers, they help teach speakers of the "athletic" techniques utilized by singers for voice production. Singing is to speaking as running is to walking. When rehabilitating someone who has difficulty walking, if the person can be helped to jog or run, leg strength and endurance improve and walking rehabilitation is expedited. The singing voice specialist applies similar principles to voice rehabilitation in collaboration with the speech-language pathologist and other voice care team members.

Acting-Voice Specialist

Acting-voice trainers are also called voice coaches, drama voice teachers, and voice consultants. Traditionally, these professionals have been associated closely with the theater. Their skills have been utilized as a part of a medical voice team only since the mid-1990s.[6] Consequently, few acting-voice trainers have any medical experience; but their contributions have proven invaluable.

Acting-voice trainers use a variety of behavior modification techniques designed to enhance vocal communication, quality, projection, and endurance in theatrical settings. They train actors to speak or scream through eight shows a week, and/or theatrical runs that may last years, without tiring or causing injury to their voices. They also teach techniques for adding emotional expression to vocal delivery, and they work with body language and posture to optimize vocal production and communication of information. They may be a great asset to the voice team in teaching people how to apply the many skills learned through the speech-language pathologist and singing voice specialist to their everyday lives. Acting-voice

trainers are especially valuable for people who speak professionally such as teachers, lecturers, politicians, clergy, sales personnel, and others concerned with effective vocal delivery and endurance.

There are no formal programs to prepare acting-voice trainers to become acting-voice specialists and work in a medical milieu. Those who do receive training generally do so through apprenticeships and collaboration with medical voice care teams under the direction of a laryngologist, and in collaboration with speech-language pathologists and singing voice specialists.

Acting-voice trainers interested in working with voice patients are generally members of the Voice and Speech Trainers Association (VASTA) and the Voice Foundation.

Voice Scientist

Many voice centers include a voice laboratory that has equipment to measure phonatory and respiratory output. The clinical voice laboratory may be directed by a clinical speech pathologist, or by a clinical voice scientist. Voice scientists usually have a doctoral degree in communication science, physics, computer science or some related discipline. Many are certified speech-language pathologists. Some voice scientists devote their entire careers to laboratory research and are not involved in patient care. Others include clinical research among their efforts and can be extremely valuable members of the voice team. They are particularly skilled at gathering and analyzing objective data in the voice laboratory, assessing outcomes, ensuring reliability and validity of data, and in designing and facilitating clinical research to advance the field of voice care.

Nurse

Nurses are indispensable assets in medical offices, and they are important members of the voice team in many centers. Nurses who work closely with a laryngologist generally have vast experience in the diagnosis and treatment of voice disorders. They are wonderful information resources for patients and frequently provide much of the patient education in busy clinical settings. These nurses are usually members of the Society of Otolaryngology-Head and Neck Nurses (SOHN). Nurses with advanced knowledge and skills can become certified (by SOHN) and are identified as such by the initials "CORLN" (certified otolaryngologic nurse) after their names.

Nurse practitioners are advanced practice nurses with master's degrees, who are licensed to provide independent care for patients with selected medical problems. They are identified by the initials "CRNP" (certified registered nurse practitioner). They work in conjunction with a physician; but they can examine, diagnose, and treat selected problems relatively independently. A few nurse practitioners specialize in otolaryngology and work with voice teams. They ordinarily receive special training "on the job" from the otolaryngologist, and they provide care within their scope of practice. Nurse practitioners can also become members of SOHN, become certified through examination by SOHN, and on certification will also use the designation CORLN after their names.

Physician Assistants and Medical Assistants

Physician assistants, like nurse practitioners discussed above, function in association with a physician. Physician assistants graduate from a training program that usually lasts 4 years and teaches them various aspects of medical diagnosis and physical examination. They use the initials "PA" (physician assistant) after their names. They practice in conjunction with physicians but can perform examinations and treat patients independently. They are licensed in many states to write prescriptions. A few physician assistants specialize in otolaryngology, and a smaller number have had extensive training and experience in voice care. In collaboration with a laryngologist and voice teams, they are qualified to evaluate and treat patients with voice disorders.

Physician assistants should be distinguished from "medical assistants" who have less training and are qualified to assist in medical care and patient education but not to diagnose and treat patients independently. Medical assistants generally are trained to perform tasks such as phlebotomy and perform electrocardiograms. In a laryngology office, a good medical assistant can be trained to perform many other tasks such as taking histories, assisting with strobovideolaryngoscopy, and assisting during the performance of surgical procedures in the office, participating in research and other activities.

Consultant Medical Professionals

Otolaryngologists often refer voice patients for consultation with other medical professionals. Other specialists consulted commonly include neurologists, pulmonologists (lungs), gastroenterologists (stomach and intestinal system), psychologists, and psychiatrists. However, physicians in virtually any medical specialty may be called on to care for voice patients. Traditional and nontraditional ancillary medical personnel may also be involved in voice care, including nutritionists, physical therapists, chiropractors, osteopaths (for manipulation), acupuncturists, and others. Within virtually all of these fields, there are a select few professionals who have an interest in and an understanding of arts medicine. Just as caring for voice professionals (especially singers) involves special considerations and challenges for the otolaryngologist, caring for hand problems in a pianist or ankle problems in dancers also poses challenges for the orthopedic surgeon. Orthopedic surgeons, neurologists, pulmonologists, and others who are accustomed to working with performing artists (dancers, wind instrumentalists, etc) are most likely to have the insight, sensitivities, skills, and state-of-the-art information needed to provide optimal care to voice professionals. Many such physicians tend to be associated with arts-medicine centers or are performers themselves. There is no certification or broad-based national or international organization that helps to identify such physicians, although some are members of the Performing Arts Medicine Association (PAMA). In most fields, there are no formal artsmedicine training programs or associations. Physicians acquire such training through their own interest and initiative and through apprenticeship or observation with colleagues. If there is no arts-medicine center in the area in which a patient is seeking care, arts-medicine physicians are identified best by word of mouth or through arts-medicine-related Web sites. Referrals can be obtained through the local laryngologist or voice specialist or by consulting with eminent performing arts teachers in the community. For example, the leading private university and conservatory violin and piano teachers often know who the best hand specialists are; the wind instrument teachers know whom to see for neurologic and pulmonary problems that affect musicians; and dance teachers know the best foot-and-ankle physicians.

A Voice Clinic: Common Models

Although not necessary, it is ideal for the core members of a voice team (laryngologist, speech-language pathologist, singing voice specialist, acting-voice specialist, and voice scientist) to practice in the same building in close proximity. This arrangement facilitates communication among members of the voice team, allows team members to see patients simultaneously during portions of the evaluation and treatment, and facilitates interchange of ideas, as well as feedback regarding clinical strategies among members of the voice team. In this paradigm, it is important for the voice team to be cognizant of the sensitivities of professionals within the community, particularly voice teachers. Generally, singing voice specialists should limit their practices to patients with vocal injuries and should make every effort to return patients to the guidance of excellent singing teachers within the community as soon as appropriate.

When a voice clinic cannot be established "under one roof," an excellent "virtual" team can be established. In some ways this arrangement requires even more work and diligence on the part of the voice team than the single-site model. It is essential for voice team members to meet and communicate on a regular basis. This may mean establishing a frequent "voice conference" at a time when everyone including the physician can be depended on to attend. The "virtual" paradigm can have some potential advantages. It may allow a team to train as singing voice specialists and work with a larger number of singing voice teachers in the community, some of whom may spend only part of their time working with voice patients. However, it is best if these singing voice specialists are provided with the same depth of diagnostic information (including an opportunity to review stroboscopic images) to which they would have access if they were in a medical office. They must also maintain medical confidentiality, write progress notes for the medical record, and perform all the other functions expected of singing voice specialists. In some practices and in many communities this level of documentation may be difficult, but the fundamental need for communication is preferred.

Otolaryngologists are accustomed to referring to speech-language pathologists who are not located in their medical offices. So, this would seem to be a routine and comfortable approach for a voice team, as well.

However, several pitfalls must be avoided. First, the speech-language pathologist (SLP) must also have access to all diagnostic information, stroboscopic images, and medical treatment plans. Second, the SLP must have easy and frequent communication with the singing voice specialist and acting-voice specialist, as well as the laryngologist. Team treatment is most effective when it is coordinated closely and when all members of the therapy team know exactly what they are doing for each patient, and how the patient is responding.

If treating professionals are not working in the same office where they can talk with each other easily, they must commit to frequent communication. Telephone calls work well. However, another good solution is preparing progress notes at the end of each treatment session and sending them by secure E-mail to the physician and other members of the voice team treating the same patient. This approach ensures that each member of the voice team will have his or her own notes in good order, that they will be in the physician's medical record, and that they will be in the hands of all members of the treatment team before the patient can move from one therapist's office to the next. Acting-voice specialists and voice scientists require the same procedures.

Third, there is one particularly important pitfall relating to speech-language pathologists that must be avoided if a "virtual" practice paradigm is selected. Strobovideolaryngoscopy is performed initially (and often primarily) to establish a medical diagnosis. Medical diagnosis is the responsibility of the physician and is outside the scope of practice of a speech-language pathologist. There have been communities in which physicians are unwilling to invest in a stroboscope for their offices and have arranged for a stroboscope to be purchased by a hospital, and for the stroboscopic procedures to be performed by the speech-language pathologist in a hospital setting (remote from the physicians' offices). This arrangement usually starts out with a marginally acceptable theory and good intentions: The physician will review each study and render a diagnosis. Unfortunately, in practice, physicians often do not review the stroboscopy and rely on the analysis provided by the speech-language pathologist. This puts the SLP in the uncomfortable position of practicing outside his or her scope of practice and being the only member of the team with experience in reading stroboscopy. This arrangement should be avoided.

However, there is no problem with having stroboscopy performed by a speech-language pathologist and read together with an otolaryngologist. It is best if this can be done while the patient is still present. If this is not practical, every effort should be made to acquire stroboscopic equipment for each physician's office in which voice patients will be treated so that the team can rely on its physician for expertise in and responsibility for medical diagnosis of voice disorders. Stroboscopy can serve to allow the SLP to follow the progress of their treatment, but this too is also best done with some physician input or supervision.

COMMUNICATION

Although the need for good communication seems obvious, inadequate communication is common in medical practice; and this problem is the source of considerable misunderstanding, anguish, and litigation, as discussed in the following chapter. It is exceedingly important for laryngologists to understand the problems and goals of every professional voice patient, and for each voice patient to understand the realistic goals, limits, and time constraints of treatment. No matter how skilled a communicator the laryngologist may be, such mutual understanding cannot be accomplished dependably in one patient visit. The collaboration of the entire voice team is invaluable in ensuring real understanding. Speech-language pathologists, singing voice specialists, acting-voice specialists, voice scientists, nurses, and other members of the team spend hours with voice patients during the analytic and therapeutic process. Relationships are established that allow team members to gain insights into professional and emotional issues that may have great bearing on outcomes in voice professionals. Each team member should be aware of the importance of this component of his or her responsibility; and there should be excellent communication among all members of the voice team (including the **patient**, who is the most important member of the team) so that these insights have appropriate influence on therapeutic decisions. This is important for patients undergoing therapy alone, as well as for those undergoing surgery. Issues regarding surgical consent are discussed at greater length in the following chapter which addresses medical legal issues.

It is often helpful for the laryngologist, speech-language pathologist, singing voice specialist, acting-voice specialist, and patient to involve the patient's singing teacher or acting teacher in the decision-making process. Everyone must understand not only the risks of surgery, but also the risks involved in deciding against surgery and relying on technical maladjustments. In many cases there is no "good" or "right" choice; and the voice care team must combine great expertise with insight into the career and concerns of each individual patient to help the voice professional make the best choice. It must also be understood fully by everyone (doctor and patient particularly) that the therapeutic choice is the patient's. The physician and other members of the health team educate, guide, and advise the patient; but ultimately, the patient decides. As voice team care proceeds, the patient ordinarily comes to understand how much the team cares about making the voice professional better, the complex and unpredictable outcomes of voice treatment, the reasons why surgical decisions are delayed until nonsurgical therapy has been tried, and that every effort has been made to improve the patient's voice without operative intervention. The insights and relationships developed during this process should communicate the voice team's concern for the patient's best interest and outcome, and make clear the patient's ultimate control of the therapeutic process.

In addition to patient communication, communication with families and referring professionals within the community are also essential in building a voice practice. Community outreach initiatives are extremely important, as discussed below. In addition, laryngologists should not underestimate the importance and value of clinical research and publication. Research activities are valuable in their own right. They help us advance our field by communicating new insights to our colleagues. As a convenient byproduct of this effort, they also constitute excellent marketing in our progressively "better educated" patient population. Many voice professionals are computer literate and concerned enough about medical intervention to research physicians before they select a doctor or a practice. If such patients have a voice problem, they are often more comfortable going to the doctor who "wrote the book" or an article on the subject than someone who simply paid for marketing.

COMPASSION

Despite the best care, communication through the laryngologist and all members of the voice team and all efforts to achieve a perfect outcome, bad results may occur. It is essential for the physician to empathize and continue communicating with the patient. Physicians should understand (and feel) that an unfavorable result is almost as troubling to the physician as it is to the patient. Surgery is our art, and patient care is our passion; any doctor is upset when results are poor. We need not hide these reactions from our patients. We also need to be sensitive to each patient's reaction to a bad voice outcome. The consequences of voice impairment or "loss" can be overwhelming, and the assistance of a psychological professional who specializes in voice problems can be extremely effective in helping the patient.[7] Psychological professionals are invaluable assets to the voice team and may provide insights not only to patients, but also to voice care providers who have to interact with angry or disappointed patients who have not enjoyed good outcomes. It is especially important for the physician and other members of the team to remain engaged with the patient who has had a bad result. They need us to see them more often and talk with them at greater length than do our many patients who have enjoyed good results. As hard as it is for us to remind ourselves frequently that we have not succeeded in a particular patient's care, we need to remember that they are reminded of the result much more frequently than we are; and we need to resist any temptation to avoid them just when they need us most. Every patient can be helped, and helping these whose final results may remain disappointing is a special challenge and ethical obligation intrinsic to good practice.

BUILDING A VOICE PRACTICE: WHERE TO START?

The information provided in this chapter so far has described the components of a good voice team, but not the practical aspects of establishing one. Dr. Michael Benninger challenged me to address this, and he posed the question "What would you do if you were starting out today or moving to another city? . . . How would you build a patient base?" In reflecting upon the interesting challenges these questions raise, I have concluded that the strategies that worked for me 25 years ago remain as appropriate now as they were in 1980. I believe that I would use all of them again if I were starting over in Philadelphia or elsewhere; and I suspect that they will be equally effective for any practitioner who applies them with diligence.

The first priority in establishing a voice practice is to truly have expertise in and commitment to voice care. Obviously, this means acquiring special knowledge and credentials (ideally a fellowship), but it also means more than that. The physician must be willing to acquire basic, essential equipment such as a stroboscope and basic voice laboratory, even when such an acquisition is financially taxing and return on investment is uncertain. The physician must be able to rest comfortably in the knowledge that he or she is providing premier care for every voice patient seen (starting on the first day), and that his or her former fellowship or residency director would be justified in referring even the most illustrious voice patient. It also means establishing working relationships with the speech-language pathology, singing, and acting communities immediately. As discussed above, it is not necessary to hire a full-time speech-language pathologist and singing voice or acting-voice specialist at the outset, but appropriate collaborators must be recruited. This can be done in several ways.

Before moving to a community, or immediately thereafter, community outreach programs should be instituted. They include lectures for music or acting programs, presentations to choirs or school assemblies, talks to groups of speech-language pathologists, singing teachers, and acting teachers; presentation of grand rounds for physicians in other specialties; educational programs for school teachers; radio and television interviews, and presentations in others venues. Ideally, a one- or two-day educational program for the voice community (speech-language pathologists, singing teachers, acting teachers, physicians, and any other interested parties) should be presented. It may be helpful to invite one's fellowship director or other luminary as a guest presenter. This may help draw attendees and establish a new doctor's credibility. I routinely offer to copresent one training program for each of my graduating fellows in his or her new locale.

Such a program should include ample time for questions and answers and ample break time during which the new physician and the community voice professionals can get to know each other. The physician should arrange to visit various singing teachers, acting teachers, and speech-language pathologists to observe a few sessions of their work and should invite voice professionals to observe in the physician's office and operating room. Such visitors should also be made familiar with appropriate HIPPA (Healthcare Information Privacy and Portability Act) requirements and should sign an appropriate document agreeing to respect confidentiality restrictions.

The physician also should look continuously for opportunities to lecture in music classes, music pedagogy courses, acting courses, and to provide health lectures for local schools, theaters, and musical organizations. This enhances the level of understanding about voice and voice care in the community, and usually improves the level of vocal health. In addition, knowledgeable voice users are an excellent source of referrals; and it is important to remember that speech-language pathologists, singing voice teachers, and acting teachers are referring professionals who appreciate a letter (as would be written to a referring doctor) about the patients they send. A laryngologist's routine HIPPA compliance document should address the issue of permission to communicate with referring teachers and SLPs so that such permission is provided (or specifically denied) by each patient.

If laryngologists have any performance talent at all, it is well worth joining a choir, community theater, or some other performance group. Such activity is fun and educational in and of itself. Moreover, it demonstrates knowledge of performance that enhances physician credibility; and it establishes contacts in the performing community. For most practices, patient-to-patient referrals and referrals from singing and acting teachers and speech-language pathologists are at least as numerous as physician referrals (especially early in a practice), and often considerably more so.

Of course, establishing contact with physicians in various specialties also is extremely important. These may include lectures or grand rounds to pulmonologists on special management of respiratory problems in singers and other voice professionals; gastroenterologists on current concepts about laryngopharyngeal reflux disease; neurologists on neurolaryngologic diagnosis and treatment, laryngeal electromyography, tremor management, and other problems; gynecologists and endocrinologists on hormonal aspects of voice disorders, with special emphasis on iatrogenic masculinization and on thyroid problems; psychologists and psychiatrists on psychological concomitants of voice dysfunction, as well as on vocal manifestations of psychological disease and on the effects of psychotropic medications on voice performance; to physiatrists on postural and pain management in performers; and other physicians. In each case, the laryngologist should emphasis that he or she will be referring frequently to practitioners in the given specialty, what special information will be sought from such referrals, and opportunities for collaboration. There is no better way to generate referrals from other physicians than by sending patients to them. Eventually, they reciprocate; and when they do, a new laryngologist has the opportunity to provide them with a report more comprehensive, insightful, and practical than any they have seen before.

Generating referrals from other otolaryngologists in one's new community is often the greatest challenge. The voice course presented with the laryngologists fellowship director or other well-known laryngologist is often helpful in establishing these relationships and credibility. Setting a one- or two-day course at a time when otolaryngologists can attend may help (such as on a Saturday). Inviting members of one's own practice or department to attend as guests (without charge) is an appropriate courtesy to a fellow department member. Presenting departmental rounds on specific aspects of voice care and commenting judiciously at academic conferences on voice matters also can be helpful. Many laryngologists will be more comfortable referring to a new doctor if he or she has established expertise in the field by having written significant papers or a book related to voice. This constitutes one of the many reasons to remain academically productive regardless of whether the laryngologist's setting is private or an academic salaried position. As with other physicians, referring nonlaryngology cases is also an excellent way to establish new relationships.

It also may be helpful to establish a special relationship with a conservatory or particularly excellent music school. When I first started in practice, I offered to see all the incoming students at our primary opera conservatory in Philadelphia at no charge to the patient. Most of them were financially challenged and had no health insurance; and without this help the students would not have been able to get laryngologic care when they needed it. I have also taught a voice pedagogy course at that institution for the last quarter of a century. There have been several interesting consequences of this policy. First, the overall level of vocal education improved noticeably, and after the first few years, I have rarely seen students from this institution who have presented with preventable voice problems; and when they do, they are embarrassed about them because they know better. Second, each student undergoes a baseline strobovideolaryngoscopic examination and objective voice evaluation as a freshman. These data have not only uncovered an impressive number of asymptomatic "abnormalities" that would have been confusing if they had been seen for the first time during an illness, but they have also provided years of longitudinal information about a population of healthy, high-level singers. Third, this policy establishes relationships with students that have lasted throughout their professional careers. Many graduates from the Academy of Vocal Arts sing with the Metropolitan Opera and other major companies; and they still come to Philadelphia for their health problems, and often send their students here, as well. Caring for the students at no charge has been a joy; but it has also helped build the practice over time.

SUMMARY

Opportunities for establishing a successful voice practice remain unlimited. With focus, commitment, and enthusiasm, any well-trained laryngologist should be able to create an environment in which voice care professionals and professional voice users can flourish together.

REFERENCES

1. Sataloff RT, Heman-Ackah YD, Hawkshaw MJ. Voice care professionals: a guide to voice care providers. In: Sataloff RT. *Professional Voice: The Science and Art of Clinical Care.* 3rd ed. San Diego, Calif: Plural Publishing; 2005:1421–1426.
2. Sataloff RT. Professional singers: the science and art of clinical care. *Am J Otolaryngol.* 1981;2(3): 251–266.
3. Sataloff RT. The professional voice. In: Cummings CW, Frederickson JM, Harker LA, et al, eds. *Otolaryngology-Head and Neck Surgery.* Vol 3. St. Louis, Mo: CV Mosby; 1986:2029–2056.
4. Sataloff RT. *Professional Voice: The Science and Art of Clinical Care.* New York, NY: Raven Press, 1991:1–542.
5. Emerich KA, Baroody MM, Carroll LM, Sataloff RT. The singing voice specialist. In: Sataloff RT. *Professional Voice: The Science and Art of Clinical Care.* 3rd ed. Vol 3. San Diego, Calif: Plural Publishing; 2005:1021–1041.
6. Freed SL, Raphael BN, Sataloff RT. The role of the acting-voice trainer in medical care of professional voice users. In: Sataloff RT. *Professional Voice: The Science and Art of Clinical Care.* 3rd ed. San Diego, Calif: Plural Publishing; 2005:1051–1060.
7. Rosen Caputo D, Sataloff RT. *Psychology of Voice Disorders.* San Diego, Calif: Singular Publishing Group; 1997.
8. Heuer RJ, Hawkshaw MJ, Sataloff RT. The clinical voice laboratory. In: Sataloff RT. *Professional Voice: The Science and Art of Clinical Care.* 3rd ed. Vol 1. San Diego, Calif: Plural Publishing: 2005: 355–393.

Chapter 25

MEDICAL-LEGAL IMPLICATIONS OF PROFESSIONAL VOICE CARE

Robert T. Sataloff
Michael S. Benninger

*B*eing a defendant in a malpractice action is traumatic for any physician; we are all at risk. Not only does a lawsuit feel like an insult and assault, but it also emphasizes the fact that we have an unhappy patient. Because all of us strive to make our patients better, this component of a lawsuit is particularly troubling, even when we feel we have done "nothing wrong." There is no formula for avoiding lawsuits. However, there are certain practices that may minimize our risk. The authors emphasize the "three Cs": competence, communication, and compassion as the most important approaches to establishing a strong relationship with the patient and preventing potential legal action.

It should be self-evident that competence is the keystone of good medical practice in all fields, including laryngology. However, all experienced laryngologists have encountered patients who have received laryngologic care that is below the current standard of practice. In many cases, this care has been rendered by laryngologists who are outstanding in their area of expertise but not familiar with the latest teachings in laryngology. All interventions should be reasonable and appropriate; and the patient should have good reasons for the recommended therapeutic course. It is helpful if those reasons can be supported by research or expert opinion cited in the literature.

Most litigation has its roots in communication, or lack thereof. In laryngology, this applies particularly to

patients who have undergone voice surgery. Prior to performing voice surgery, it is essential to be certain that patient selection is appropriate and that the patient understands the limits and potential complications of voice surgery. Appropriate patients for voice surgery not only have voice abnormalities, but also really want to change their voice quality, effort, and/or endurance. For example, not all people with "pathological" voices are unhappy with them. Sports announcers, female trial attorneys with gruff voices, and others sometimes consult a physician only because of fear of cancer. If there is no suspicion of malignancy, restoring their voices to "normal" (eg, by evacuating Reinke's edema) may be a disservice and even jeopardize their careers. Similarly, it is essential to distinguish accurately between organic and psychogenic voice disorders before embarking on laryngeal surgery. Although a breathy voice may be caused by numerous organic conditions, it is also commonly found in people with psychogenic dysphonia. The differentiation may require a very skilled voice team.

Although all reasonable efforts should be made to avoid operative intervention in professional voice users, particularly singers, there are times when surgery is appropriate and necessary. Ultimately, the decision depends on a risk-benefit analysis. If a professional voice user is unable to continue his or her career, and if surgery may restore vocal function, surgery certainly should not be withheld. Sometimes, making such judgments can be challenging. A rock or pop singer with a vocal fold mass may have satisfactory voice quality with only minimal technical adjustments. Pop singers perform with amplification, obviating the need to sing loudly and project the voice in some cases (depending on the artist's style). Such a patient may be able to "work around" pathology safely for many years. However, even much more minor pathology may be disabling in some classical singers. For example, if a high soprano specializing in Baroque music develops a mild-to-moderate superior laryngeal nerve paresis, she may experience breathiness and instability. If she gives in to the temptation to compensate by slightly retracting her tongue and lowering her larynx, the breathiness will be controlled because of increased adductory forces, but she will lose the ability to perform rapid, agile runs and trills. Similar problems may occur from compensatory maladjustments in response to other lesions such as vocal fold cysts. In such instances, the artist may be served better by surgical correction of the underlying problem than by long-term use of hyperfunctional compensation (bad technique) that can itself cause other performance problems, as well as vocal fold pathology. The patient must understand all of these considerations clearly, including the risks of surgery. He or she needs to acknowledge the risk that any voice surgery may make the voice worse permanently, and the patient must consider this risk acceptable in light of ongoing vocal problems.

Even in the best hands, an undesirable scar may develop, resulting in permanent hoarseness. Hence, the patient must be aware that there is a possibility that the voice may be worse following surgery. Naturally, other complications also must be discussed including (among others) complications of anesthesia, dental fracture, recurrence of laryngeal lesions, airway compromise, vocal fold webbing, and other untoward occurrences. This discussion and documentation should include all the relevant risks, benefits, and alternatives, with a thorough documentation of that discussion in the formal medical record. In addition to the hospital's standard surgical consent, the authors provide patients with additional written information prior to surgery. The patient keeps one copy of the "Risks and Complications of Surgery" document, and one signed copy remains in the chart. Specialized informed consent documents are used also for other selected treatments such as injection of Cidofovir and injection of botulinum toxin, even though such documents are not mandated. If medications are used for treatment purposes (rather than research purposes) and are off-label uses of medicines approved by the FDA for other purposes, their use does not necessarily require institutional review board (IRB) approval or a special consent. However, these authors believe it is helpful and prudent to provide patients with as much information as possible and to document that they have been so informed.

Preoperative objective voice assessment and documentation are essential in addition to routine documentation of informed consent discussions. As a bare minimum, a high-quality tape recording of the patient's voice should be obtained before surgery. Auditory memories of physicians and patients are not good in general, and both the doctor and postoperative professional voice user are often surprised when they compare postoperative and preoperative recordings. Frequently, the preoperative voice is worse than either person remembers. In addition, such documentation is invaluable for medical-legal purposes. Photographs or videotapes of the larynx obtained during strobovideolaryngoscopy are extremely helpful, as well. Ideally, complete evaluation by a voice team should be performed. Proper documentation is essential for assessing outcomes, even for the physician who is not interested in research or publication; as such information can be invaluable in a medical-legal context.

Clearly, the most important measure that a voice professional can take to prevent litigation is establishing a strong and appropriate relationship with patients and, at times, also with their families. Although this is clearly important in all performers, surgical patients require a subtle additional level of trust and confidence in the surgical judgment, skills, and expertise of the laryngologist. Being honest about our experience and about our prior results allows the patient to determine whether or not he or she is willing to entrust the operation to us. Overselling such skills and experiences will increase dramatically the potential for a less-than-optimal outcome leading to litigation. We have found that patients greatly appreciate feeling as if they have continuous access to their surgeon. We will give them multiple ways to reach us and our staff through the office, answering service, and E-mail. They will rarely, if ever, call, and if they do it is almost always something significant enough that the surgeon would want to know about it. This ready access goes a long way in alleviating any concern and furthering the strength of the relationship.

Despite excellent care, bad results may occur. It is essential for the physician to continue communicating with the patient and to empathize.

It is important that we not hide from our patients the fact that we are also concerned that their outcome is not perfect, and that we be honest with them in all other ways. It is imperative that the medical record be complete and nonopinionated. The record should never be modified without a clear notation that the record has been changed. The provider should bring together the appropriate resources and people to help resolve the problem, if possible. If there is any concern that litigation may occur, it is not unreasonable to discuss this with your institution and your legal counsel, even before any suggestion of litigation is present. It may allow for help with "damage-control" and will help focus the plan for alleviating any potential legal issues.

Despite the best efforts of the voice team, a poor result may persist. In such cases, "communication" and "compassion" become critical. Good listening skills are important as it is often difficult to know what patients are most concerned about. In many cases, their perception of a less-than-expected outcome may not be based on the actual results but rather on either unrealistic expectations or some emotional aspect of their lives or careers. They may have hoped that all their career difficulties were based on this one problem and that everything would be terrific once they were treated. In many cases, supporting their emotional and psychological health is important. In such cases, it may be worthwhile considering professional psychological intervention.[1] The assistance of a psychological professional who specializes in voice problems can be invaluable in helping the patient, facilitating the efforts of the voice team, and channeling the patient's frustration into therapeutic effort rather than extensive litigation. A psychological professional can be especially helpful if concerns or extraordinary stresses are detected by the laryngologist or voice therapy team prior to surgery, allowing for preoperative psychological intervention and support that may be invaluable not only if there is a bad operative outcome, but even when the surgical result is good. Attending to our patients' emotional needs and reactions to vocal injury

and vulnerability is part of optimal laryngological care and invaluable in preventing anger and misunderstanding that can lead to litigation.

Although the risks of legal action may seem more significant for the surgeon, any member of the voice team could be at risk. It is important to remember that the three "Cs" are relevant to all aspects of professional voice practice. Making the wrong medical decision or not paying close attention to medications prescribed can result in a poor outcome. Not recognizing an early vocal hemorrhage and allowing a patient to perform may be more risky than a controlled surgical procedure. Voice pathologists and music teachers may be liable if they participate in the care of patients who develop a complication or bad outcome. Fortunately for these professionals, it is much more likely that a suit will be directed at the "deeper pockets" of the surgeon and/or hospital.

The voice care team professionals need to be very cognizant of informedconsent and confidentiality issues, and be aware of the legal ramifications of the Healthcare Information Privacy and Portability Act (HIPPA) in the United States. It is often particularly difficult to maintain confidentiality for performers as there are so many people competing to obtain information about the status of their care and health. These include managers or agents, directors, promoters, the patient's family, the media, and the public. In each of these cases, no information about the patient should be divulged without explicit written consent from the patient. Pictures and videos should remain within the confidential relationship of the patient and provider, unless expressly released for wider exposure by written patient consent. The voice care team must make extra efforts to protect the confidentiality of the patient. With the aggressiveness of the media in obtaining any information on celebrities, the medical records need to be carefully protected. Moreover, secretaries and other personnel must be trained not to discuss patients (including celebrities) with anyone, including their families. Although we all realize how much the performer's illness may have an impact on all the people involved with his or her production, explicit direction and formal release of information should be obtained from the patient prior to any discussion of their status or care. Failing to do so may not only draw malpractice litigation, it may also result in other civil or regulatory action and fines.

WHAT SHOULD BE DONE IF THERE IS A LAWSUIT?

Fortunately, it is uncommon that an adverse result will lead to litigation. Much of this has to do with the quality of the voice care that is currently available. However, there may be times when, despite appropriate care and diligence, compassion and communication, the patient is unhappy with his or her voice or other outcome and might consider bringing a lawsuit. In such cases, one of the first questions that must be asked is whether or not we can continue with fair, unbiased, and supportive clinical care of the patient. If the answer is no, and if he or she has not been able to establish contact with another provider or team, it is important to help the patient identify other providers who can continue to care for him or her. This is important not only from a medical standpoint, but also shows our care and concern for the patient and may play a positive role should a claim be made.

It is also very important to not develop an adversarial relationship with the patient or his or her family. All communication should be unbiased and balanced. A patient who is trying to find out if he or she has a case might be convinced to pursue one if it is felt that he or she has been treated poorly or disrespectfully. If there are issues that we are unsure how to handle, it may be helpful to stay in close contact with legal counsel. Similarly, disparaging comments should never be made about the patient as others, including office staff, may be asked to testify. The chart should include no negative commentary and should be limited to an objective assessment of the clinical aspects of the patient's care.

The last important thing to remember is that most laryngologists will experience at least one lawsuit in their careers. Such cases do not suggest that the laryngologist is a poor doctor. In most cases, the outcome may have been unavoidable, or the decision was one that most others would have made. In other cases, it truly may have been a poor decision. Every doctor has made a wrong decision at some point in his or her career. The best doctors are the ones who critically evaluate the cause for the bad outcome and then take steps to prevent such occurrences in the future.

SUMMARY

The care of the professional vocalist may be fraught with potential legal and litigation risks. In most practices it is highly unlikely that even a poor outcome will lead to legal action. The three Cs of "competence, communication, and compassion" are important not only in optimizing clinical care and outcomes, but they are also the best protection against litigation. Taking time to establish a strong relationship with patients, supporting them with our knowledge and expertise, and being accessible for them should they have concerns and questions are all important components of the high-quality, low-risk voice practice. In the rare occurrence of an adverse outcome, it is important that the laryngologist, voice pathologist, or voice professional identify the key issues that have impacted the outcome, make every effort to mitigate their sequelae, and take appropriate steps to prevent them from occurring again in the future.

REFERENCE

1. Rosen DC, Sataloff, RT. *Psychology of Voice Disorders*. San Diego, Calif: Singular Publishing Group; 1997.

Appendix

VOCAL HYGIENE

Vocal hygiene is a daily regimen to achieve and maintain a healthy voice. Vocal hygiene includes maintaining adequate rest and hydration (6 to 8 glasses of water per day), minimizing exposure to noxious chemicals, no smoking of cigarettes or other tobacco substances, and avoiding excessive shouting, screaming, or other nonessential loud voice use.

Proper nutrition is also part of a good vocal hygiene program. Excessive weight may lead to faulty use of the respiratory muscles that are important for generating the power of the voice. In addition, excessive weight adds to overall body fatigue and may restrict a singer or actor from certain roles that require a high level of physical activity.

The following tips apply to keeping and maintaining a healthy voice:

- Good general health.
- Regular exercise to maintain adequate muscle tone.
- Rest when fatigued or injured.
- Use a reduced voice usage schedule when tired.
- Rehearse only after warming up.
- Use ear protection when the sound level is high.
- Have your hearing checked regularly.
- Review past recordings of your voice; note the changes if any.
- Avoid long telephone conversations prior to rehearsals or performances.
- Warm up your voice prior to singing.
- For school children—adequate hydration prior to after school rehearsals. A few minutes of stretching also helps.

Do's and don'ts of vocal hygiene

- Drink 6 to 8 glasses of water per day (there is no substitute for plain water).
- Reduce or eliminate caffeine and caffeinated drinks—coffee, tea, colas, and so forth.
- Rest before performances. Allow plenty of time between long airplane flights and rehearsals or performances.
- Eat a balanced diet. Avoid crash diets. They may contain substances that change the way you feel and produce voice.
- Examine the details of food supplements. Excessive vitamin E may cause blood vessels in the vocal folds and other parts of the body to rupture.

continues

- Do not clear your throat. Excessive throat clearing is an indicator of a problem and should be addressed by an otolaryngologist.

- Laugh. The muscles of the body relax during laughter.

- Do not shout.

- Do not whisper with strain.

- Eliminate and avoid all tobacco products.

- Avoid areas of noxious chemicals/fumes.

- Do not smoke cigarettes, cigars, or pipes.

- Avoid second-hand smoke.

- Do not use recreational drugs.

- Do not share the prescription medications of other performers (such as antibiotics).

- Avoid over-the-counter medications. Your voice is too important. Consult an otolaryngologist who specializes in the care of performers.

- Review all prescription medications with your doctor in relationship to potential impact on your voice.

- Minimize alcohol. Like caffeine, it dries out the mucous membranes that cover the vocal muscles, inside the mouth and throat.

- Be cautious about weight lifting that requires grunting or straining. Use lighter weights and more repetitions if possible.

- Eat light meals with plenty of water before rehearsals and performances.

- Take steps to reduce stress. Exercise, rest, and counseling are proven ways to reduce stress.

- Humidify your studio and bedroom during winter months. If you have mold allergies, try not to let the humidity get too high.

- Be cautious about voice use in environments with loud background noise, such as clubs or airplanes.

- After an injury or sickness, consult your vocal coach or singing teacher to see if you have modified or changed your vocal techniques.

- Women—select birth control medications with the help of a physician who understands the effects of hormones on the voice.

- ***Do not sing when sick***—A cold or upper respiratory infection changes the way you use your breathing muscles, may cause the vocal folds to swell, and may affect the way you hear your voice.

- ***A hoarse voice, change in the sound of the voice, or noticeable voice fatique for 2 weeks requires attention by a qualified voice care team—otolaryngologist, voice pathologist, and voice teacher.***

Glossary

abduction: the action of bringing the vocal folds apart. Vocal folds abduct during the act of inhalation.

acoustic analysis: evaluation of the sound properties of voice. Measures considered important to acoustic analysis are fundamental frequency (F_0), jitter, shimmer, signal-to-noise ratio, and maximum frequency range.

adduction: the action of bringing the vocal folds together to produce voice. Vocal fold adduction may occur at voice onset, during the production of voiced consonants such as /b/, /d/, and /z/, and during coughing or throat clearing. The vocal folds also adduct during swallowing.

aerodynamic analysis: evaluation of the amount of air and rate of airflow available to set the vocal folds into vibration. Measures include flow or phonation volume, phonation time, and airflow rate. Subglottic pressure, glottic resistance, and glottic efficiency are also measures that can be extracted using equipment designed for aerodynamic analysis. Pulmonary function tests, which measure an individual's amount of lung capacity and use of air for breathing, could also be considered parts of aerodynamic analysis.

airflow rate: a measure of speed of airflow between the vocal folds during voice production. This generally is measured in millimeters per second (ml/sec) or cubic centimeters per second (cc/sec). The value is obtained by dividing the total amount of air expelled, for example, while saying "ah" (/a/) by the amount of time it took to produce that sound. Higher airflow rates (>200 ml/sec) are associated with "breathy" or "weak" voice, and low airflow rates (<80 ml/sec) may indicate tight, strained voice. Trained singers are able to maintain steady airflow rates across various fundamental frequencies.

apron: the part of the stage that extends from the curtain to orchestra pit.

aria: a song usually from an opera for solo voice with instrumental accompaniment. Arias also are found in oratorios and cantatas. Arias provide lyric interludes that draw the listener away from the primary action of the opera.

arpeggio: the notes of a chord sung (or played) in succession. Arpeggio exercises have many uses, but among the more common ones are range extension, flexibility, and legato singing (the negotiation of intervals in a smooth and connected manner).

articulation: in speech-language pathology, the shaping of resonated tones into vowels and consonants by the tongue, lips, and jaw. It is considered to be the "endpoint" of a model of the process of speech production. Musically, articulation refers to the way a phrase is executed. In vocal pedagogy, it is the production of consonant sounds. Proper articulation in singing is achieved when the production of consonants is accomplished without tension and the process does not interfere with the production of tone. The result is good tone quality with clear diction.

attack: in speech-language pathology, the onset of sound or the act of bringing the vocal folds together to produce sound. A *hard glottal attack* is a voice onset in which the vocal folds are brought together and pressure is built up beneath them so that on release there is a popping sound. This usually occurs at the beginning of a sentence or breath group and is most noticeable on initial vowels. When used habitually, this is an abusive method of producing voice. An *easy attack* or *easy onset* is a method of voice production in which the vocal folds come together more gently.

The coordinated attack (simultaneous release of air and onset of voice) is considered ideal for singing.

baritone: a male voice with a range higher than a low bass voice and lower than a high tenor voice.

baroque: the period of music that begins in the early 1600s and extends to about 1750. This period saw the birth of opera.

bass: the lowest range of the male voice. There are bass profundos who sing serious roles, bass fuffos who sing comic roles, and bass bel cantos who sing art songs.

bel canto: an Italian term meaning "beautiful singing," which became associated with a vocal style in the 18th century. Bel canto style emphasizes phrasing, tone, and technique, valuing beauty and purity of voice and considering beautiful tone to be more important than any other aspect of interpretation.

belting: a style of singing used in several types of popular music, generally by female voices, where the chest voice or chest register is pushed upward, often beyond its limits. The effect is a dramatic sound, is relatively loud, and sounds pushed. A similar manner of production in classical music is referred to as *chesting*.

blocking: when the director moves people around the stage by the stage prior to singing during the preliminary phases of rehearsal.

break: a sudden, audible shift in register, also referred to as a *crack*.

breathy: In speech-language pathology, this is a vocal quality associated with the release of excessive air during phonation. Breathiness occurs as a result of inefficient vocal fold closure. Breathiness can be "functional," meaning produced as a result of inappropriate voice production, or "organic," meaning produced as a result of vocal fold weakness or paralysis or due to a mass interfering with vocal fold closure. In vocal pedagogy, a breathy tone is the opposite of a *focused* tone. It is like a picture out of focus—unclear, lacking definition. It may be used consciously as an interpretive effect, but with that exception it has a negative connotation in the vocal studio. Pathologic causes include edema, nodules, and polyps. Where no pathology is present, the cause is likely to be inefficient *breath support*, inefficient laryngeal control, poor vocal *placement*, or a combination of the above. Although breathiness is not harmful to the singing voice, it indicates inefficient use of air and is generally considered to be esthetically unpleasant. It is the lack of breath support that may cause more serious vocal problems.

bridge: the transitional area between vocal registers.

Camarata: a group of 16th century Florentine philosophers who argued against the polyphony of the times for a more classical presentation that emphasized the words and emotional content of a composition.

cantabile: a musical expression that results in singing or playing in a tuneful manner.

cantata: a musical form, generally for chorus and soloists, based on a primarily narrative text; the most famous cantatas are those written by Bach, all of which take scriptural texts as their starting points—some are even for solo voice and instrument.

cantilena: a lyrical melody line, obviously meant to be sung or played "cantabile."

canzone: a short, lyrical operatic song; the term itself may have originated in Provence and could have referred to arias, which have no narrative quality at all, but simply reflect the singer's state of mind. Cherubino's "Voi che sapete" in Mozart's *The Marriage of Figaro* is called a canzone.

canzonetta: literally, a little "canzone;" Mozart used the words "canzone" and "canzonetta" frequently to differentiate between the more serious (and longer) arias and the shorter (and more conversational) solo works in his operas.

cavatina: a short, simple solo song, occasionally instrumental rather than vocal, that was popular in 18th century Italian operas.

chest voice: used to describe the lower notes of a vocal range, thus named because of the sympathetic vibrations produced in the chest while singing with the thicker vocal configuration required to produce those tones.

classical: the period in music that comes after the baroque period and before the romantic; the dates are roughly 1756 (which is the birth of Mozart) to 1830 (3 years after the death of Beethoven). Although the period is not as long as the baroque period, it represents the greatest standardization in orchestral form and sonority; even composers who lived beyond 1830 continued to use the standard "classical" orchestra of pairs of flutes, oboes, clarinets, and bassoons, four horns, two trumpets, three trombones, strings, and timpani.

coda: the last musical thoughts in a composition; in strict formal terms, a piece might contain exposition (which sets forth the principal themes of the work), development (which uses that material in new and varied fashions), recapitulation (where the principal material is restated almost verbatim), cadenza (for a last-minute vocal improvisation, sometimes based on the early materials in the work), and coda (where one last little idea is put forward by the composer).

coloratura: a type of soprano, generally, but also the description of singing that pertains to great feats of agility—fast singing, high singing, trills, embellishments, and so forth. Some coloratura sopranos during this century have been Lily Pons, Roberta Peters, Joan Sutherland, and Beverly Sills. An example of coloratura is Marguerite's "Jewel Song" from Gounod's *Faust*.

commedia dell'arte: a style of dramatic presentation popular in Italy from the 16th century on; the commedia characters were highly stylized and the plots frequently revolved around disguises, mistaken identities, and misunderstandings. The principal commedia characters are Pierrot, Harlequin, and Colombine. Operatic spoofs of the commedia characters can be found in Leoncavallo's *Pagliacci* and Strauss' *Ariadne auf Naxos*.

compass: refers to the total range of a piece of music or to a singer's tone range.

comprimario: a singer who takes the secondary character roles in an opera; from the Italian which means "next to the first"; confidantes, maids, servants, messengers, and medical personnel generally fit under the heading of comprimario roles.

continuo: the small group of instruments that accompanies the recitatives in baroque music; as a general rule, the continuo group comprises cello and harpsichord or organ, although in some of the larger works of Monteverdi (*Orfeo, The Coronation of Poppea*), the continuo group can comprise a dozen or more instruments.

contralto: the lowest female voice; the term comes from two Italian words, which signify against ("contra") the high ("alto") voice. In baroque operas, the contralto generally represented a certain character type on stage: either comic (a sort of female basso buffo), or spooky and other worldly, or just plain matronly. Marian Anderson and Maureen Forrester have been legendary contraltos in the concert and operatic world.

counterpoint: the putting together of two or more independent musical lines; when the same musical tune is repeated several times, in different vocal ranges, the result can be a fugue or a round.

countertenor: a high male voice, generally singing within the female contralto or mezzo soprano range; popular in the baroque period, the countertenor frequently portrayed young, virile men or innocent, blushing adolescents—the voices were

generally quite powerful, and not considered effeminate. This vocal range is sometimes referred to as "male alto."

covering: a technique of making the transition through vocal registers that aids in maintaining an evenness of vocal quality and color. Used primarily by men, this technique involves vowel modification, generally rounding and darkening the vowel (/a/ to /o/ or /ɔ/, for example) to prevent the sound from becoming "spread" or "white."

crack: see **break.**

crescendo/decrescendo: increasing/decreasing. Primarily relating to increases and decreases in loudness.

cul-de-sac resonance: a voice quality in which the tone appears to be "caught" in the back of the mouth. This can occur when there is nasal blockage. Often, tongue retraction can give the voice this muffled quality.

deus ex machina: literally, "god out of a machine," a literary or staging device that refers to some last-minute salvation of a tricky situation by a god or goddess who has been watching the entire plot unfold from afar. In the baroque period, elaborate scenery was devised whereby a particular god (more often than not Amor, the god of love) would descend from above the stage in a little cloud or carriage.

director/producer: depending on the locale of the producing company, the person who creates the staging for a play or an opera; in America, this person is called the director, or the stage director, as opposed to the conductor who leads the orchestra. Throughout Europe, this person is known as the producer and the orchestra conductor is frequently called the director!

diva: a female opera star of great rank or pretension; the original Italian word means "goddess."

dramma giocoso: an opera that combines serious elements, enacted by aristocratic personnages, with comic relief, played out and commented on by earthier peasant stock. The most famous example of dramma giocoso is Mozart's *Don Giovanni*, although the composer himself never actually called it such—only Lorenzo da Ponte, the librettist, did.

"drinking in the tone": imagery that conveys the feeling that the tone reverses its direction and comes back to its source. This concept is used by some to aid in sustaining the tone.

duet: a musical composition for two performers.

dynamics: varying degrees of loudness and softness, and intensity of a sound.

dysphonia: a disorder of voice production resulting in poor voice quality. Occasionally, adjectives are added to this term such as *functional, musculoskeletal tension,* or *spasmodic,* which refer to qualities of the dysphonia or to its suspected cause.

edema: a medical term for *swelling.* When referring to the vocal folds, this usually occurs as a result of infection or as a reaction to irritation or vocal abuse.

embellishment: the addition of extra notes to an already established melody line; in the days of Handel, and again in the flourishing of 19th century Italian bel canto, the process of embellishing a vocal line whenever it is repeated was the standard practice. Some composers, like Bach and Mozart, wrote out their own embellishments—others trusted the instrumentalists and singers to add their own.

entr'acte: a musical composition played between acts or between scenes within an act of an opera.

entrée: a musical composition, used mainly in the French baroque period by its greatest practitioners, Rameau and Lully, which has a martial, aggressive quality; the entrée generally was played to introduce an important character or group of characters. In some French baroque works, such as Rameau's *Les Indes galantes,* each act was called an entrée.

erythema: a medical term for *redness* occurring as a result of infection and in cases of contact irritation, especially at the vocal processes of the arytenoids or in the posterior commissure of the larynx.

falsetto: the diminutive of the Italian *falso,* "false." This is the lightest and highest vocal register, produced with extremely thin vocal folds. It also enables a bass or a baritone to imitate a female voice. Some voice teachers use the term interchangeably with *head voice.*

fioritura: understandably confused with coloratura but meaning almost the same thing; taken from *fior,* which means "flower" in Italian, fioritura refers to the actual flowery, embellished vocal line within an aria. All coloratura sopranos have to sing fioritura at some point or another, but there is no such thing as a fioritura soprano.

flow volume (or phonation volume): The amount of air (in liters or milliliters) expelled during one phonation after a maximum inhalation.

formant: the resonant frequency of a speech sound. It appears as a prominent band of energy on sound spectrography. There are four or five formants in most speech sounds (including fundamental frequency). Researchers have identified a "singer's formant" that is present in Western-style classical singing. This appears as a clustering of energy in the high frequencies. In the male voice, this can vary between 2.3 and 3.8 kHz.

full voice: to sing with complete breath support and resonance at a relatively loud volume, as opposed to *half voice,* which implies a lighter, less supported and often unfocused tone. *Full voice* can indicate either volume level or the technical effort made to produce the tone.

fundamental frequency: the number of times per second that the vocal folds vibrate (in hertz). Although there are several frequencies or harmonics in a sound recorded at the lips, the fundamental frequency (F_0) reflects the tone generated at the vocal folds. For women, average conversational fundamental frequency is approximately 220 Hz. For men, average conversational fundamental frequency is 125 Hz.

glissando: sliding rapidly up or down a musical scale.

glottal fry: a type of voice production in which the vocal folds are vibrating in a rhythmic, but abnormal fashion. The sound to the ear is one of a popping, bubbling sound. Glottal fry occurs due to a reduction in airflow and subsequent decrease in *subglottic pressure.* It is often heard at the end of a sentence when a speaker runs out of air and drops pitch; however, it can be produced over a range of frequencies.

glottis: the area of opening between the vocal folds. Occasionally, this term is used to refer to the general area of the vocal folds.

grand opera: opera that is sung from start to finish, as opposed to opera that may have spoken dialogue; grand opera frequently treats serious, dramatic subjects and, in French operas, of the 19th century, was generally epic in scale with a full scale ballet inserted in the middle of the work.

harshness: a quality of voice that is heard as a grating or "hard" sound. There is an aperiodic sound to harshness. Sometimes used interchangeably with *hoarseness.*

hauptstimme: this refers to the principal musical material of a work. In the operas of Schoenberg or Berg, early 20th century German composers, the main melodies are marked with an "H" to indicate that the composers considered those the principal tunes.

head voice: most voice teachers use this term interchangeably with *falsetto*. Others use it to denote the upper part of the range when produced with relatively light registration, but still fully supported, as differentiated from pure *falsetto*.

heldentenor: a type of tenor voice that harkens back to the golden age of Wagnerian singing; the typical heldentenor has an unusually brilliant top register (high notes) combined with a muscular lower voice, almost like a baritone, and is capable of long passages that require great vocal stamina. Tristan and Siegfried are great heldentenor roles. One of the great heldentenors of the century was Lauritz Melchior.

hoarseness: a quality of voice that is heard as harshness with breathiness. Hoarseness is often differentiated between *dry*, that generally heard in cases in which the vocal folds are not closing adequately, and *secretions* (eg, saliva) are pooling in the region of the vocal folds.

hooking: a technique that combines vowel modification (usually a more open vowel moving to a more closed one) with pushing lower registration to higher notes. This is generally thought to be esthetically unpleasant and bears a negative connotation in the voice studio.

hypernasal, hyponasal: to the speech-language pathologist, *hypernasality* refers to a disorder of resonance in which too much sound is escaping through the nasal cavity during speech. This is due to velopharyngeal incompetence (the soft palate is too short or too weak to seal off the oral from the nasal cavities). *Hyponasality* refers to a vocal quality in which sounds that should be nasalized (/m/, /n/, and /ŋ/) are not; these sounds become (/b/, /d/, and /g/). There is a great deal of variation in the degree of nasality across the dialects of English. *Excessive nasality* (beyond considerations of dialect) usually denotes a structural, neurologic, or functional abnormality. These terms are not common in the vocal studio, but their meaning is. Hypernasality is often referred to as *nasal twang* or simply *too nasal*, whereas hyponasality or insufficient nasal resonance is often referred to as *too far back* (placement), *too dull, too dark, too covered*. Although what is "right" is as much an esthetic and expressive choice as it is anything else, the singer is generally trying to balance nasal resonance with oral and laryngeal resonance. When control of nasal resonance is primarily a problem with function of the velum, hyper- and hyponasality are regarded as relatively minor vocal problems.

imbroglio: operatic scene in which diversity of rhythm and melody create chaos and confusion; the original meaning of the Italian word was "intrigue."

intensity: a measurement of the amplitude of a sound, expressed in decibels (dB). Intensity is the acoustic correlate of loudness. *Dynamic range* refers to the range of intensity an individual can produce, from softest to loudest sound.

intermezzo: a short musical entertainment, which in its earliest manifestation might be played between the acts of a longer, more serious operatic work; the intermezzo was almost always of light-hearted character, and never involved more than three or four singers. One well-known operatic intermezzo is *La serva padrona* (The Servant as Mistress) of Giovanni Pergolesi (1733), which was sung between the first and second acts of a much larger, and quite forgotten, work *Il prigioner superb* (The Model Prisoner).

jitter: frequency perturbation or the cycle-to-cycle variations in the frequency of vibration of the vocal folds. There are several ways to measure jitter and various types of equipment use different methods to extract this value. In general, high jitter values are correlated with a decrease in the quality of the voice.

legato: from the Italian meaning "to tie" or "bind together." As a musical direction, it is one way of performing a musical phrase, meaning to connect the notes smoothly and evenly in a musical line. It is also used conceptually in vocal technique, based on the fact that the voice is an instrument intended to change pitch smoothly, without articulating or punctuating the change with movement of the larynx. It also implies the unbroken connection of breath, vibration, and resonance. The opposite of legato is marcato (in a marked punchy style) or even staccato (in an even shorter, more aggressive style).

leitmotiv: a short musical passage, sometimes no more than three or four notes, that instantly calls to mind a character or situation in a musical drama; although Wagner may not have invented the device, he is certainly the best-known user of it. This example is the glance motive from Wagner's *Tristan und Isolde*.

libretto: the text of an opera; the literal translation is "little book," which reminds us that, in a Broadway show, the texts of the songs are called the "lyrics" whereas the spoken text of the rest of the play is called the "book."

lied: a German song; the pronunciation is "leed" and the plural is lieder (pronounced "leader"). In some pre-Wagnerian German operas, the songs that the characters sing are called "lieder" as opposed to "aria," which would be the Italian determination.

lift: the note at which transition from one register to another register occurs.

maestro: a title of courtesy given, especially in Italy, to conductors, composers, and directors; translation (from the Italian), "Master."

manufactured sound: tone that lacks ease and "naturalness" of production, sounds labored or overly technical.

marking: a rehearsal technique intended to save the voice, marking can be done in a variety of ways, including singing very softly, singing up or down an octave to make the range more accessible, and speaking words in rhythm.

mask: the area of the face around the nose and eyes where one might wear a mask. This is often used in teaching the concept of *placement* as a student may be directed to "sing in the mask" or "feel the vibration in the mask."

masque: a staged performance in which music, poetry, song, and dance are blended; although the word is French, and pronounced "mask," the form is more frequently associated with English works that appeared in the time of Queen Elizabeth I.

mean phonation time: the average time to produce a sustained vowel. Often used in assessment as a measure of the "health" of the respiratory and phonatory systems, the average value ranges from 18 to 20 seconds, although this can vary greatly with age.

messa di voce: as a musical direction, the meaning is to *crescendo* and *decrescendo* on a single note. Also used as a vocal exercise. Historically, a singer who could execute *messa di voce* successfully on every note in the range was considered to have complete mastery of vocal technique.

mezza voce: the Italian term for half voice, or literally "medium voice," as contrasted with full voice. When singing mezza voce, the singer reduces the volume to intensify the emotion. This may be a musical directive intended to achieve a certain dramatic effect in performance. It is also a method of singing used in marking.

mezzo-soprano: the female voice range that lies between the soprano, which is the highest, and the contralto; the tone of a mezzo-soprano can either be voluptuous (in the case of Delilah or Carmen) or it can be thinner and more agile (which might describe Rosina in *The Barber of Seville*).

mixed voice (voice mixte): a tone sung with mixed registration, but with a preponderance of head voice.

opera buffa: a style of opera that revolves almost entirely around comedy; perhaps an outgrowth of the Italian intermezzo, the opera buffa as a form was popular in the baroque days as well as in Italy of the early 19th century. Its counterpart is *opera seria,* which implies opera almost entirely about lofty ideals or with tragic consequences.

opéra comique: a misleading term, French in origin, which would seem to describe opera that was funny; in fact, opéra comique describes opera in which there is some spoken dialogue as opposed to grand opera in which there is none. As a matter of fact, both Gounod's *Faust* and Bizet's *Carmen* were originally conceived with spoken dialogue and are, thus, opéras comiques even though their subject matter would seem to make them "grand" operas.

operetta: light, frothy musical entertainments that generally do not pertain to terrifically important subject material; spoken dialogue, dancing, practical jokes, and mistaken identities seem to be the trademark of the operetta form, most popular in late 19th century Vienna or France, under the hands of the Strauss family or Offenbach. *Die Fledermaus, The Merry Widow, La Périchole,* and Noel Coward's *Bitter Sweet* are all operettas.

optimal pitch: the ideal habitual speaking pitch for a certain individual. Optimal pitch was thought to be located approximately one-fourth from the bottom of one's total range. This concept now is considered to be outdated, and speech-language pathologists tend to help people find their "comfortable" range of habitual pitch.

opus: a single work or composition; from the Latin; the plural form of "opus" is "opera" and it was that term that the Camarata (see above) adopted as their new stage presentations combined the musical work, the dramatic work, and the staging work—thus making "works."

oratorio: a musical composition (generally not staged) for chorus, orchestra, and soloists, whose text is generally religious, serious, or philosophical in nature; a long version of a cantata. It was to oratorio that Handel turned when the English public turned sour on his staged operas, although the story line and characterization of the oratorios are often totally operatic. *Messiah* and *Israel in Egypt* are oratorios; *Julius Caesar* and *Rinaldo* are not.

orchestra: the group of musicians which accompanies a staged presentation; in early operas (from 1600 to about 1750); the orchestra might consist of a few strings, pairs of oboes, bassoons, flutes, trumpets, and continuo (see above). The orchestra grew from the time of Mozart through Beethoven, Berlioz, Wagner, Verdi, Puccini, and Richard Strauss so that nowadays an opera orchestra can easily consist of 90 to 100 players. In America, the first floor of a theater is called the orchestra, whereas in England that area is called the stalls.

ornamentation: the extra notes, like appoggiaturas, scales, trills, or cadenzas that can enhance a melodic line when it has to be repeated. Ornamentation and embellishment are probably interchangeable terms.

overture: the instrumental introduction to a musical drama or oratorio; frequently the overture will incorporate musical themes that will later be heard in the course of the opera. In *Don Giovanni*, the ominous theme of the Stone Guest (from Act II) is heard as a premonition at the beginning of the overture, thus setting an emotional tone as well as providing musical structure to the entire work.

parlando: literally, "speaking"; this Italian term directs the singer to imitate speech in singing. The "patter songs" of Gilbert and Sullivan operettas frequently employ a great deal of parlando singing.

partial: a component of sound sensation that is usually distinguished as a single tone and cannot be further distinguished audibly, but contributes to the timbre of a complex sound. This may be higher or lower than the audible frequency and may be either harmonic or inharmonic.

passaggio: the Italian word for *passage*, which describes the area of the voice between registers where preparation for a change in registration should take place.

phonation: the process of the production of voice. To the speech-language pathologist, it may be described as "breathy," "strained," or "normal." The singer's main concern is to initiate sound so that the vibration of the vocal folds is coordinated exactly with the release of supported air and perceives that the tone is initiated by the air.

pitch: the location of a sound on a scale ranging from high to low.

placement: a process of the imagination by which the voice is directed to a certain area of the body (usually the head) and the subsequent awareness of resonance in that area.

polyphony: literally, "many voices"; the mixing together of several melodic lines in a pleasant fashion. Counterpoint is certainly an element that creates polyphony.

portamento: the smooth movement in singing or playing a stringed instrument from one note to the next, effectively sliding over all of the notes in between; a portamento can only be achieved in legato singing or playing and is frequently compared to "glissando," which literally means sliding from one note to the next.

prelude: the instrumental introduction to an individual act within a musical drama, whether opera or operetta; some composers use the words overture, prelude, and entr'acte interchangeably.

prima donna: the female star of an opera cast; in Verdi's time it was considered a matter of course to differentiate the roles in terms of their dramatic and vocal importance, such as "Prima Donna," "Seconda Donna," "Terza Donna," and the like. It did not until recently come to describe the personality of the singer, rather than the importance of her role in the opera.

projection: the quality of vocal production that refers to the ability of the voice to travel through space and be heard over the musical accompaniment.

prompter: a member of the musical staff of many large opera houses; the prompter sits in a small box practically invisible to the audience, under the apron of the stage, and gives singers and choristers the vocal cues seconds before they are required to sing them. In many international houses, where singers perform without benefit of long musical rehearsal periods, a prompter can be invaluable as a memory aide for a jet-lagged singer.

proscenium: a misunderstood term; most performers, even designers, refer to the proscenium when they actually mean the proscenium arch. The proscenium, to be technically exact, is the part of the stage between the curtain and the orchestra pit—and the architectural arch that encloses the curtain is called the proscenium arch. Even so, proscenium is used in a larger, more general sense, in the meaning of a stage constructed with a curtain, as opposed to a thrust stage where the stage has no formal enclosure.

prosody: the pattern of stress or inflection of a sentence or utterance. Prosody is the contribution of voice to language through the use of pitch, loudness, and duration.

prova: rehearsal; from the Italian word for "test"; often in Italy, one hears of a "prova generale," which means the final dress rehearsal. In Germany, a rehearsal is called "probe" (PROE beh); in German houses, one frequently hears of a *sitzprobe* (a rehearsal with orchestra where the singers sing seated on chairs at the front of the stage instead of moving about) or *wandelprobe* (where the singers actually go through the motions of their acting while the orchestra plays the music) or *generalprobe* (which is, in essence, the last dress rehearsal).

raked stage: a stage that slants upward away from the view of the audience; in the earliest opera houses, the stage was so slanted so that the audience member sitting in the back of the theatre could have an easy view of someone standing at the back of the stage. Many opera houses in Europe today have stages that are permanently sloped like this.

range: the division of the human voice according to six basic types: soprano, mezzo soprano, contralto, tenor, baritone, and bass.

rasp: a tone quality that sounds harsh and gravelly, somewhat like a protracted throat clearing, while maintaining a semblance of pitch. Thought of by some rock singers as a vocal style.

recitativo: a musical form within an opera that, by imitating rapid speech, advances the plot; this is not the same as parlando, which is a style of singing, but rather a formal device that links together the arias and choruses. Those forms generally express states of mind, whereas the recitative describes a course of action.

recitativo accompagnato: is accompanied by the full orchestra. The introduction to Donna Anna's "Or sai chi l'onore" in *Don Giovanni* is an example of the "accompagnato" style, where the orchestral sonorities are capable of varying the mood of the narration more than the simple harpsichord accompaniment could.

recitativo secco: is accompanied by the continuo instruments. Numerous passages abound in the operas of Mozart and Rossini of the "secco" style.

register: a group of notes produced with similar laryngeal function, yielding like quality of sound. Opinions among singers and teachers vary as to how many registers there are (from one to three) and whether to call the lowest *chest* or *pulse*, the middle *middle* or *modal*, and the highest *head* or *loft*.

resonance: the amplification of certain components of the tone produced at the vocal folds along the vocal tract (above the vocal folds and including the oral and nasal cavities). An individual's vocal resonance is determined by the shape of his or her anatomy and by the way this configuration is changed during speaking or singing. Often used mistakenly in the voice studio as interchangeable with such terms as *timbre, tone, color,* or *quality of voice,* the singer is concerned with esthetic result of achieving a good balance of resonation among the naso-, oro-, and laryngopharynx.

respiration: the process of breathing. For speaking, we use a relatively small proportion of our available lung capacity to produce voice. People with quite impaired respiration (reduced lung capacity and ability to move air in and out of the lungs) can produce voice without severe difficulty. However, breathing for singing is much more dynamic, more athletic, and more exaggerated than it is for speaking. Breath control is achieved through the development and coordinated interaction of the abdominal and intercostal muscles in an opposite manner from the way they are used in everyday speech. That is, instead of inhalation being active and exhalation passive, the process is conceptually reversed. On inhalation, the abdominal muscles "relax" outward and downward, aiding the contraction of the diaphragm while the rib cage expands. *Breath support* occurs when, as opposed to a passive release of air, exhalation becomes an active and dynamic force by engaging the lower abdominal muscles and moving the air through the expanded rib cage. The rib cage should remain expanded as the process is repeated.

ring: vibrant tone quality with a predominance of high partials in the frequency range of approximately 2800 Hz.

ritornello: the instrumental prelude to an individual song within a cantata, concerto, or aria; in baroque Italian operas, the ritornello (which comes from Italian meaning "a little return trip") could be heard not only at the beginning and the end of the aria, but as a dividing mark between stanzas.

romantic: the period of music between 1830 and the turn of the 20th century; composers of romantic music frequently found inspiration in other than musical ideas, such as nature, painting, birdcalls, or rainstorms. Beethoven was probably the first romantic opera composer, although the most famous are Wagner and Verdi.

scooping: an upward slur, most often defining an attack that begins below the pitch. Scooping may also occur within a vocal line, and is differentiated from the *portamento* by the fact that it is usually not a conscious act. Generally considered by voice teachers to be unmusical and technically detrimental.

shimmer: for the speech-language pathologist, it is intensity perturbation or the cycle-to-cycle variation in the amplitude of the sound signal. As with jitter, the methods for measuring shimmer vary, and shimmer may be expressed as a percentage, in decibels, or in some other value. Increased shimmer values generally correlate with hoarseness. To the voice teacher, shimmer is a tone quality that is highly desirable. The voice is used properly, has a good vibrato rate and projects well.

signal-to-noise ratio: the ratio of the periodic signal produced at the vocal folds to the "noise" or aperiodic signal. Someone with a great deal of hoarseness would have a low signal-to-noise ratio; that is, the "signal" and the "noise" might be very similar in loudness.

singspiel: early German musical drama, which employed spoken dialogue along with musical numbers; Mozart's *The Abduction from the Seraglio* and *The Magic Flute* are both examples of this genre, as are Weber's *Der Freischutz* and Beethoven's *Fidelio*. The singspiel is very similar to English ballad opera or French opéra comique.

"sitting on the breath": a sensation of the voice resting on the supported breath, achieved by maintaining constant breath pressure, a relaxed throat, and an expanded thorax.

soprano: the highest range of the female voice; the soprano voice ranges from lyric (a light, graceful quality) to dramatic (obviously fuller and heavier in tone).

sotto voce: a musical direction that asks the performer to sing, or play "under the voice," or in a subdued manner. Singing sotto voce can be compared to declaiming in a stage whisper and can be very effective in a large theatre.

soubrette: a lightweight soprano voice or type of soprano role, frequently found in comic operas or operettas; the soubrette usually possesses a flirtatious demeanor and street-wise manner, as in the case of Adele in *Die Fledermaus*, or is a particularly fetching country innocent, like Adina in *The Elixir of Love*.

spin: describes tone quality that is free and apparently effortless in production and projects or carries well. Implicit is the presence of true vibrato.

spinto: a kind of voice that is "pushed" toward another; from the Italian "spingere" (to push); thus a "lirico spinto" soprano is a lyric voice that has some qualities of the heavier dramatic range. Frequently, sopranos who have essentially light voices will take on the role of, say, Mimi in *La Bohème* (to portray her youthfulness and frailty) and push their voices to ride over the orchestra, thus developing a "spinto" sound. Licia Albanese, the great Italian soprano, would be a prime example of this type of soprano.

sprechstimme: literally, "speak voice"; a kind of vocal instruction often found in the operas of Schoenberg and Berg, where the singer half speaks and half sings a note. The declamation sounds like speaking, but there is a duration of pitch that makes it seem almost like singing.

staccato: Italian for "detached," "separate," "short." A type of singing or playing that is characterized by short, clipped, rapid articulation; the opposite of staccato is legato.

stage right/stage left: the division of the stage from the performer's point of view; thus, when a singer goes stage right, he or she moves to his or her right but to the audience's left.

straight tone: a tone produced without *vibrato*. Because vibrato is normally present in a mature, well-produced voice, a straight tone is considered symptomatic of some constriction in the throat, of a problem with breath support, or both. Straight tone singing can be executed at will and is used by some singers for stylistic effect, and in that case is an esthetic choice.

subglottic pressure: the amount of pressure just below the vocal folds. An adequate amount of subglottic pressure is crucial for the regular vibration of the vocal folds. Subglottic pressure is created by a steady stream of air originating from the lungs and regulated by the amount of tension and mass of the vocal folds. Subglottic pressure is raised to produce increased loudness.

supernumerary: a performer who appears in a nonsinging role; a "super" might have a solo walk-on to deliver a message or might be included as part of a large processional, for example. In the old days, supers were often referred to as "spear carriers."

swallowed tone: tone that is constricted in the throat and therefore lacing high partials and forward placement.

s/z ratio: a value obtained by dividing the amount of time an individual produces the sound /s/ on a maximum inhalation by the amount of time to produce the /z/ on a maximum inhalation. If the vocal folds are healthy, then the times should be roughly equivalent, or equal to 1.0. The upper limit for "normal" is considered to be below 1.4.

tempo: the speed of a musical passage or composition; the tempo may range from very slow ("largo" in Italian, "langsam" in German) to extremely fast ("presto" in Italian, "schnell" in German).

tenor: the highest natural male voice.

tessitura: Italian for "texture." When referring to a song or role, *tessitura* means that range wherein the majority of pitches lie; for example, the tessitura of Lucia di Lammermoor is quite high, that of Santuzza in *Cavalleria rusticana*, although it is still a soprano role, is low enough that the role could be sung by a mezzo soprano. When referring to a singer, *comfortable tessitura* describes that portion of the singer's range produced with the greatest ease and beauty.

timbre: the distinctive quality or "color" of a voice produced by the combined effect on the ear of the listener of the fundamental tone and its harmonic overtones.

tremolo: describes undesirable vibrato, whether too fast, too slow, or too wide.

trill: two adjacent notes rapidly and repeatedly alternated.

twelve tone: a system of composition put forth in the early part of the 20th century by Arnold Schoenberg whereby (in very simple terms), each note of the chromatic scale should be used as part of a melody before any other note gets repeated. Many composers have used this system, which is also called "serialism," but the best known operas in this style are Berg's *Wozzeck* and *Lulu*, Schoenberg's *Erwartung*, and Roger Sessions's *Montezuma*.

upstage/downstage: the position on stage farthest or nearest the audience; because of the raked stage that was so prevalent in early opera houses, the farther "back" a singer went on the stage, the "higher" he seemed to become in stature—thus the distinction of being "up"-stage. When a singer is directed to move downstage left, he goes toward the audience and toward his left side; to the audience, he seems to be coming forward and moving to the audience's right.

verismo: literally, "truth"; a style of theatre made popular in the latter part of the 19th century in which ordinary events and characters participate in melodramatic situations. Bizet's *Carmen* was considered an early and powerful example of verismo and so are most of the operas of Puccini and Mascagni.

vibrato: a regular and relatively even pattern of oscillation above and below a pitch, which occurs naturally at a frequency of approximately six to seven times per second in a mature, well-produced voice; the slightly wavering quality that a singer has in his or her voice while sustaining a tone; if the vibrato becomes terribly pronounced, it is pejoratively called a wobble. Though beauty is subjective, most voice teachers agree that vibrato adds warmth and beauty to tone. It is also one of the measures of the health and function of the voice. Some singers will drain their voice of any vibrato for a particularly haunting effect.

videostroboscopy: a technique to visualize the vocal folds under full light and under "strobed" or flashing light. In stroboscopy, a light flashes onto the vocal folds at a rate slightly slower than the rate of vibration of the vocal folds. When seen by the human eye, this gives the illusion of slow motion. The images are recorded on videotape and can be reviewed as often as necessary. An otolaryngologist or speech-language pathologist may use a rigid endoscope or a flexible fiberoptic scope for this procedure.

vital capacity: the maximum amount of air that can be exhaled after a maximum inhalation.

vocal abuse: encompasses a range of behaviors, from poor vocal hygiene (smoking, inadequate hydration) to misuse and overuse of the voice. For the speaker, this is the etiology of most "benign" voice disorders. For the singer, overuse will become apparent sooner in an untrained or poorly trained voice, but also occurs in well-trained voices that are doing too much: too long, too loud, too high, and so forth. Misuse may be the result of poor vocal technique or the conscious imitation of unhealthy vocalism. It may also result from an improper or insufficient warm-up/cool-down period, singing in an inappropriate tessitura (that part of the vocal range within which lies the majority of pitches as opposed to the total range), or singing beyond one's natural range. Unfortunately, some forms of vocal abuse have come to be considered stylistically acceptable, even desirable among certain vocal styles.

vocal focus: *focus* describes a tone that, through correct production, effectively turns all of the air used to produce it into clear, vibrating singing or speaking sound. Although often used interchangeably in the vocal studio with the term *vocal placement*, focus is better described as the result of good vocal placement and its unencumbered connection to breath support.

vocalise: a vocal exercise.

voce di capra: Italian for "voice of the goat." Characterized by a quick, bleating pulsation of the tone.

whistle register: the female equivalent of male falsetto. The highest notes in a female voice.

wobble: uneven and unusually slow fluctuation of pitch.

zarzuela: a Spanish popular musical presentation that blends dialogue and music in skits and dramas ranging from one to three acts that deal satirically with aspects of daily life. The derivation of the name is intriguing: early zarzuelas were performed in the Palacio de la Zarzuela in Madrid, so named because it was surrounded by a field of brambles ("zarza" being Spanish for bramble).

Index

GER (gastroesophageal reflux) *(continued)*
  overview, 117–118
  and Reinke's edema, 189
  as "supine" reflux, 119
Gingko biloba, 168
Ginseng, 167, 171
Globus pharyngeus, 118, 120
  and assessment, 63
Glottography, *See also* FLOG (flow glottography)
Goldenseal, 167, 171
Gonadotropins, 158
Gould, Wilbur J. (1919–), 10
Granuloma, laryngeal, 118
GRBAS (grade, roughness, breathiness, asthenia, strain) scale, 74, 181
Guaifenesin, 154, 155
Guarana, 168

H

Haemophilus influenzae, 159
Haloperidol, 155
Hawthorne, 168
H2-blockers, 124, 159
Herbs
  aconite, 171
  astragalus membranaceus, 171
  black cohosh, 169
  Chinese, 172–173
  contraindications, 167–169
  cordyceps sinensis, 171
  echinacea, 167, 170
  feverfew, 168
  garlic, 169
  gingko biloba, 168
  ginseng, 167, 171
  goldenseal, 167, 171
  guarana, 168
  hawthorne, 168
  kava kava, 167
  ma huang, 169
  pulsatilla, 169, 171
  pygeum africanum, 168
  saw palmetto, 168
  St. John's wort, 169
  uncaria tomentosa, 171
HIPPA (Healthcare Information Privacy and Portability Act), 286, 291
Histamine blockers, 123
History, patient, 171, 181, 233
History, phonomicrosurgery, 246–247
History, voice care

Albrecht, Rosemarie (1915–), 10
American Laryngological Society, 7–8, 10, 11
autoscopy, 9
Babington, Benjamin G. (1794–1866), 7
Czermak, Johann (1828–1873), 7
García, Manuel Patricio Rodríguez (1805–1906), 7
Gould, Wilbur J. (1919–), 10
Hirano, Minoru (1932–), 10
Jackson, Chevalier (1865–1958), 9
Jako, Geza, 10
Kirstein, Alfred (1863–1922), 9
Kleinsasser, Oskar (1930–2001), 10
Knight, Frederick, 7–8
laryngeal examination, 7–9
laryngoscopy, 7
Lawrence, Van, 10
Liston, Robert (1794–1847), 7
Moses, Paul (1897–), 10
objective assessment, 12–13
pharmacology, 12
photography, laryngeal, 8, 9
surgery, 9–10
therapy, 12
vocal tract knowledge, 10
Voice Foundation, 10
von Leden, Hans, 10
Hoarseness, 120, 158
  and assessment, 63
  from medications, 156
  persistent, 234
Homeopathy, 170
Hormones, *See also* Oral contraceptives; Thyroid
  androgens, 157–158, 158
  antiprogestin, 158
  estrogen, 158
  female voice, 38–45
  gonadotropins, 158
  and larynx, 35
  male voice, 45
  as medications, 157–158
  menopause, 43–45, 49, 158
  menstrual cycle, 42–43
  overview, 34
  and pregnancy, 43
  premenstrual voice syndrome, 38–43
  prostaglandins, 157
  puberty, 35–38, 158
  testosterone, 158
  and voice development, 34–35
H1-receptor antagonists, 153
Hypertonicity, 174
Hypnotherapy, 173–174

Z